Cardiovascular
Risk Factors
in Children

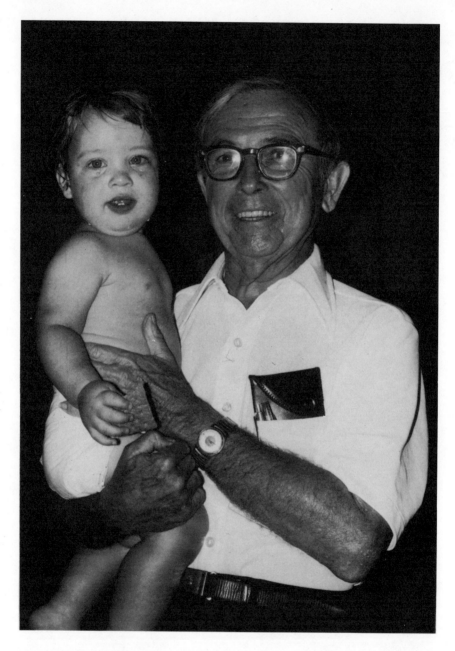

A dedicated staff member and a young participant
in the Bogalusa Heart Study

Cardiovascular Risk Factors in Children

The Early Natural History
of Atherosclerosis
and Essential Hypertension

GERALD S. BERENSON, M.D.

and

C. A. McMahan, Ph.D.   Antonie W. Voors, M.D., Dr.P.H.
Larry S. Webber, Ph.D.   Sathanur R. Srinivasan, Ph.D.
Gail C. Frank, R.D., M.P.H.   Theda A. Foster, M.S.
Caroline V. Blonde, M.D., M.P.H.

With the editorial assistance of
Caroline Andrews, B.A. and Helen E. Hester, M.A.

Louisiana State University

New York   Oxford
OXFORD UNIVERSITY PRESS
1980

Library of Congress Cataloging in Publication Data

Berenson, Gerald S
  Cardiovascular risk factors in children

  Bibliography: p.
  Includes index.
  1. Atherosclerosis in children—Louisiana—Bogalusa—
Longitudinal studies.   2. Hypertension in children—Louisiana—
Bogalusa—Longitudinal studies.   3. Hyperlipoproteinemia
in children—Louisiana—Bogalusa—Longitudinal studies.
4. Children—Medical examinations—Louisiana—Bogalusa.
5. Health surveys—Louisiana—Bogalusa.   I. Title.
RJ426.A82B47   618.9'21'36   79,13775
ISBN 0-19-502589-X

Acknowledgments for figures and tables appear on pages 451–453.

Printed in the United States of America

Foreword

There is every scientific reason to think that atherosclerosis has its origin early in life. Even though the lesions may develop at an accelerated pace only in adulthood when environmental conditions, especially nutritional and other living habits, are unfavorable, the formation of these very habits certainly begins in childhood and, once formed, they are difficult to change. Actually, pending further research, the odds are that even the earlier lesions are decisively under environmental control. Thus, whatever the eventual answer, the prevention of premature atherosclerosis must begin in youth.

This book on the findings of the Bogalusa Heart Study deals, of necessity, with risk factors—the precursors of coronary heart disease—or rather, the links between risk factors and the disease itself. The latter kind of study, the evolution of clinical disease, would have to encompass at least four or five decades. It should be remembered that the history of coronary heart disease epidemiology only started around 30 years ago, that its spectacular results relate mostly to "middle aged" adults, and that the need to include children in such investigations was actively recognized only at a later stage in the course of epidemiological research. But it is not necessary to conduct a "cradle-to-grave" study in order to provide evidence for a causal relationship between risk factors and disease. If such a relationship exists in middle-age and beyond, the impact of risk-factor control is bound to be even greater if started in youth, when lesions are beginning to form.

Therefore, population studies to determine the characteristics of children destined to become high-risk adults are a key to the control of cardiovascular disease. The Bogalusa Heart Study is neither the first nor the only risk-factor study in children, but probably no other study of this kind is as equally community-based, as encompassing in the variables under investigation, and as promising in terms of the potential of looking at children as members of the whole family. Moreover, the biracial character of the town of Bogalusa makes it possible to gain insights into ethnic determinants of early risk. The Bogalusa Heart Study already has made its mark amongst its companion studies and will serve as a guide and reference for similar investigations around the world. The lead taken by the World Health Organization in encouraging and coordinating risk-factor studies in the young underlines the significance of these investigations at the level of international health.

This monograph deals with susceptibility—the susceptibility of children to cardiovascular disease later in life, a model, incidentally, for the major chronic diseases in general. Why, it may be asked, are some investigators particularly "susceptible" to certain kinds of research? In this case, why did Dr. Berenson undertake the Bogalusa Heart Study? No doubt, as with the causes of coronary heart disease, there are many reasons. At Louisiana State University in New Orleans, where he studied and worked, the most decisive pathological groundwork for the belief that atherosclerosis starts in youth was convincingly laid. As a clinical and experimental investigator, Dr. Berenson had already made his name amongst atherosclerosis researchers. Finally, the choice of Bogalusa as the site for this new venture into epidemiology and preventive cardiology was not accidental. Dr. Berenson's family helped found the town. Presumably Dr. Berenson himself would be able to tell the tale of his development into an epidemiologist and his deep commitment to preventive cardiology. However, creative ideas have a tendency to escape explanation!

Reading between the lines, one will possibly sense that this is not only a scientific report but the saga of a serious and exciting venture. Visiting Bogalusa and seeing the team in action is an unforgettable experience. The children in the study are received and treated with the now proverbial but not always practiced "TLC" (tender, loving care).

They feel good will and attention, but not the tightness of the statistical design and the rigorous quality control guiding the examination schedule. There is a quiet and matter-of-fact devotion and identification with the project on the part of all those involved, from the strictly professional staff to the volunteer health workers.

Research in community medicine is the pacesetter for community prevention programs. It is recognized more and more that motivation toward sensible patterns of everyday living is the prerequisite of success in reducing the risk factors predisposing to disease. The Bogalusa Heart Study, apart from its scientific merit, represents a statement of faith in disease prevention, a model for the creation of a working relationship between the people in the community and the "health team," and an action program true to the call, "from epidemiology to prevention."

Frederick H. Epstein, M.D.

Professor of Preventive Medicine
University Zurich, Switzerland

Formerly: Professor of Epidemiology
University of Michigan
School of Public Health
Ann Arbor, Michigan, USA

Preface

It is now clear from anatomic studies, necropsies on soldiers killed in Korea and Vietnam, and studies of coronary arteries from all age groups that atherosclerotic coronary artery disease exists early in life. Although it is considered that essential hypertension begins in the young, the early onset of this disease is not distinct. Determining the early phases of atherosclerosis and essential hypertension in children is a critical step in preventing the major cardiovascular diseases of our time.

Over the past 20 to 30 years, outstanding epidemiologic studies such as those in Framingham (Mass.), Tecumseh (Mich.), and Evans County (Ga.), have clearly shown the importance of relating risk factors to coronary heart disease and morbidity from hypertension.But this information has been obtained mostly from adult populations, and often from an age group in which advanced disease already exists.

The large epidemiologic studies of the past have been significant in that they outlined our attack on the major cardiovascular diseases occurring in the United States and many other Western countries. Our findings in the Bogalusa Heart Study on 5,000 children, reported in this text, begin a serious attempt to collect risk-factor data in childhood—a period when these diseases are developing. While developing, these diseases produce no pain or disability; young people are asymptomatic. These are aptly referred to as the "silent diseases."

Major aspects of our study on children have followed the design of the epidemiologic programs on adults. With time, we will be able to link findings in children with those in adults, especially adults who have suffered heart attacks, strokes, and heart failure.

Although some risk-factor data, that is, levels of blood pressure and serum cholesterol, have been previously collected from children, carefully standardized techniques have not been followed, nor have those data been collected simultaneously to provide an opportunity to examine interrelationships of the variables, such as weight and cholesterol, or diet and lipids. The Bogalusa Heart Study has attempted to survey overall risk-factor data in a total community of children. This is different from studying selected children or individual patients seeing physicians and being admitted to hospitals for diagnosis and treatment. The Bogalusa Heart Study information is relevant to the general adult population—to the 10–20% who will develop hypertension, and ultimately suffer strokes and heart failure, and to the 50–75% who will develop arteriosclerotic heart disease.

We have described methods by which health personnel can obtain useful information on risk-factor variables in children, with the hope that the application of these methods in childhood will help to prevent cardiovascular diseases in adulthood.

One of the book's main purposes is to aid the physician in predicting a child's health care needs at a time when prevention can have optimum effects. The data will be particularly helpful to physicians interested in preventive health measures for the two major cardiovascular diseases: coronary artery disease and essential hypertension.

The Bogalusa Heart Study findings presented here will be a framework for future studies. The observations can be used for a single child under medical care or can serve as a comparison to observations from other populations of children. For such comparisons, the Appendix contains resource information in the form of grids on (1) growth and maturation, (2) blood pressure, and (3) lipids: cholesterol, triglycerides, and concentrations of α (high density), β (low density), and pre-β (very low density) lipoproteins.

Diet will be a main target in future efforts to alter a child's susceptibility to heart disease in adulthood. Nutrition studies and observations on eating behavior in Bogalusa children are presented here as a first approach in defining this major environmental factor.

Our last chapter is a summing up of general recommendations for the care of children, and our impressions of the work being done on cardiovascular risk factors in children.

We know there are certain discrepancies and inconsistencies within the book—some because many of the chapters have been published earlier in somewhat different form, others because of our limitations. We hope they will not necessarily distort the information or the message.

G.S.B.
New Orleans
September 1979

Acknowledgments

Obviously, our acknowledgments must first recognize the children of Bogalusa. They comprise this study.

The research which formed the basis for this book was supported by funds from the National Heart, Lung and Blood Institute of the U.S. Public Health Service (HL 02942) and Specialized Center of Research —Arteriosclerosis (SCOR-A) (HL 15103).

The implementation of an epidemiologic study such as the Bogalusa Heart Study involves the contribution of many persons. Some stand out significantly. Others involved in supporting services receive little or no recognition from the accomplishments of the study—for example, laboratory technicians, computer personnel, and secretarial staff. They are just as important, for without their help the daily implementation of our program would falter.

We have formally and informally drawn upon the experience and expertise of many consultants. The standards we set for the Bogalusa Heart Study were taken from previous epidemiologic programs such as Framingham, Tucumseh, and Evans County. Consultants from these programs and other professionals interested in cardiovascular epidemiology were used freely, and we appreciate their help in designing our studies.

A number of individuals at Tulane and LSU Medical Schools have helped through their encouragement, frequent consultations, and support of the program. Dr. Jack P. Strong has been a continual advisor to the program. One colleague deserves particular mention. Although not a coauthor in the clinical research, Dr. Bhandaru Radhakrishnamurthy has been a coinvestigator in all of our laboratory work for many years. He served as a daily contributor, not only to the biology of the program but to the administrative decisions we faced. His patience and reassuring guidance are a continual support to this research.

Mr. Edward R. Dalferes, Jr. has also been part of our family for many years. He is the first person we turn to for everything. Dr. Ralph R. Frerichs was an epidemiologist with our program and we owe him a great deal of thanks for his help in conducting the first phase of our study and publication of much of the material in this text. Recognition must also go to Dr. John L. Harris (deceased) and Dr. Lawrence J. Cohen, our first pediatricians.

In Bogalusa, appreciation is given to the field staff. Not only has this group performed as a closely knit team, responsible in their research and training duties, but their dedication to the program and faith in our leadership has been inspiring. They and the many volunteers who helped with the screening really represented this program to Bogalusa. The staff's direction has come from Mrs. Imogene W. Talley, but we cannot appropriately fit her role to the title we have given her—community coordinator. Her patience and dedication molded the program into part of Bogalusa itself. Without her tireless efforts and mature insight into the needs of the study, our degree of success could not have been accomplished. Imagine finding someone with Mrs. Talley's capability (along with eleven nurses and other staff, all of whom volunteered to join the group), in a small community like Bogalusa and transforming them into a well-trained group to collect research data! We refer to our research team as "ordinary" nurses (but nothing is ordinary about a good nurse). Their willingness to be monitored and repeatedly trained according to the same protocol reflects their desire that the study be conducted properly and their commitment to the program's importance. What blessings were given to this study from such a mixture of talent—people within a small community who accepted an unproven program on a trial basis, worked part-time, and struggled to do something that seemed worthwhile.

From a personal standpoint, thanks must be given to my parents, who lived in Bogalusa over many years. Respect for them in Bogalusa made our task easier. The acceptance shown to us by Bogalusa convinces me that the community had that respect, and that we chose the right place for the study.

In every investigator's career there are those who help shape his approach to research. First, I must thank Dr. George E. Burch, who helped excite within me an interest in research and who emphasized the importance of research in clinical medicine. I am grateful to Dr. Albert Dorfman and his team, Martin B. Mathews, John A. Cifonelli, and Saul Roseman, who showed me the unlimited horizons of applying biochemistry and biochemical research to medicine, and who supported and encouraged me over many years to continue in academic medicine. And, I am also grateful to Dr. C. A. McMahan, whose insight into clinical research design guided me in conducting research involving large numbers of people and helped me understand the necessary methods involved in obtaining reliable information in an epidemiologic study. His penetrating comments, "The award of a grant only provides a hunting license," "the importance of standing on the shoulders of others," "the need for development of protocols," "the Director has to set the standards," and "when you stand in front of the scientific public," have served as guidelines for the conduct of this program.

Finally, we are especially grateful to the Bogalusa children and their parents, who have had such tremendous faith in the Heart Study. Their unusually high participation has made our program a success. Without them and their support this study would not have been possible. This contribution will be to children all over the world.

Contents

I. Introduction to studies on the early natural history of arteriosclerosis

1. Cardiovascular risk factors in children

For thy children we shall have visions.

Although coronary atherosclerosis was recognized much earlier, it was just 60 years ago that James Herrick related myocardial infarction to the anatomic obstruction of a major coronary artery and alerted the medical profession to this clinical syndrome (Herrick, 1912; Lie, 1978). From that time our understanding of the clinical features of coronary heart disease and the underlying arterial lesions has advanced considerably. Although the precise phenomena accounting for the complete occlusion of coronary vessels are still being debated, there is little doubt that in Western countries the fat-laden, raised, intimal fibrous plaque of atherosclerosis occludes most of the lumen of coronary arteries. Despite the need for further study, our understanding of coronary artery disease has now provided insight into ways of approaching the clinical problems and their prevention. Studies of children are just beginning to show directions for prevention at an optimum time. Clearly, it is at the early stages of disease that efforts to limit the ravages of atherosclerosis and primary hypertension have potential to be most fruitful.

It hardly seems necessary to emphasize the significance of the major cardiovascular diseases that occur in adults in this country. Coronary heart disease, essential hypertension, and diabetes mellitus are so common that we almost accept them as expected morbidity in the middle aged and in the elderly. Even though recent national health

3

statistics (Levy, 1978) are beginning to show a decline in death from these diseases, they still overshadow all our other medical problems.

PATHOGENESIS OF ATHEROSCLEROSIS AND CORONARY ARTERY DISEASE AS IT RELATES TO STUDY OF CHILDREN

The pathogenesis of atherosclerosis is a frustrating area to review because of the extensive research and literature on the subject. Still, many areas remain as blindspots in our understanding of the evolution of the vascular lesion. It is clear that many factors are involved; in fact, we are probably studying not one disease but manifestations of several. Furthermore, the interrelationship of hypertension, accelerating atherosclerosis, and the ultimate development of coronary heart disease is becoming apparent. (For the most part in this text the term *arteriosclerosis* will be used to refer to vascular disease related to both atherosclerosis and hypertension. The interrelationship is so close that they must be studied together to understand the development of coronary heart disease.)

Three general areas will be discussed briefly to indicate how the need for studies in children evolved. These are: 1. pathogenetic considerations in development of atherosclerotic lesions; 2. efforts to link

Table 1–1. Factors to be considered in the pathogenesis of atherosclerosis

Anatomic	Hemodynamic	Hematologic
Vasa vasorum	Mechanical stress (wear & tear)	Clotting mechanism
Microvasculature	Vascular site	Platelet aggregation
Interstitial space	Hypertension	Thrombosis
Lymphatics		plaque formation
		clot formation
Intrinsic	*Metabolic*	*Inflammatory*
Cellular function	Genetic	Inflammation–repair
Structural proteins	Hormonal	Viral infection
Macromolecules	Nutritional	*Temporal*
lipid-carbohydrate-protein	Smoking	Accumulation of factors
Enzymes	Physical activity	Aging?
	Ponderosity index	
	Metabolic disorders	
	Mental stress	
	Type A behavior	

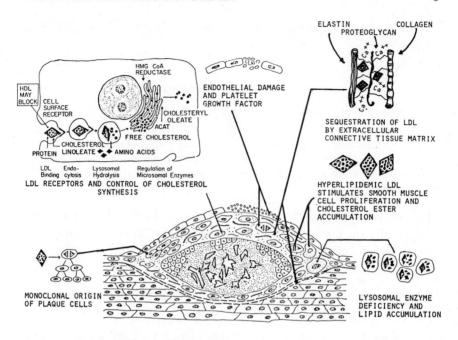

Figure 1–1. A diagrammatic representation of the various physiological mechanisms and biochemical mechanisms hypothesized to be involved in the pathogenesis of atherosclerotic lesions. (Adapted from Wissler, 1978.)

anatomic lesions with clinical observations; and 3. clinical considerations of coronary artery disease—the development of the risk-factor concept.

Pathogenetic considerations in the development of atherosclerotic lesions

Factors thought to be involved in the development of atherosclerotic vascular lesions may be grouped under several headings, as in Table 1–1. The anatomic, hemodynamic, hematologic, intrinsic, metabolic, inflammatory and reparative, and temporal factors need not be discussed here since they have been reviewed in detail in the literature (Wissler, 1978; Berenson et al., 1971a; Berenson et al., 1973 and others). The significance of these factors in the pathogenesis of atherosclerosis at the vascular level seems obvious. More recently, specific mechanisms leading to the formation of atherosclerotic lesions are now being elucidated (Fig. 1–1). The complexity of the problem can be appreciated from a statement by McMillan (1973) that apparently:

there is no exclusive or unique early lesion for all atherosclerosis but a variety of initial changes such as endothelial injury, platelet adhesion, altered endothelial permeability with insudation of blood proteins, infiltration of lipoproteins, and the like which can lead to injury–repair reactions and, in some circumstances, to plaque building. Such initial events can be brief, episodic, repeated, evanescent, cumulative and synergistic. They are not conceived to be confined to one period of life and, indeed, one very often finds lesions like those of childhood among the more advanced lesions of arteries from adults.

This description and the mechanisms shown in Figure 1–1 illustrate the variety of interacting influences that occur over a lifetime in the genesis of atherosclerotic lesions, beginning at birth.

Efforts to link anatomic lesions with clinical observations

Clinicopathologic studies (McGill, 1968) have provided a link between mechanisms of atherosclerotic plaque formation and the clinical observations of risk factors in individuals. Epidemiologic studies of the early natural history of atherosclerosis have attempted to describe the relationship of individual characteristics to the existence and extent of atherosclerotic lesions of the coronary and other arteries. Figure 1–2 illustrates the presumed risk factors and various clinical manifestations that are encountered. This is not, of course, the same as an anatomic study of the underlying arterial lesions. McGill, Strong, and their colleagues in the International Atherosclerosis Project (McGill, 1968) attempted to relate risk factors specifically with atherosclerotic lesions:

Data from the International Atherosclerosis Project and other recent autopsy surveys are used to illustrate the association of risk factors for coronary heart disease to coronary atherosclerotic lesions. Coronary atherosclerosis (anatomic disease) is found to vary with age, sex, geographic location, and race. Lesions seem to be related to serum cholesterol and dietary fat when comparing populations, but insufficient data are available to confirm such associations on an individual basis within a population. Lesions are greater in hypertensive and diabetic individuals than in those without these conditions. Lesions are also greater in heavy cigarette smokers than in nonsmokers. No consistent association of atherosclerotic lesions is observed with physical activity or obesity. There is much variability in extent of coronary athero-

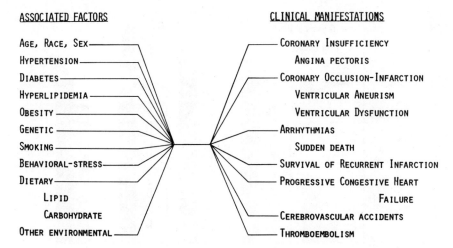

Figure 1–2. A spectrum of the variables linked to coronary artery disease and hypertension. Figures 1–1 and 1–2 indicate the multifactorial aspects of arteriosclerosis and clinical cardiovascular disease.

sclerosis among individuals of similar race, sex, age, geographic location, disease, and smoking habits. Thus, there are other important factors involved in development of atherosclerosis that have yet to be determined. (Strong and Eggen, 1969)

The important finding that atherosclerotic lesions are associated with cigarette smoking (Strong and Richards, 1976) is illustrated in Figure 1–3. Unfortunately, the relationship between blood pressure or serum lipid and lipoprotein levels and the extent of early vascular lesions has not been as consistent. The complete lack of correlation of anatomic disease with risk-factor observations at a young age remains a major gap in our knowledge. Without such correlation it will be difficult to determine the significance of the variations in risk factors observed in children as they relate to the development of cardiovascular disease later in life.

Clinical consideration of coronary artery disease—the development of the risk-factor concept

The growth of cardiovascular epidemiology seems to have paralleled the progress in our understanding of the events preceding the morbid

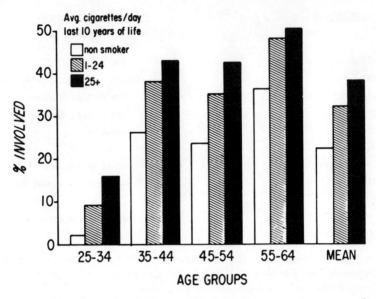

Figure 1–3. Coronary artery disease in white men at autopsy according to cigarette smoking history, according to percent of coronary surface exhibiting raised lesions. Intimal surface disease increases with the degree of smoking in all age groups. Note the considerable difference observed in young nonsmokers as compared to heavy smokers (courtesy of J. P. Strong). One can visualize the problem of smoking from our observations on the incidence of smoking in Bogalusa children, see Chap. 26, Fig. 26–4.

manifestations of coronary heart disease. The superb epidemiologic studies conducted in Framingham, Tecumseh, Evans County, Chicago, and elsewhere have established the risk-factor concept as a means of predicting morbid events related to coronary heart and hypertensive disease (Kannel, 1972). Corollary studies of diet, both nationally and internationally, linked environmental factors with the varying expression of these diseases in different geographic areas. Consequently, much attention has been given to the relationship of dietary fat, exogenous cholesterol, and serum total cholesterol levels with cardiovascular disease in populations. Figure 1–4 gives an international picture of the relation between cholesterol intake and death rates from coronary heart disease (Connor and Connor, 1972). Similar relationships can be shown between hypertension and stroke and the consumption of sodium chloride.

Once atherosclerosis and hypertension were recognized as the leading cardiovascular diseases, at least in the industrialized Western countries, attention turned to methods of prevention, mainly by modifying diet, controlling hypertension, attempting to decrease cigarette smoking, and controlling other risk factors.

Although risk factors do not explain the occurrence of all coronary heart disease, their recognition has allowed physicians to identify individuals with high risk, appreciate differences in these diseases in populations around the world, and ultimately to decrease the occurrence of such diseases. The background needed to study these diseases in their early natural history, in childhood, has now been provided.

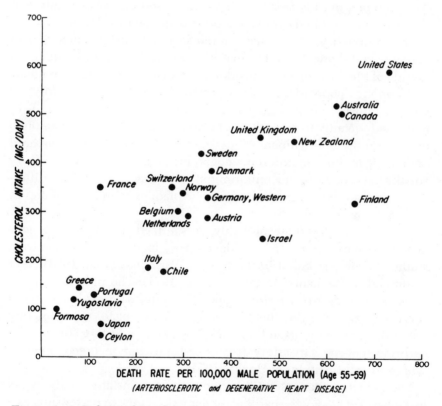

Figure 1–4. Relationship of death rates in various populations with cholesterol consumption in the respective countries (courtesy of W. E. Connor).

EVOLUTION OF STUDIES PROVIDING EVIDENCE OF ATHEROSCLEROTIC AND HYPERTENSIVE DISEASE BEGINNING IN CHILDHOOD

Russell Holman and his colleagues McGill, Strong, and Geer (1958) developed methods for quantitating the anatomic changes of atherosclerosis in New Orleans in the 1950's. In those studies Holman emphasized the occurrence of lesions in infants and drew attention to the fact that atherosclerosis begins in early life. Years before, Zeek (1930) had pointed out that lesions occurred in the aortas of children, which were similar to or possibly precursors of adult disease. These observations began to question the concept of coronary artery disease as a result of aging.

Holman suggested that atherosclerosis might be a pediatric nutrition problem, but his farsightedness was based on rather scanty evidence about the initial events related to pathogenesis. His team, however, continued to stress that arterial lesions could be detected in early life and showed that the severity of disease progressed with each decade of life, though with considerable variability among individuals and among populations. They divided the natural history of atherosclerosis into subclinical and clinical changes (see Fig. 1–5) and used quantitative methods to assess the degree of anatomic changes in the International Atherosclerosis Project, which compared pathologic findings in different geographic areas (McGill, 1968). Fatty streaks have been found uniformly at young ages, but major differences arise in the progression of fibrous plaques in individual and in different populations.

The observations that probably crystallized a national concern about coronary artery disease developing in early life came from studies of soldiers killed in the Korean War (Enos et al., 1953), later confirmed in Vietnam (McNamara et al., 1971). The presence of significant coronary artery lesions in healthy young soldiers killed in the service clearly showed that the early lesions began as completely asymptomatic disease (see Fig. 1–6). The need for further study of the early onset of coronary artery disease became a national recommendation (National Institutes of Health, 1971).

The evidence that essential hypertension begins at an early age is less clear. Yet among the cardiovascular risk factors, hypertension, as a disease itself and a contributor to accelerated coronary artery disease,

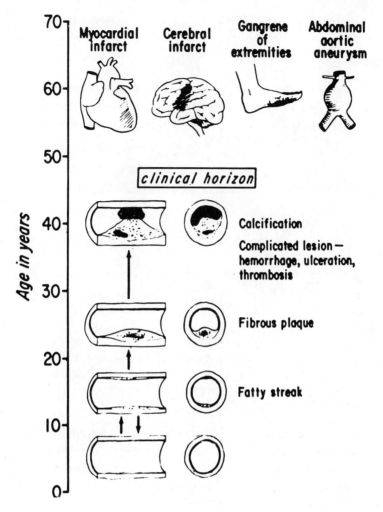

Figure 1–5. Natural history of atherosclerosis divided into two phases, the subclinical and clinical horizon (courtesy of J. P. Strong).

plays a major role. Although among young patients in pediatric clinic populations, secondary hypertension has been traditionally considered the major form (Loggie, 1971; 1975), a survey of medical students indicated an unexplained elevated diastolic pressure in almost 10% (Berenson et al., 1971b). In a more recent study, no causes were found to account for elevated blood pressure in a majority of children screened from a school population (Londe and Goldring, 1976). Our

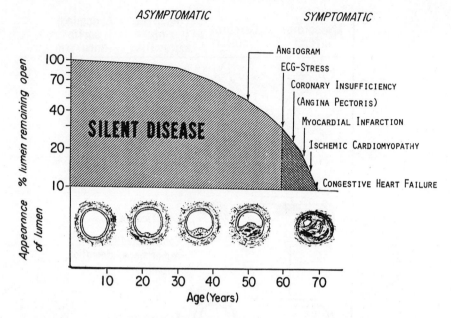

Figure 1–6. A schematic presentation of the natural history of coronary artery disease progressing from the long asymptomatic period to the occurrence of various clinical manifestations following the narrowing of coronary vessels. The thrust of the Bogalusa Heart Study is on the "Silent" phase of atherosclerosis. Essential hypertension could be depicted similarly in its early natural history.

investigations support the notion that essential hypertension, like atherosclerosis, begins early in life, although its occurrence has not yet been documented by anatomic changes. Hypertension seems to be a more quantitative abnormality, more easily interpretable clinically than levels of serum lipids, but the precise definition of abnormality of all risk-factor parameters will require equating them with vascular disease and their anatomic correlates. The silent or subclinical phase of essential hypertension needs parallel investigations at both the clinical and the anatomic level similar to the studies outlined for understanding the early natural history of atherosclerosis.

EARLIER EPIDEMIOLOGIC STUDIES OF CHILDREN

Most early observations of cardiovascular risk factors in children were cross-sectional studies which considered only one parameter such as blood pressure or serum cholesterol. Little effort has been made to correlate body development and maturation with serum lipids and lipoproteins, blood pressure, diet, and other factors in an attempt to trace the early onset of coronary artery disease or hypertension. A major limitation of earlier studies is they did not provide an opportunity to observe correlation among the various risk factors, especially over time. Blood pressure studies of children at school and in an office setting have been conducted in different ways, resulting in considerable variation in the levels observed. Further, the indirect approach of extrapolating criteria for abnormal levels of blood pressure from experience with adults to children is not appropriate. Amid these difficulties the notion has arisen that hypertension is quite rare in children and that most of those who do have hypertension acquire the disease as a result of secondary causes (Dustan, 1976).

During the past few years several large-scale community studies of "healthy" free-living children have been initiated. Three communities have been pinpointed for cardiovascular multi-risk-factor studies, and preliminary observations have been published in a monograph (National Heart, Lung, and Blood Institute, 1978). The three communities are Bogalusa, Louisiana; Rochester, Minnesota; and Muscatine, Iowa. Longitudinal studies are ongoing in Bogalusa and Muscatine and will begin to provide data on changes in risk-factor variables in children over time. The Muscatine Study (Lauer et al., 1975) has pinpointed levels of risk factors in white children from a midwestern farming community, and the studies from Rochester (Ellefson et al., 1978) present serum lipid and lipoprotein levels in white children from a middle to high social class in Minnesota. Certain differences in levels among the three study groups await confirmation by eliminating methodologic differences: for example, lower blood pressure levels in Bogalusa than noted in Muscatine and Rochester (Blumenthal et al., 1977; Berenson et al., 1978b).

A National Health Survey (National Center for Health Statistics, 1970, 72, 73, 74, 77) was conducted on 7,000 children from selected areas around the United States and has also provided cross-sectional data. The survey included observations on growth, height and weight, skinfolds, maturation, blood pressure, and serum cholesterol. Notable studies abroad have also been conducted in the Netherlands (Van Der Haar and Kromhout, 1978) with a particular emphasis on nutrition. A summary table of serum cholesterol for selected international pediat-

Table 1–2. Mean and standard deviation of serum total cholesterol[a] for selected international pediatric populations

Population	Blood Source	Boys N	X̄ ± S.D.	Girls N	X̄ ± S.D.
United States					
HANES (4–17 years)[1]					
White	Serum	2006	165 ± 31	1986	168 ± 32
Black	Serum	639	169 ± 33	683	175 ± 34
Bogalusa (5–14 years)[4, 8, 11]					
White	Serum	1142	161 ± 29	1030	164 ± 27
Black	Serum	669	169 ± 31	605	171 ± 30
Cincinnati (6–17 years)[7]	Plasma	477	159 ± 26	450	161 ± 23
Muscatine (6–18 years)[6, 8]	Serum	3765	160 ± 29	3824	164 ± 30
Rochester (6–18 years)[3, 8]	Serum	1193	158 ± 39	1228	163 ± 41
Latin America					
Guatemala (7–12 years)[10]					
Urban Private School	Serum	48	187 ± 27	48	188 ± 30
Urban Public School	Serum	48	143 ± 29	48	156 ± 30
Rural Public School	Serum	48	121 ± 24	48	128 ± 24
Mexico (Tarahumara Indians)[2]					
5–18 years	Plasma	118	115 ± 19	104	117 ± 25
Europe					
Netherlands (4–13 years)[5]	Serum	490	176 ± 30	413	180 ± 30
Finland (5–13 years)[9]	Serum	761	234 ± 40	735	238 ± 40
Africa					
South Africa (Blacks)[13]					
10–12 years	Serum	40	120.0 ± 23	40	123.9 ± 25
16–18 years	Serum	50	130.1 ± 22	50	138.2 ± 27
Asia and Australasia					
India (Punjab) (5–18 years)[14]	Serum	299	133.5 ± 4[b]	226	130.0 ± 3[b]
Japan[15]					
13 years	Serum	55	157 ± 27	66	167 ± 27
14 years	Serum	48	155 ± 30	57	171 ± 27
New Zealand (Adolescents)[12]	Serum	—[c]	175.6 ± 2[b]	—[c]	182.6 ± 2[b]

[a]Determined by different laboratory methods
[b]Assumed to be the standard error
[c]N = 653 (number of children by sex not available)

1. Abraham, 1979
2. Connor et al., 1978
3. Ellefson et al., 1978
4. Frerichs et al., 1976
5. Kromhout et al., 1977
6. Lauer et al., 1975
7. Morrison et al., 1978
8. National Heart, Lung and Blood Institute, 1978
9. Räsänen et al., 1978
10. Scrimshaw et al., 1957
11. Srinivasan et al., 1976a
12. Stanhope and Sampson, 1977
13. Walker and Walker, 1978
14. Werner and Sareen, 1978
15. Hatano, 1979

ric populations is presented in Table 1–2. All of these programs are beginning to document levels of risk-factor variables at a young age. The major contributions thus far are the development of methods to obtain risk-factor levels in children and to provide observations on large numbers of children in different populations. Further studies must be conducted in order to understand the significance of the observations being made and on how these factors might be altered when needed.

AN APPROACH TO STUDYING CARDIOVASCULAR RISK FACTORS IN CHILDREN

Clearly, most medical attention given to atherosclerosis is directed toward its clinical aspects and particularly treatment of the complications shown in Figure 1–6. Although prevention of atherosclerotic and hypertensive heart disease is what we desire, how do we accomplish this? To begin the Bogalusa Heart Study, our major question was: How do we describe the early natural history of arteriosclerosis in children? It is obvious that we must first obtain more clinical and anatomic information on the origin of the disease process. Several observations underscored this need:

1. In adults, risk factors such as hypertension, obesity, and hyperlipoproteinemia that increase the probability of morbid events have been defined. But disease also occurs without clinical evidence of risk, and the role of other risk factors, such as genetics and emotional stress, remains ill-defined. Furthermore, there appears to be an interaction among the various factors (Fig. 1–7).

2. Marked individual variability in the severity of arteriosclerosis occurs—but reasons for variations in the expression of disease both anatomically (Fig. 1–8) and clinically are not established.

3. Anatomic evidence indicates that atherosclerotic vascular lesions occur in youth—but the initiation of lesions and the evolution of the disease are not clear.

4. Anatomic correlates of early essential hypertension are not yet known (Heptinstall, 1976). More sensitive methods for studying cardiovascular changes associated with early hypertension are needed.

5. Clinical and anatomic manifestations are not fully equated— often morbid events (complications of the disease) do not necessarily

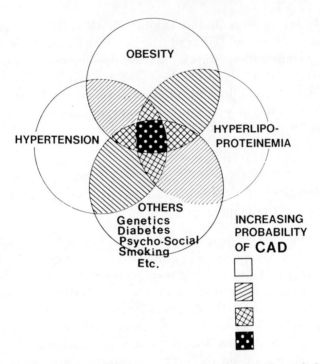

Figure 1–7. The concept of an interrelationship among the risk factor variables with the probability of coronary disease (CAD). A major objective of the studies on children is to show the interrelationship of hypertension, obesity, hyperlipoproteinemia, and other conditions. As will be discussed in several chapters, the precise definition of hypertension in children, for example, is not possible at this time. Therefore, we will provide data that show the interrelationships of blood pressure levels, relative weights, and serum lipid and lipoprotein levels.

mean that extensive or severe vascular lesions have developed, and vice versa. Reducing clinical problems by altering risk factors may not reflect actual regression of the vascular lesions.

6. Marked international differences in atherosclerotic vascular disease and hypertension exist, but the precise environmental or genetic factors involved remain unknown.

These observations indicate large gaps in our knowledge which may be addressed by careful studies in children. But, such studies are handicapped by the lack of noninvasive methods of assessing asymptomatic vascular lesions, by our inability to observe vascular changes over time, and by the lack of morbid events or end-points of disease in children. If, however, risk factors defined in adults do indeed relate to the progression of disease from childhood, clinical and anatomic studies of children over time can begin to fill in some of the information gaps. The characterization of risk factors in a well-described and total population of children would be a good start.

MAJOR INITIAL STUDY QUESTIONS

Several immediate questions emerge from the above discussion which help guide the design of clinical studies of children:

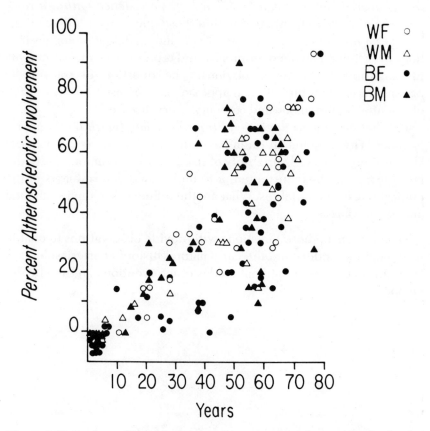

Figure 1–8. Surface atherosclerotic involvement in human aortas of individuals dying in New Orleans. Note the considerable variation in the degree of atherosclerosis at any given age, especially after age 30. It might also be noted that after age 30 almost all individuals in our population have significant atherosclerotic involvement.

1. *What are the distribution and prevalence of risk factors in children from a well-defined population?* Simply, what are they in the general population of young people? Hidden in this apparently straight-forward question is another: How do we define hypertension or hyperlipidemia or obesity in children? At what levels do these factors become a risk?

2. *What are the interrelationships of these factors in children?* Are they similar to those in adults? When do the interrelationships become apparent?

3. *How do these risk factors change with time? What are the trends over time? And can "tracking" or persistence within a rank order be observed?* Contained within these questions is still another: Are measurement techniques precise enough to detect biologic variations over time? The need for precise and reproducible measurements in longitudinal studies is obvious. The question of tracking is paramount to the future clinical approaches to be used for prevention of essential hypertension and coronary artery disease.

4. *What are the etiologic conditions associated with levels of risk factors?* Why do some children have high values, others low values? Why is there a marked variability of risk-factor levels among individuals? Further studies must attempt to understand determinants of the clinical risk factor variables. What are the influences of environmental and genetic factors?

The answers to these questions will provide observations to enable us to begin to understand the early natural history of arteriosclerosis. With this background, rational modes of intervention can then be developed.

2. A community approach to study the cardiovascular risk factors in children—objectives, design, participation, and quality controls

> If I have seen further it is by standing upon the shoulders of
> Giants.
> SIR ISAAC NEWTON, 1676

> . . . a dwarf standing on the shoulders of a giant may see farther
> than a giant himself.
> ROBERT BURTON, ca 1621

> Pigmies placed on the shoulders of giants see more than the
> giants themselves.
> LUCAN, ca AD 39

Although numerous studies of cardiovascular disease are now being conducted on children, many select their sample based on a specific risk-factor variable, such as hypertension or hyperlipoproteinemia. But we must appreciate that the majority of the general population, not just a select group, is at risk for the two major cardiovascular diseases, atherosclerosis and hypertension. Consequently, an epidemiologic study of *all* children within a geographic and well-defined population has merit in the study of the early natural history of arteriosclerosis.

A study of an entire population within a given community has the advantage of characterizing and defining specific parameters related to the objective of that study. Although the observations will apply only to that population, they will serve as a comparison to others. The Bogalusa Heart Study was initiated in 1972 to observe the patterns of cardiovascular (CV) risk-factor variables projected over time in a group of free-living (i.e., not institutionalized) children within a defined geographic area. These children are destined to be the next generation of adults with coronary heart disease and essential hypertension, the major CV diseases in the Bogalusa community, as well as in the United States. The Heart Study is a major program of the Specialized Center of Research in Arteriosclerosis (SCOR-A) of the Louisiana State University Medical Center in New Orleans. Bogalusa, Louisiana, and the immediate surrounding area, designated Ward 4, was selected for this community study. Training programs and pilot studies were conducted in Franklinton, Louisiana, 20 miles west of Bogalusa.

The overall study consists of clinical and laboratory observations to obtain both research and service information. The observations include 1. a blood sample from children (with fasting requested) for lipid, lipoprotein, and hemoglobin analyses; 2. several anthropometric measurements; 3. a physical examination; 4. replicate blood pressure readings; and 5. daily rescreening of a sample. For each type of observation an effort is made to obtain an estimate of measurement error as a guide to the reliability of the data being generated.

Study objective

The objective of the Bogalusa Heart Study is to describe the distribution, interrelationships, and course-over-time of hypothesized risk factors that may relate to beginning arteriosclerosis in children. This chapter is a report of the first phase of the study, a cross-sectional evaluation of children from birth to 14 years of age.

Mixed epidemiologic design

A four-year plan was developed for examining children in two cross-sectional studies linked with four longitudinal (age cohort) studies (Fig. 2–1). The mixed cross-sectional and longitudinal design, although incomplete, allows an efficient means of obtaining information over a broad age range in a short time. The repeat cross-sectional study allows a duplication of the original set of data, provided that the original protocol is adhered to and no great changes occur within the community that might influence the observations.

The first year of general screening began in September 1973 and ended in May 1974. As seen in Figure 2–1, the first cross-sectional

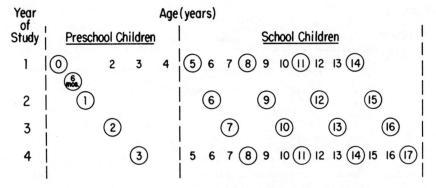

Figure 2–1. The experimental design is to yield information for the period from birth through 17 years of age. A mixed longitudinal and cross-sectional study allows this over a four-year period. Methods need to be sufficiently precise to observe changes of variables from one year to the next. The design will allow us to observe whether tracking of risk-factor variables occurs. For a single person, it is difficult to observe blood pressure and serum lipid changes over this short period of time, but group tendencies are revealed.

study included all children 5 through 14 years old (Frerichs et al., 1976; Srinivasan et al., 1976a; Voors et al., 1976; Foster et al., 1977). All children attending kindergarten through the ninth grade were examined. Enrollment lists were obtained from all schools, which included elementary, junior high, and high schools (through ninth grade), and a parochial and a private school. Ninety-three percent (3,524) of the 3,786 eligible children, ages 5–14, residing in the community were examined during the first school year of the study. During the following summer months 714 preschool-age children, approximately 80% of those identified, were transported to and examined at a central location (Berenson et al., 1978a). From January 1974 through June 1975, clinical and laboratory information was obtained on 440 infants, 98% of all babies born in Bogalusa from Ward 4, to begin a newborn-infant cohort study.

During the second, third, and fourth years, the school children in the four age cohorts were examined at one-year intervals and the infants were followed at the designated intervals (Fig. 2–1) in order to observe changes with time and to note if a child was *tracking* with respect to any of the selected variables. (Tracking occurs when a child remains over time in the same general position in a frequency distribution based on his age, race, and sex cohort. For example, a 5-year-old black girl with a blood pressure between 80th and 90th percentiles

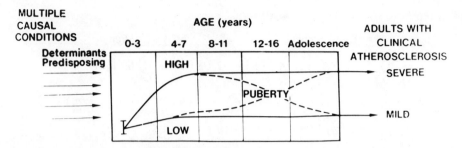

Figure 2–2. A schematic presentation of the change of risk-factor variables over time. The important question is how these variables tend to change, ultimately resulting in clinical disease.

based on all 5-year-old black girls would be tracking if she remained at that high percentile when her age group was 6 years old, or 7, or 8).

The longitudinal information is designed to show changes of variables in a given individual with time and provide information on the question of tracking (Fig. 2–2). Will a child at a high level persist into adulthood with a high level? How much regression toward the mean for the population will occur? It is likely that interpretation of longitudinal information over this period of time will be limited, but such information is urgently needed. Many problems are inherent in a research program seeking to obtain longitudinal observations which ideally may never be obtained.

Over the four years, we are attempting to observe changes over time with respect to anthropometric characteristics, blood pressure, and blood lipids for each of the age cohorts. In addition, by comparing the cross-sectional data in years 1 and 4, we have tried to assess reproducibility of observations and determine if our presence in the community (Levine and Cohen, 1974) or other factors has greatly altered the distribution of the indicated risk-factor variables.

INHERENT LIMITATION OF THE COMPRESSED DESIGN
In comparing observations over time, an interpretation of biologic changes will be limited in part by imprecise measurements. To aid these interpretations, observations which would enable us to estimate measurement error were therefore incorporated into the design. For example, on a cross-sectional basis the annual increment of systolic blood pressure per year of age is 1.3–1.7 mm Hg. Based on our measurement error studies, an approximate 95% confidence interval for a single measurement of systolic blood pressure is 4 mm Hg. Obviously,

estimates of tracking will be limited over a short period. We also found from our studies that three to four serial observations are required to obtain consistent levels of blood pressure.

The community

GEOGRAPHY

Bogalusa is a semirural, biracial community 69 miles north of New Orleans. Ward 4, a political subdivision surrounding and including Bogalusa, was designated as the geographic boundary for children eligible for the study. Certain characteristics make the community useful as a practical epidemiologic laboratory.

POPULATION AND INDUSTRY

Founded in 1906 in the center of virgin pine forests, Bogalusa grew as a lumber town encompassing one of the world's largest lumber mills. With depletion of virgin timber in the 1920's, reforestation led to the development of mills to use rapidly growing pine for manufacture of paper and containers. Small farming operations were the other major activities in this rural area. Substantial migration to the city during the 1940's and 1950's resulted in a 20% population growth rate per decade. Besieged with the integration problems of the times and a recurrent labor strike, this growth ceased in the 1960's when Ward 4 lost 9.4% of its population.

Even with these changes the community has been more stable than neighboring communities and many other regions of the United States (Christou, 1973). Almost 89% of Bogalusa's population lived in the same parish (county) from 1965 to 1970, while for inhabitants of similar-size U.S. communities and the country in general, the percentages were only 71.1 and 76.3 respectively. In 1970, the population of Ward 4 was 22,371 with 82.3% residing in Bogalusa. Racially, the 1970 population was 29.5% black, 70.4% white, and 0.1% of other racial heritage. The Caucasian population arose mostly from a mixture of English, German, and Italian immigrants. The proportion of blacks in Bogalusa has remained relatively stable at 30–35% since the 1940's. Bogalusa was one of the first southern communities to become racially integrated and to develop a federally acceptable program (1969) for school integration.

The Bogalusa lumber mill still dominates the city's economy and employs almost half (49.2%) of the city's work force. Essentially, the populace is conservative and has remained oriented around a major industry of timber and paper production and rural small farms.

Bogalusa is a poor community relative to national standards, but it is comparable to many southern semi-rural populations. In 1970, the median family income was 31% less than the U.S. national average ($6,582 vs $9,590). Over one sixth of all white families (15.5%) and almost one half of all black families (45.3%) had incomes below the U.S. poverty level. Of those below the poverty level, female heads of families comprised 40.6%.

SELECTION OF THE COMMUNITY

Bogalusa was selected as the site for this study for several reasons. The population is biracial and is readily accessible by transportation, communication, and temperament. Church and organizational structures are strong, and according to 1970 U.S. Census, emigration is relatively low. The community respects its physicians and is served by two hospitals, a community private medical center and a charity hospital that is part of a statewide network related to the large medical center in New Orleans. Additionally, smaller adjacent communities were available for development of protocols, testing, and training personnel. Finally, the program director has family ties in the community and has maintained excellent rapport with the citizenry.

Efforts to gain support from community structure

The most important step in initiating the study was obtaining support from *all* local physicians. In approaching the community, the SCOR-A director first contacted the physicians to gain their cooperation, and assured them that the project would not increase their work, compete for patients, infringe on their practice, or lure any medical personnel currently working in Bogalusa away from their present employment. The director solicited advice on procedures and promised continued communication about the study.

With aid from business and social acquaintances, endorsement was obtained from the city officials, key civic leaders, and school administrators. Support was also obtained from the local newspaper and radio stations. A total of 47 meetings was held with various medical, civic, religious, labor, and educational groups, as well as the administration and faculty of each school. (This approach was chosen rather than public announcement of the program through the news media.) Meetings to improve the understanding and appreciation of the importance of the program were continued.

An Advisory Group was formed, consisting of parents, teachers, physicians, ministers, and members of other community related disciplines. At all times SCOR-A has emphasized that this study belongs to the community and is being conducted by individuals from the community.

Preparations for conducting the program

An administrative office was established in Bogalusa with a laboratory area for preparing blood samples for shipment to the New Orleans laboratory for analyses. A full-time member of SCOR-A's Planning and Analysis section was placed in the community to implement the program and a knowledgeable and dedicated Community Coordinator, highly respected in Bogalusa, was employed. After the initial field staff was hired in mid-1972, training sessions began in preparation for feasibility studies in nearby Franklinton. A mobile research unit (MRU) was converted from a three-bedroom house trailer to aid examination of the children in conjunction with facilities at each of the 14 Bogalusa schools. Three preparatory studies involving over 450 school children were conducted in Franklinton between November 1972 and May 1973, and a final pilot study was performed in August 1973. These studies advantageously popularized the program and created an interest in the upcoming studies in Bogalusa. Most importantly, however, they were needed to establish the methods and to train the staff before beginning in the study population.

Extensive studies of paired testing, Graeco-Latin Square designs (Snedecor and Cochran, 1967) and field tests were made at LSU Medical School and in Franklinton to compare seven blood pressure instruments and to select a design conducive to obtaining reliable indirect blood pressures of children (Webber et al., 1975) (Chapter 5). After a year spent developing protocols* and conducting preliminary field studies, the SCOR-A field unit, trained to follow a designated protocol, was considered ready to start the Bogalusa Heart Study.

---

*Detailed protocols of SCOR-A are unpublished but available for cost of reproduction. Some are outlined in *Cardiovascular Profile of 15,000 Children from Three Communities*, DHEW publ. No. (NIH) 78-1472, 1978.

Consultation in planning

Throughout the study, consultation continued at three levels: 1. within the project staff at weekly one-hour meetings, 2. by cross-disciplinary consultation—formal, funded, and unfunded consultations were organized with other departments of the local universities and medical schools, covering a wide range of subjects, and 3. with selected national experts, some of whom visited the field operation. Besides aiding in planning, these efforts served an in-service training function and fostered a widespread sense of responsibility.

Collection of information and examinations

LETTERS, FORMS, AND HEALTH HISTORY

Letters were written to parents or guardians and delivered through teachers to students selected for study. Parental consent was obtained for each participant along with a health history. Since a 12- to 14-hour fast was required for the lipid determinations, fasting instructions were sent to the parents the day before the child's screening session. Brochures explaining various studies were made available to parents and teachers. Additional letters were developed to send to parents and physicians of the parent's choice when warranted by clinical and laboratory observations of a child.

The health history form sent to each child's parents requested selected information about 1. possible heart, lung, or kidney disease; high blood pressure; diabetes; or anemia, 2. special medication or physician-prescribed diets, and 3. smoking habits and source of the child's drinking water (well or city).

RECORDING OF DATA AND FLOW OF EXAMINATION

A detailed data pack which included color-coded forms for keypunching was developed on which to record observations for each child. The data packs accompanied each child through the series of stations designated for specific examinations. The outside cover was clearly marked for confidentiality along with the code number and identification of the child, and for review follow-up when required. All data were entered by trained staff assigned daily to each of the stations (Figs. 2–3 to 2–15).

When possible, all examinations were conducted in the school au-

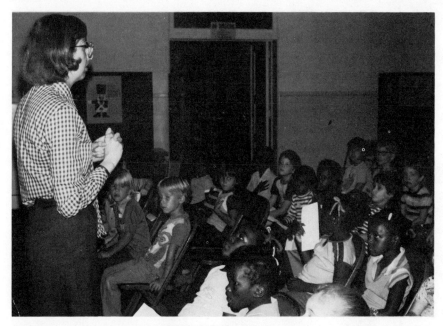

Figure 2–3. Dr. Caroline Blonde, a pediatrician and epidemiologist, speaks reassuringly to elementary school children as they wait to begin screening. Dr. Blonde explains the procedures they will be following, including venipuncture, anthropometric measurements, examination by a physician, and blood pressure measurements. Confidentiality is stressed to older children. Shortly afterwards movie cartoons are shown.

ditoriums and in the SCOR-A MRU. The auditorium was used for assembling and identifying children, drawing the initial blood sample, and later for housing six blood pressure stations. The MRU contained facilities for conducting physical examinations, making selected anthropometric measurements, and editing for completeness of data packs.

All children (up to 50 per day) were examined between 8:30 a.m. and 12 noon. The field personnel for screening included two or three physicians, five registered nurses, six licensed practical nurses, one physician's assistant, six other staff members, and several volunteers. The staff wore regular clothing or colored SCOR-A jackets rather than white uniforms. Physical examinations, largely a service function, were conducted by part-time physicians and occasionally by medical students. Three or four volunteers from the Bogalusa Civic League

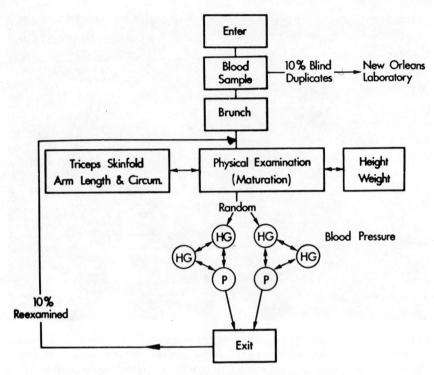

Figure 2–4. The flow of examination of the children to obtain information on risk-factor variables. The specific function(s) at each station is indicated. Note blind duplicate blood samples and reexamination of children as part of daily quality controls.

complemented the staff. Movie cartoons were shown to the children as they waited.

Figure 2–4 shows the flow of the examination, which included:

1. *Communication with children*—The children were assembled and then addressed by the day's senior physician, who discussed the procedures, importance of the screening, and confidentiality. The children were escorted by volunteers in an organized (strictly at random) order to each of the stations.

2. *Blood sample*—Fasting or nonfasting was designated by the time of the child's last meal in order to obtain a reported account. This information was gathered by probing questions, often related to television viewed the evening before. Two blood samples from the antecubital site were taken from each child, an anticoagulated sample for

hemoglobin and a clotted sample for lipid analyses. Only two attempts at venipuncture were allowed. The clotted blood samples were centrifuged in Bogalusa and the separated sera and samples of anticoagulated whole blood were sent in a cold pack box on the evening of screening by bus to New Orleans. The samples were received by laboratory personnel and refrigerated at 4° C. On the following day, serum total cholesterol and triglycerides were measured by a Technicon AutoAnalyzer II, the operation of which follows the standardization and control program of the U.S. Center for Disease Control in Atlanta (Lipid Research Clinics Program, 1974). In addition, α-lipopro-

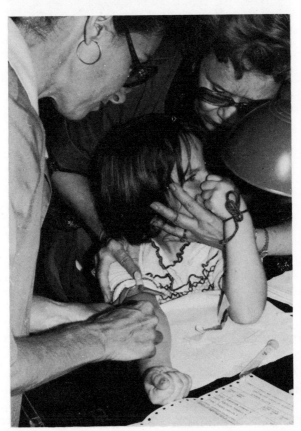

Figure 2–5. Susan Marie Stephens, a first grader, is at a venipuncture station. Susan has been randomly selected to have duplicate blood samples drawn. The samples are identified with different numbers and are given fictitious names from the telephone book to begin the flow of "blind duplicates."

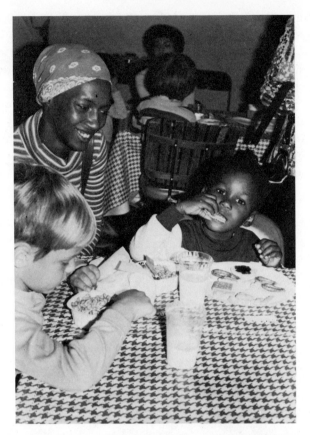

Figure 2–6. Walter Curney, a 4-year-old participant, enjoys the brunch he selected to eat after his venipuncture fast, while his mother, Mrs. Genester Curney, looks on. By allowing Walter to choose between different foods, Heart Study nutritionists are observing beginning dietary habits.

tein, β-lipoprotein, and pre-β-lipoprotein concentrations were determined for each serum sample by methods described elsewhere (Berenson et al., 1972a; Srinivasan et al., 1975a). For a research study, the measurement of lipoprotein macromolecules was considered necessary as a better index of the metabolic state than cholesterol and triglycerides alone. An additional set of blood samples for blind duplicate analyses was collected daily from four randomly selected children for assessment of measurement error. Budgeting limitations prevented duplication of all blood samples.

    3. *Brunch*—A light breakfast of cereal, milk, fruit, and graham

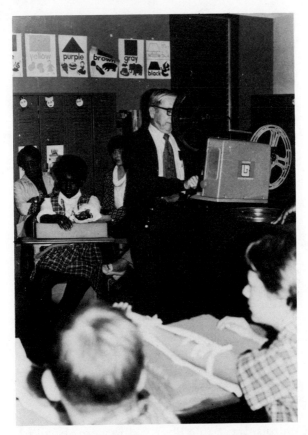

Figure 2–7. After venipuncture, Melissa Frazier and Alan Theriot are about to view a movie cartoon to keep them relaxed while waiting for another blood sample—the arm is partially immobilized and a heparin lock is used when a glucose tolerance test is given. Mr. E. L. Burrus runs the projector while staff member Brenda Burris, clerk, and Linda Anderson, volunteer, look on.

crackers was served to the children immediately after venipuncture.

4. *Anthropometric measurements*—Once the children entered the MRU and changed into uniform dressing gowns, measurements were made of their height, weight, upper-arm length (acromion-olecranon), upper-arm circumference (mid-point), and triceps skinfold thickness. Height was measured manually on a height board constructed by the University of Iowa and weight on a standard platform scale. An electronic height board* and electronic weight scale with a digital printer

*Constructed locally, modified from plans from Mayo Clinic.

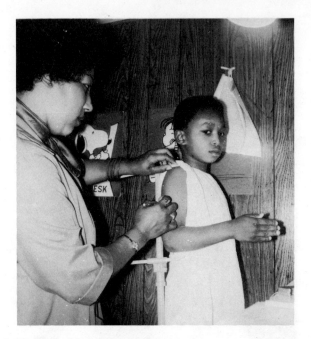

Figure 2–8. Maevella Moore, LPN, follows the protocol hanging on the wall as she prepares to make skinfold measurements at the center of the arm on Eric Bolton. Protocols are visible and available at each station. At this station arm length and circumference are measured to determine cuff size for blood pressure measurements later in the examination.

(National Controls, Inc. Santa Rosa, Calif.) were also used to test their utility in mass screening programs to help eliminate observer bias. Upper-arm lengths and circumferences were measured with an anthropometric caliper and a cloth tape measure, respectively. These values were used to select the proper size cuff for blood pressure determinations. The triceps skinfold was measured three times by the same examiner with Lange skinfold calipers (Cambridge Scientific Industries, Cambridge, Mass.). Observations were recorded after each single measurement.

5. *Physical examination*—A physician gave each child a physical examination. The observations were recorded by a staff member, usually a licensed practical nurse, on forms listing essential points of each organ system. Special attention was given to suspicious or abnormal findings. The detection of suspected or definite abnormalities was noted on the data pack for review at final editing and later by a physi-

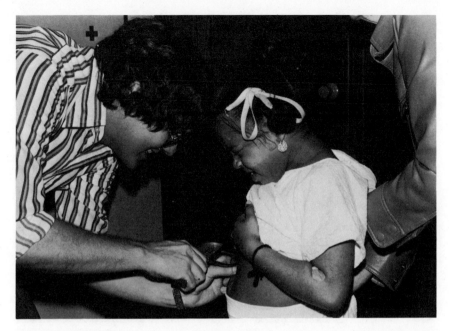

Figure 2–9. Multiple precise anthropometric measurements were performed on some children. Here David Harsha, a graduate student in anthropology, takes an abdominal skinfold measurement from Tamanthea R. Ford.

cian. Only summary reviews were recorded for coding later. Each child was graded for maturation according to the criteria of Tanner (1962), and the adolescent girls were asked for the date of onset of menarche and the use of contraceptive pills. When physical abnormalities were found, a description of the observations or the tentative diagnosis was sent to the child's family physician or to the Charity Hospital in Bogalusa, and another letter was sent to alert the parents.

6. *Blood pressure*—At the completion of the examination in the MRU, the children dressed, returned to the auditorium where six stations had been assembled for recording blood pressures, and were encouraged to urinate before their blood pressure was recorded. Each child was randomly rotated through a team of observers at three stations. Blood pressure readings were recorded three times at each of the three separate stations (Fig. 2–16). For the number of children being studied, two teams were needed to minimize ear fatigue and decrease examination time. For each team, two stations were equipped with the standard mercury sphygmomanometers (Baumano-

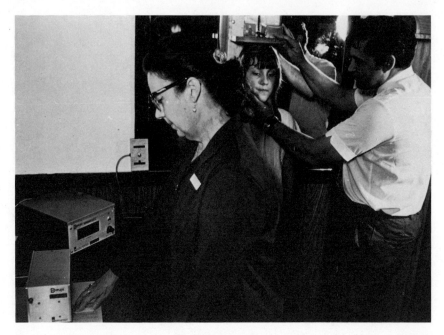

Figure 2–10. Height measurements are made not only with a manual board, seen over the shoulder of staff member Herbert Temple, but with an automatic electronic height board. The measurement is recorded on a data form by Barbara Henderson, technician.

meter, W. A. Baum Co., Inc. Copiague, N.Y.) and the third with a Physiometrics automated blood pressure instrument (Sphygmetrics, Inc., Woodland Hills, Calif.). The first (systolic), fourth (diastolic), and fifth Korotkoff sounds were recorded at the mercury sphygmomanometer stations. The records generated by the Physiometrics were equivalent to the first and fourth phases. To avoid examiner bias, both the team and the order of stations within the team were assigned strictly at random for each child. Only trained observers were used for blood pressure measurement. In an effort not to compress these readings, serial training sessions were conducted for *all* members of the team simultaneously without personal review of their performance in collecting research data.

7. *Reward*—At the completion of the examination, each child was awarded a colored metallic "Mardi Gras" doubloon, emblematic of the study. Children who participated in special substudies (not de-

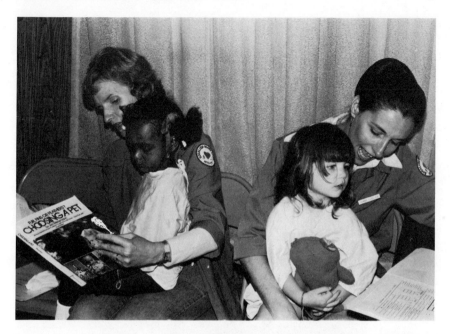

Figure 2–11. Rhondalynne Hogan (child on the left) is kept amused by Doris Sorey, RN, while Amy Stewart and Donna Lee, RN, look at a data pack. These children are waiting for physical examinations in the Mobile Research Unit. Shortly afterward these nurses will be recording blood pressures for the completion of the examination. The relaxed mood enables obtaining more reproducible blood pressures.

scribed here) received embroidered blue-jean patches and hand-lettered certificates.

8. *Data by rescreening*—Information on rescreenees was obtained daily to observe reproducibility of observations and estimates of measurement errors. At the end of each morning, an independent sample of four children was selected strictly at random, for a second complete examination (except for venipuncture and brunch). Since boys and girls could not be processed through the MRU at the same time, all children selected for replicate examinations on a given day were of the same sex.

9. *Nutrition survey*—the collection of dietary information on a total population of children is difficult and practically not feasible. Dietary data were collected on a 50% random sample ($n = 185$) of all

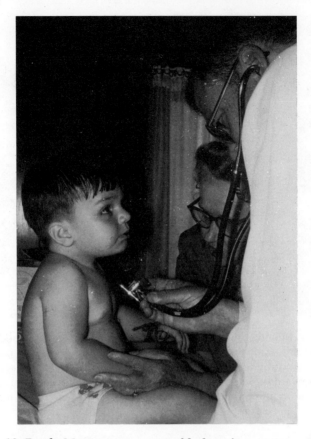

Figure 2–12. Randy Maness, a two-year-old, doesn't seem to appreciate the thorough examination he is receiving from Dr. John Harris. Mae Abrahamsen, LPN, assists and records observations in the data pack. Note the mark on the right arm, site of skinfold measurement and colored ribbon on left wrist that matches ribbon on outside of child's data pack folder.

children born in 1963 (ages 10–11 years) with a 24-hour dietary recall method slightly modified for use in children (Frank et al., 1977a; Frank et al., 1978). The method included a computer analysis of some 1,800 food items in the Extended Table of Nutrient Values (Moore et al., 1974). Similar information was collected on a small sample of preschool-age children and efforts were made to obtain dietary information on the infant cohort by a questionnaire and recall studies with the mothers.

    10. *Socioeconomic status*—A questionnaire was sent to all parents

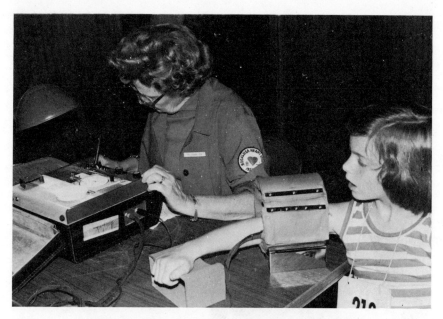

Figure 2–13. Blood pressure is being recorded on Lisa Paige Erwin with an automatic instrument by Peg Graham, LPN. Blood pressure measurements follow a random sequence, shown by the numbered card worn by Lisa. All discs with blood pressure recorded are read later by one observer. If desired, the influence of observer–child interaction on blood pressure can be obtained.

asking the education and occupation of the head of the household. These data, based upon a 75% response, were converted to a social scale using the Duncan Index (Reiss et al., 1961; Hunter et al., 1979).

Quality controls

LABORATORY BLIND DUPLICATES
In order to note limitations associated with each of the various measurements, the Planning and Analysis section established a system for replicate blood samples and examinations. Each day, 4 out of about 40 blood samples were randomly sampled and drawn in duplicate. Each duplicate sample was individually processed for subsequent laboratory analysis with a new ID number and a name from the New Orleans telephone book. The error of measurement included the capability to measure for a given child the level of the blood lipids and included er-

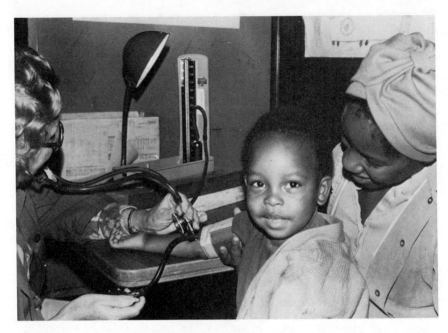

Figure 2–14. Frederick Fland, a 4-year-old participant, is held by his mother, Mrs. Marsha M. Fland, as his blood pressure is taken by Mae Abrahamsen, LPN. Because resting, relaxed blood pressure readings are sought, the children are kept calm and quiet. Younger children are held by their parents to allay their fears. Note well-lighted manometer placed at eye level to avoid parallax.

rors compounded by collection, centrifugation, analysis, and computer processing. Additional quality controls were conducted in the New Orleans laboratory by its own internal standardization program and its participation in a lipid surveillance program of U.S. Center for Disease Control in Atlanta (Lipid Research Clinics Program, 1974). Internal quality controls were also conducted in the laboratory in an effort to prevent drift.

TRAINING STAFF

Criteria for trained observers were established and extensive training programs were conducted throughout the year for all field observers to assure adherence to protocols. Errors of individual observers were not identified,* and when needed, the team of observers was retrained.

*The purpose of this procedure was to avoid bias in the future performance of the individual, which could lead to an artificial "compression" of his data.

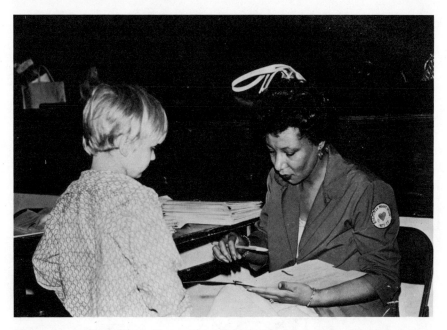

Figure 2–15. The edit desk is an important part of the quality control. One is placed in the mobile research unit and another at the end of examination flow. Here Connie Harry carefully checks the data pack for completeness.

For blood pressure, training included special movies, split stethoscope readings on a single subject, and rotation programs where each of a group of subjects was measured by each examiner. The same rotation method was used to train and test observers taking anthropometric measurements. For example, each examiner at the training sessions was asked to measure ten children and the results were analyzed to determine the deviation of the individual examiner from the group mean.

INSTRUMENT CHECKS
The manual and electronic scales were calibrated daily with uniform test weights, and the skinfold caliper was checked weekly with three standard wedges of known width. The electronic height board was periodically checked against a set of 26 standards of varying lengths and with the manual height board. Regression curves for the electronic board were calculated periodically during the study.

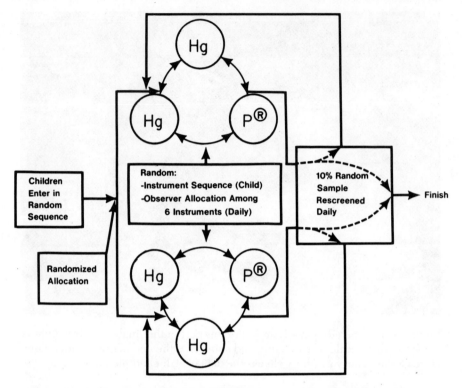

Figure 2–16. The pattern for blood pressure measurements. The randomization, reexamination, and use of an automatic instrument allows detailed study of indirect blood pressure.

MONITORING

Members of the Planning and Analysis section periodically made unannounced site visits to observe adherence to protocols at each station. While developing protocols and training personnel, for later review, we photographed activities at the stations. Once the study was begun, deviations from protocols were corrected at a later time through a scheduled training session directed at the team of observers. On occasion, data from a randomly selected week were extensively analyzed by statisticians, independent of SCOR-A support, to observe the quality of data being generated. Preliminary data were similarly analyzed on the first two school cohorts. Blind duplicate laboratory data were checked monthly without altering stored data. These checks permitted us to detect incipient aberrations from the protocol which were subsequently corrected. More frequent monitoring of selected data would have been desirable but was not feasible. No other analyses were allowed until completion of an entire phase of the study.

Study participation

PARTICIPATION OF SCHOOL-AGE CHILDREN

Almost 95% of the eligible children, whose names were supplied by school enrollment lists, originally consented to participate in the study. Each child in the respondent group was given three opportunities to be examined. These children were 3 through 18 years old, with the younger and older ages included to obtain the target population, 5 to 14 years of age.

NONRESPONSE

Of the 4,288 children, 316 (7.4%) were not examined because they either refused, did not respond, moved, or died. Several parents indicated they did not wish to force their child to participate or subject him to blood drawing and the examination. Some refused examination because of illness and close medical supervision already received.

In the summer of 1974, the staff and local school teachers determined the number of children living in Ward 4 who were not accounted for in the Bogalusa school census. Adding these children and deleting those less than 5 years old, those older than 14, and those who lived outside Ward 4 during the 1973–74 school year, we estimated a total eligible population of 3,786 children. Of the eligible population, 93% (3,524) were subsequently screened, 37% of whom were black and 63% white. Almost 97% of the black children participated in the study compared to 91% of the white children. The youngest and oldest age groups had the greatest percentage of nonparticipants. White girls had the lowest participation percentage (89.5%) among the four race-sex groups and black girls had the highest percentage (98.1%). Using chi-square analysis, a highly significant difference ($p < 0.0001$) was found in the race-sex distribution between the participants and nonparticipants. This difference was mainly due to an under-representation of white children in the examined population, and over-representation of black children, especially girls.

Preschool-age children

To identify the children of preschool age, we utilized birth records and information on relationships to the school children. Of the estimated 898, 714 were examined. We modified the examination of this age cohort, especially in observing blood pressure levels (Berenson et al., 1978a).

Newborn-Infant Cohort

The beginning of the Newborn-Infant Cohort Study was much simpler than the studies of children, since all but seven deliveries occurred in two hospitals. With the aid of physicians and nurses in the obstetrical units, we collected 95% (419 of 440 consents) of the cord bloods from infants residing in Ward 4. Serial clinics were conducted at the Parish (county) Health Unit to follow the infants according to the study design.

Efforts for and reflections on continued community support

The first year of the Bogalusa Heart Study brought 91% participation from the eligible population. This high participation reflected the enthusiasm with which the community received the Heart Study, recognizing its service aspects and its overall research contributions. Most of the success is attributed to thorough preparation and public relations efforts during the year prior to beginning screening. Informing and soliciting the cooperation of both the lay and medical communities were continual efforts. Talks to organizations were given as often as requested, and feedback from the community was welcomed. A weekly column by the SCOR-A staff writer appeared in the Bogalusa Sunday News. Entitled "What's the SCOR?", this human-interest column featured photographs of local children, discussed program-related material, and gave a running account of the number of children screened. In general, the local staff created a climate of confidence surrounding the program's intent. Continued communication with the field staff on the importance of the data being collected also indirectly furthered community support.

We added a service aspect by incorporating a physical examination, a hemoglobin analysis, and reporting of abnormalities. These services were beneficial to our image, and the reporting of abnormalities was consistent with good medical practice, especially since the importance in children of high percentiles of risk-factor variables is still unknown.

Finally, our general guiding principle was to conduct the study professionally, as a physician/single patient relationship transposed into an epidemiologic research setting for 5,000 children. Significant findings or potentially abnormal observations from the clinical examinations or from laboratory data based on clinical standards were communicated to parents and physicians. Support by SCOR-A professional staff was given to Bogalusa or Franklinton physicians when requested.

GENERAL GUIDELINES FOLLOWED DURING THE STUDY

Attempts to collect reliable information

Since products of research ideally should be based on facts free of emotional bias, the measurements of children of all ages were intended to be objective, reliable, accurate, and reproducible. To achieve the model, as discussed above, we established protocols; trained observers as teams and periodically retrained them without attempts to "compress" the observations of specific individuals; monitored all observations (when possible, within limits of staff availability); randomized procedures; and adhered to confidentiality of data. Electronic equipment was incorporated when possible as a control of manual equipment. Monitoring of data was conducted on blind and random samples of data. These analyses served as a preliminary indication of data being generated and assessed our adherence to protocols. For studies being conducted over time (longitudinal studies), it obviously becomes necessary to follow a fixed protocol and minimize deviations in collection of information. Estimates to obtain measurement errors within the laboratory were made by daily blind duplicate blood samples and for the clinical observations by daily rescreening of children.

Attempts to maintain population and data uncontaminated

In initiating the study, we avoided the study population. Pretesting and pilot studies were conducted elsewhere. Similarly, data remained intact until completed and were not released to investigators. These approaches served to limit distortions of the data base and to decrease premature judgment.

Confidentiality

Confidentiality was stressed throughout the study. For example, all data packs were clearly marked CONFIDENTIAL, and information on an individual child was reviewed and reported only by a designated pediatrician. Such information was not made available to the general staff in the community or to parents unless deemed appropriate. For data handling purposes, each subject was identified by a code number, and laboratory blind duplicates were reported by real and fictitious code numbers. All field observers were identified by code numbers; efforts were made not to identify specific observers. All data for analysis by investigators were handled by the statistician in charge of the Planning and Analysis section, and tapes for computer analysis were identified by a code not available to computer personnel outside the SCOR-A staff. Finally, the director assumed responsibility for all treatment and observations on each child and for the handling of all data.

SUMMARY

The Bogalusa Heart Study is an epidemiologic investigation of a total community of children for cardiovascular risk factors for coronary artery disease and essential hypertension. The approaches used to solicit community support and participation, gather reliable information on entire population, and maintain rigid quality controls are outlined in detail. We have particularly tried to obtain reliable information on clinical and laboratory variables that are likely to play a role in cardiovascular diseases. The findings form a base for future observations. Extended observations over time will be critical to understanding the natural history of these diseases. Through combined efforts, this study of children transposes a community into a useful laboratory for research on the major cardiovascular diseases occurring in this country's population.

II. Methodology

3. A simple method of quantitating serum lipoproteins

Because increased concentrations of certain serum lipoproteins relate to susceptibility to coronary artery disease, practical methods for quantitation are needed to obtain baseline data in the general population, especially in children. The minimum requirement for the diagnosis and classification of hyperlipoproteinemia is an estimation of both serum cholesterol and triglyceride concentrations and electrophoresis of serum lipoproteins. Although serum cholesterol can be measured easily, estimates of serum triglycerides and electrophoretic separation of lipoproteins are done only in specialized laboratories. In many instances, neonates and children for example, if only serum cholesterol is determined, lipid deviations of abnormalities may not be detected (Kwiterovich, 1974; Srinivasan et al., 1976a; Frerichs et al., 1978a).

The reports of Gofman and co-workers (deLalla and Gofman, 1954) emphasize differences in serum lipoproteins which could be characterized by ultracentrifugation. Although the techniques of analytical or preparative ultracentrifugation are generally accepted as the standard methods, they cannot be applied to large-scale studies because of their complexity and expense. Several simple methods are currently in use to assay serum lipoproteins for clinical purposes. Most commonly used are the electrophoretic-based phenotyping system for the differential diagnosis of hyperlipoproteinemia. For detecting subtle

47

lipoprotein differences or abnormalities in a group of individuals, quantitative rather than qualitative methods are required, which include selective precipitation by polyanions in the presence of divalent cations, quantitative agarose-gel electrophoresis, and membrane ultrafiltration (Hatch and Lees, 1968; Burstein et al., 1970; Stone et al., 1970; Friedewald et al., 1972; Hatch et al., 1973).

Recent studies in our laboratory indicate that the characteristics and concentrations of polyanions (glycosaminoglycans), the lipoproteins in serum, and the divalent metal ions (e.g., Ca^{2+}, Mg^{2+}, Mn^{2+}) are all critical for quantitative and selective precipitation of the lipoproteins (Srinivasan et al., 1970b; Srinivasan et al., 1975b). From these observations, a simple method for measuring lipoproteins was developed that is adaptable for easy laboratory use and does not require expensive equipment. The method uses only 0.5 ml serum and is a combination of a heparin-Ca^{2+} precipitation and an agarose-gel electrophoresis of serum (Srinivasan et al., 1970a; Lopez-S, et al., 1971; Berenson et al., 1972a; Berenson et al., 1972b; Srinivasan et al., 1975a).

PROCEDURES

β- plus pre-β-lipoprotein cholesterol

Briefly, the method consists of mixing serum (0.2 ml), distilled water (3.2 ml), beef lung heparin (0.1 ml of 0.25 g/100 ml solution, $\simeq$ 140 units/mg Upjohn Co., Kalamazoo, Mich.), and $CaCl_2$ (0.5 M, 0.5 ml) in the order given and measuring the turbidity obtained after 15 min at 600 nm against a blank containing a similar mixture but omitting heparin. (Plasma is not suitable for this method.) The precipitate obtained after centrifugation can be analyzed for the corresponding β- and pre-β-lipoprotein cholesterol content by dissolving it in 0.2 ml of 0.15 M NaCl. The cholesterol content in β + pre-β-lipoprotein can also be related to turbidimetric measurements by constructing a standard curve. This curve is obtained by measuring turbidity with increasing amounts of serum (0.05–0.4 ml), the addition of distilled water to make the total volume 4.0 ml, and analyzing the cholesterol content of the precipitate as described above. From this standard curve (Fig. 3–1) the β + pre-β-lipoprotein cholesterol value of any given serum can be calculated by turbidimetry alone. In the analysis of individual serum samples for those giving higher values (above 0.5 O.D.), less than 0.2 ml should be used.

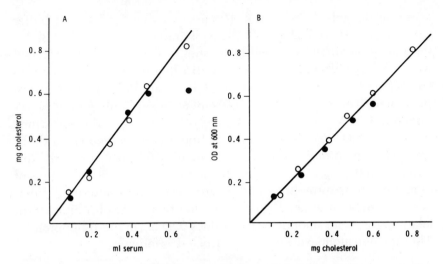

Figure 3–1. Relationship between turbidity and cholesterol of serum β- plus pre-β-lipoproteins. Cholesterol values are plotted against serum volume (A) and turbidity (B). It is apparent from the figure that 250 μg heparin is adequate for precipitation. The cholesterol of β- plus pre-β-lipoproteins of a given serum can be determined from the curve by measuring the turbidity alone, for example, to express as mg% β- and pre-β-lipoprotein cholesterol:

$$\frac{100 \times \text{mg cholesterol (turbidity curve)}}{\text{ml serum}}$$

Heparin: ● 250 μg; ○ 750 μg.

α-lipoprotein cholesterol

The value for α-lipoprotein cholesterol can be obtained by subtracting β + pre-β-lipoprotein cholesterol from serum total cholesterol (Srinivasan et al., 1975a; Srinivasan et al., 1976a). Although this is an indirect measure of α-lipoprotein, the observations compare favorably to those obtained by ultracentrifugation (Srinivasan et al., 1978a).

Electrophoretic ratios of β- and pre-β-lipoproteins

Electrophoresis of serum lipoprotein is performed according to the techniques described by Noble (1968) with some modifications (Srinivasan et al., 1970a). (Any commercial agarose-gel electrophoresis system should be adequate.) Serum (10–20 μl) is electrophoresed on agar-agarose gel plates (8.3 × 10 cm), with use of barbital buffer (pH 8.6, 0.05 M) and 22 mA per plate. Staining is done with Oil Red O for 6 hr or overnight followed by washing successively with alcohol/water (5/3 by vol) for 5 min and then distilled water. The lipoprotein bands are scanned in a densitometer (Quic Scan, Helena Laboratories, Beaumont, Texas). We set the instrument to scan only β- and pre-β-lipoprotein as $X\%$ and $Y\%$, respectively, keeping $X + Y = 100$. Since the dye uptake (per unit weight of lipoprotein) is known to differ among the lipoprotein classes (Hatch et al., 1973), because of the differences in their protein and lipid content, the densitometric ratios of β- and pre-β-lipoprotein (X and Y) are corrected as described previously (Srinivasan et al., 1975a), assuming that 1 mg of β-lipoprotein takes up the same amount of dye as does 0.86 mg of pre-β-lipoprotein. Thus the densitometric ratios are corrected as follows:

$$\% \ \beta\text{-lipoprotein,} \ X' = \frac{100X}{X + 0.86Y} \qquad (1)$$

$$\% \ \text{pre-}\beta\text{-lipoprotein,} \ Y' = \frac{86Y}{X + 0.86Y} \qquad (2)$$

where X and Y represent the original densitometric ratios of β- and pre-β-lipoproteins based on lipid stain; X' and Y' represent the corrected ratios. Although the staining capacity of the individual lipid fractions may not be identical and the relative lipid contents of the lipoproteins may vary in some instances, a reasonably good estimate of lipoproteins can be obtained by this method.

Estimation of β- and pre-β-lipoprotein concentrations

Serum β- and pre-β-lipoprotein concentrations are calculated as previously described (Srinivasan et al., 1970a, Lopez-S., 1971). These quantitations are based on the densitometric (electrophoretic scanning) ratio of β- to pre-β-lipoprotein, the β- plus pre-β-lipoprotein cholesterol content, and fractional cholesterol content of β- and pre-β-lipoprotein molecules. (Variations of 5–10% in fractional cholesterol content of lipoprotein molecules will only change the β-lipoprotein estimation to the same magnitude and do not appreciably change pre-β-lipoprotein estimation.) The following equations were used to quantitate these lipoprotein classes:

$$\text{mg\% } \beta\text{-lipoprotein: } \frac{100XZ}{46.9X + 22.2Y} \qquad (3)$$

$$\text{mg\% pre-}\beta\text{-lipoprotein: } \frac{100YZ}{46.9X + 22.2Y} \qquad (4)$$

where X = % β-lipoproteins (uncorrected densitometric ratio)
     Y = % pre-β-lipoprotein (uncorrected densitometric ratio)
     Z = mg% β- plus pre-β-lipoprotein cholesterol (heparin-Ca^{2+} precipitation method)

Combining Eqs. 1–4, we can make the following derivations:

$$\text{mg\% } \quad \beta\text{-lipoprotein: } \frac{126.1XZ}{59.1X + 24.2Y}$$

$$\text{mg\% } \quad \text{pre-}\beta\text{-lipoprotein: } \frac{108.8YZ}{59.1X + 24.2Y}$$

The lipoprotein values can be easily converted into the corresponding lipoprotein cholesterol as follows: β-lipoprotein cholesterol = mg% β-lipoprotein × 0.469; pre-β-lipoprotein cholesterol = mg% pre-β-lipoprotein × 0.222.

Estimation of α-lipoprotein

Serum concentrations of α-lipoprotein are obtained by multiplying α-lipoprotein cholesterol by a factor of 5.9, assuming that the cholesterol content of the α-lipoprotein molecule is 17%.

VALIDATION OF THE LIPOPROTEIN METHODOLOGY

A comparison of β- plus pre-β-lipoprotein cholesterol values obtained by turbidimetric (indirect) and chemical analyses (direct) shows a very good correlation between direct and indirect estimation (Table 3–1). In a group of "normal" individuals, the difference between the two methods (3.5 mg) is less than 2%. (Statistically, the difference is not significant, $p > 0.05$.) A somewhat greater difference was observed in patients with diabetes, myocardial infarction, and renal disease, as might be expected. This greater variability is probably due to the increase in pre-β-lipoproteins, which contain relatively less cholesterol. Values above an O.D. of 0.24 or β- plus pre-β-

Table 3–1. Comparison of β- and pre-β-lipoprotein cholesterol values
obtained by turbidimetric and chemical analyses of precipitated lipoproteins

			Cholesterol		
		Absorbance [1]	Turbidity [1] (mg/dl)	Precipitate [1] (mg/dl)	t [2]
"Normals"	(69)[3]	0.24 (.14–.33)	127.1 (75–175)	130.6 (75–175)	−1.76[4]
Diabetes	(21)	0.32 (.22–.53)	169.8 (115–280)	159.4 (79–270)	2.85
Mycoardial infarction	(14)	0.28 (.17–.45)	148.9 (90–240)	139.5 (72–218)	2.77
Liver disease	(16)	0.23 (.18–.49)	124.9 (95–260)	124.9 (90–301)	1.00[4]
Renal disease	(14)	0.34 (.10–.57)	178.5 (55–305)	146.5 (67–285)	3.74
Xanthoma	(4)	0.39 (.23–.62)	207.5 (120–330)	201.8 (129–350)	

[1]Mean and ranges
[2]Test of significance for the difference between the two methods (calculated from individual values)
(Berenson et al., 1974a)
[3]Number of subjects
[4]The difference is not significant ($P > 0.05$), i.e., there is good agreement between turbidity
and analyses of precipitate.

lipoprotein cholesterol over 130 mg% are considered above normal
limits. Individuals having such levels should be studied in more detail for serum total cholesterol, triglyceride levels, and lipoprotein patterns.

Beta- and pre-β-lipoproteins estimated by the present method
were compared with estimates using the analytical ultracentrifuge
method: eight sera (five normal adults and three patients with diabetes) were analyzed in blind duplicates. Ultracentrifugal analyses of
low-density lipoprotein (S_f 0-12) and very low-density lipoproteins
(S_f 12-400), which correspond to β- and pre-β-lipoprotein, respectively
(Noble, 1968), were performed according to the method of deLalla and
Gofman (1954). Table 3–2 shows results with good reproducibility
using the present method as compared to data obtained by use of the
ultracentrifuge. Duplicate analyses by the present method gave percent mean variations of ± 1.3 for β- and ±3.7 for pre-β-lipoproteins,
compared to ±5.4 (S_f 0-12) and ±9.3 (S_f 12-400) fractions. Significant
differences were observed in some samples, e.g., Number 5, where
the pre-β-lipoprotein value obtained by the present method was low

Table 3–2. Comparison of lipoprotein analyses by ultracentrifuge and turbidimetric methods

| | mg/dl lipoprotein | | | | | |
| | Turbidimetry and electrophoresis | | Ultracentrifuge | | Serum triglycerides (mg/dl) | Serum cholesterol (mg/dl) |
Sample[1]	β	pre-β	S_f 0-12 (β)[2]	S_f 12-400 $(pre\text{-}\beta)$[2]		
1	376	220	359	209	235	310
	390	250	359	231		
2	275	49	266	44	81	210
	268	55	318	49		
3	318	163	370	196	280	185
	312	169	281	194		
4	320	125	423	99	163	215
	306	119	453	140		
5	296	61	308	132	110	195
	300	62	338	171		
6	215	138	223	91	140	172
	219	123	234	102		
7	273	135	341	123	120	210
	—	—	316	87		
8	273	91	246	43	118	218
	—	—	—	—		
Mean percent difference (±) between duplicates	1.3	3.7	5.4	9.3	—	—
	(0.63–2.2)	(0.8–6.3)	(0–14.0)	(0.51–17.6)	—	—

[1] Duplicate analysis
[2] F. T. Hatch, and R. S. Lees, (1968)

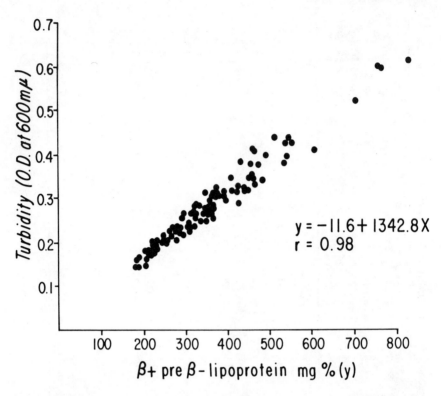

Figure 3–2. Relationship between turbidity (x) and serum β- plus pre-β-lipoprotein (y) concentrations in sera from 100 individuals (85 "normal" and 15 diabetic patients). Regression equation: $y = -11.6 + 1,342.8x$. Correlation coefficient: $r = 0.98$. Standard deviation from regression 27.6.

compared to the S_f 12-400 fraction. The low serum triglyceride value correlated better with the lower pre-β-lipoprotein value obtained by the indirect method.) These comparisons are in adequate ranges for clinical use.

The validity of the lipoprotein methodology was further tested for children by sending samples to Dr. Ralph Ellefson (Lipid Research Laboratory, Mayo Clinic, Rochester, Minn.) for independent analysis by ultracentrifugation of pre-β-lipoprotein, dextran sulfate-Ca^{2+} precipitation of β-lipoprotein and dextran sulfate-Mn^{2+} precipitation of α-lipoprotein (Srinivasan et al., 1978a). Analysis of split specimens of sera from 32 children gave the following values (mg/dl, mean ± S.D.): β + pre-β-lipoprotein cholesterol: 99 ± 16 by the present method

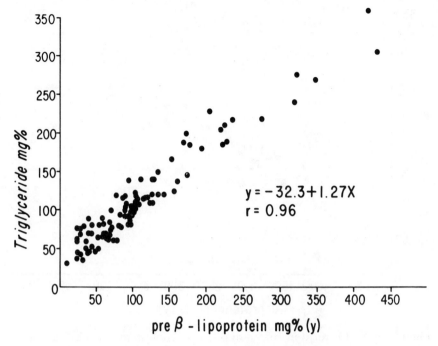

Figure 3–3. Correlation between serum triglycerides (x) and pre-β-lipoprotein (y) concentration as determined by the turbidimetric and electrophoretic methods. The individuals studied were same as in Figure 3–2. Regression equation $y = -32.2 + 1.27x$. Correlation coefficeint: $r = 0.96$. Standard deviation from regression 23.6.

compared to 98 ± 18 by the Mayo method; α-lipoprotein cholesterol: 64 ± 10 and 65 ± 11 by the respective methods. Analyses using the paired t-test revealed no significant differences between the two methods in determination of either β + pre-β-lipoprotein cholesterol or α-lipoprotein cholesterol.

In order to evaluate the relationship between turbidity and the values obtained for serum β- and pre-β-lipoprotein concentrations in different individuals, a series of 100 serum samples, mostly from "healthy" individuals (85 "normals", 15 diabetics), was studied. Diabetic sera were introduced in this series to extend the range of values. Figure 3–2 illustrates an excellent relationship (correlation coefficient $r = 0.98$, standard deviation from regression 27.6) between turbidity values and β- plus pre-β-lipoprotein concentrations. It should be mentioned that the total β- plus pre-β-lipoprotein concen-

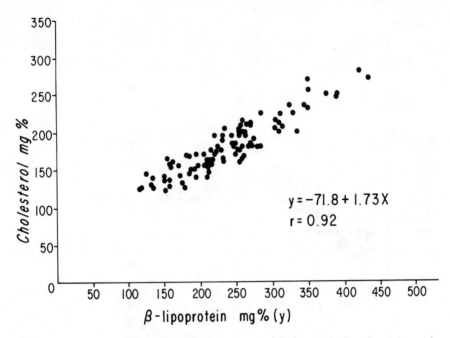

Figure 3–4. Correlation of serum total cholesterol levels (x) with β-lipoprotein (y) levels in the same group of individuals shown in Figure 3–2. Regression equation $y = -71.8 + 1.73x$. Correlation coefficient $r = 0.92$. Standard deviation from regression 27.1.

tration is the summation of individual lipoprotein concentrations calculated separately. It was obvious that two samples of sera with different proportions of β- or pre-β-lipoprotein could give similar turbidity values. Since β- and pre-β-lipoproteins are the major carriers of serum cholesterol and triglycerides, respectively, correlation coefficients were also determined for these two classes of lipoproteins and serum lipids (total cholesterol, triglycerides). The results are presented in Figures 3–3 and 3–4. A very good correlation ($r = 0.96$, standard deviation from regression 23.6) was obtained between pre-β-lipoprotein determined by the present method and level of serum triglycerides. A good correlation ($r = 0.92$, standard deviation from regression 27.1) for β-lipoprotein measurements and serum total cholesterol was also observed.

These results indicate turbidity to be a good measure of the total of the two lipoproteins, exclusive of α-lipoprotein. Simplicity of the method in determining β- plus pre-β-lipoproteins indicates another procedure which could be used clinically. The turbidity measurement is easier to perform than serum cholesterol or triglyceride determinations and is more reproducible. It could aid as a rapid initial screening procedure in small laboratories to select individuals requiring further study of serum lipoproteins.

APPLICATION

Clinical application of the present method

Applications of the present method to evaluate serum β- and pre-β-lipoprotein concentrations in a group of normal individuals and in patients with different diseases is shown by the several scattergrams in Figure 3–5. Quite arbitrary divisions of normal values were made for β- and pre-β-lipoprotein determinations. These divisions were based on earlier studies from this laboratory (Srinivasan et al., 1970a; Lopez-S., 1971) and the suggested normal limits for serum lipoprotein concentrations (Fredrickson et al., 1967) as ideal values are in the lower left quadrant; high values of pre-β-lipoprotein are in the upper left quadrant; high β-lipoproteins are in the lower right quadrant; and mixed elevations are in the upper right quadrant. The graph serves as a quick reference to the nature of serum lipoprotein abnormalities. For example, a significant number of the supposedly "normal" individuals have serum β- and pre-β-lipoprotein values which can be considered above ideal values. It is interesting to note that the mean values for β- and pre-β-lipoprotein (β 240 mg/dl; pre-β 90 mg/dl) in the case of normals are still contained in the lower left (ideal) quadrant, whereas mean values for diabetes (β 288 mg/dl; pre-β 180 mg/dl), kidney disease (β 275 mg/dl; pre-β 145 mg/dl), and myocardial infarction (β 260 mg/dl; pre-β 130 mg/dl) are contained in the upper right quadrant. Patients with such diseases lie predominantly in the upper right quadrant (representing mixed hyperlipoproteinemia), while a few of the values fall in the upper left quadrant (elevated pre-β-lipoproteins). In patients with liver disease (mostly advanced cirrhosis), the serum profile of β- and pre-β-lipoproteins showed significantly low pre-β-lipoprotein values. This information is important for therapeutic purposes and would be helpful in observing metabolic changes at a macromolecular level. In our survey a large number of lipoprotein ab-

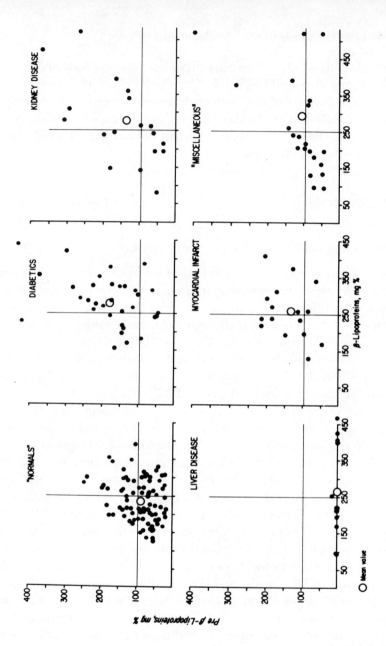

Figure 3–5. Serum β- and pre-β-lipoprotein profiles in "healthy" individuals and patients with different diseases. It can be seen from the scattergram that mean values (○) for β- and pre-β-lipoproteins in the case of "normals" are contained in the lower left quadrant, whereas mean values for patients with diabetes, kidney disease, and myocardial infarction are contained in the upper right quadrant and show elevations in both β- and pre-β-lipoproteins. Patients with advanced liver disease show significantly lower values of pre-β-lipoproteins.

normalities seem to fall into a class of mixed hyperlipoproteinemia, with elevated pre-β-lipoproteins occurring as frequently as, if not more frequently than, elevated β-lipoproteins. The significance of this common occurrence needs to be evaluated further in its relationship to the high incidence of coronary artery disease in our population.

Application in population studies

Serum cholesterol and triglycerides were determined simultaneously in a Technicon AutoAnalyzer II according to the protocol developed by Lipid Research Clinics in collaboration with Center for Disease Control (CDC), Atlanta (Lipid Research Clinics Program, 1974). A serum calibrator provided by the CDC was used to convert the cholesterol value obtained by the AutoAnalyzer II to the reference standard method of Abell-Kendall (Abell et al., 1952).

Serum lipoproteins were measured as described above with the following modifications to suit a large-scale population study (Srinivasan et al., 1976a). On every screening day, approximately 10% of the serum samples were randomly assigned for direct determination of β- plus pre-β-lipoprotein cholesterol. At the end of a study the direct determination of cholesterol in the β- and pre-β-lipoprotein fractions (chemical analysis of the precipitate obtained by heparin and Ca^{2+}) was related to the β- plus pre-β-lipoprotein index (turbidity measured at 600 nm). A factor was obtained by constructing a regression line through the origin, and the cholesterol content of these two classes of lipoproteins in a given serum (for the entire population group) was indirectly obtained by multiplying the β- plus pre-β-lipoprotein index to this factor. We have observed that the fasting status of the individual is extremely important in obtaining a valid factor for the analyses.

A comparison between the direct and the indirect methods for measuring serum β- plus pre-β-lipoprotein cholesterol was made in sera from a random sample of 349 children to test the validity of applying the indirect method for all of the children studied. Quantitative differences between the direct and indirect method were determined as described by Friedewald et al. (1972) and Glueck et al. (1973), and are shown in Table 3–3. The direct determination of cholesterol in β- and pre-β-lipoprotein fractions obtained by heparin-Ca^{2+} precipitation is considered the standard. A mean difference of -0.73 mg/dl be-

Table 3–3. Statistics on the measurement of β- plus pre-β-lipoprotein cholesterol levels utilizing direct and indirect analytical methods on 349 children

	β- plus pre-β-lipoprotein cholesterol (mg/dl) (direct method – indirect method)[1]				
Number of samples (N)	Mean difference ($\bar{X}_d$)	S.D. of difference	95% confidence interval of mean difference[2]	Mean of absolute differences[3]	Percent error[4]
349	−0.73	13.5	−2.15, 0.68	9.8	10.5

[1]Direct method (standard): heparin-Ca^{2+} precipitation method. Indirect method: β- plus pre-β-lipoprotein index × 500.
[2]Calculated as $\bar{X}_d \pm$ (t value (0.025, $n - 1$) S.D. $\sqrt{n}$).
[3]Absolute value of (direct method – indirect method), irrespective of sign.
[4]% error = (mean of absolute differences between the methods)/(mean β- plus pre-β-lipoprotein cholesterol by direct method) × 100.

tween the two methods indicates that the indirect method gave slightly higher β- plus pre-β-lipoprotein cholesterol values than the direct method. However, the difference was not statistically significant. The percent error, which is an estimate of the error of the indirectly estimated value as compared to the directly measured value, is well within the range obtained by previous investigators for their indirect estimation of β-lipoprotein cholesterol using the Friedewald formula (Glueck et al., 1973). The indirect method was applied, therefore, to measure the lipoprotein concentrations in all children. The methodology appears to be satisfactory for the majority of the population. (Perhaps extreme lipid disturbances and aberrant forms of lipoproteinemia, e.g., Type III, may not be detected.)

COMMENT

A simple method for quantitating serum lipoproteins which is adaptable for small clinical laboratories is described. The method appears to be quite useful in the study of children and can be used for a few samples as easily as for large numbers. Most reproducible are the quantitations of β-lipoproteins, but satisfactory assays of pre-β- and α-lipoproteins can be obtained.

The determination of concentrations of the individuals lipoproteins, rather than serum lipids alone, will aid in a more accurate assessment of the state of the individual.

4. An assessment of laboratory measurement error of lipids and lipoproteins for a total community study*

Time-course observations of certain factors, such as lipids, are obviously fundamental in studying how atherosclerosis begins. Inasmuch as biologic variation and technical error in measurement intermingle, knowledge about the precision of measurements is critical to the usefulness of such observations as they relate to individuals.

The estimation of serum lipid levels is a primary aspect of the Bogalusa Heart Study. In such a large-scale community study, laboratory performance, to a great extent, determines whether or not specified goals of the study can be attained.

It is the primary purpose of this chapter to describe an external (statistical) quality control (Youden, 1951) of clinical analytical lipid methods, to discuss the reproducibility of reported laboratory values of the various lipids, and to specify how well an investigator might expect to track lipid levels in the individual over time. A secondary purpose is to present the basic statistical techniques used in terms that can be understood by a specialist who is not a practiced statistician (see Appendices at end of chapter).

In addition to studying the research variables, the investigators collected data on service variables, such as hemoglobin, for which estimates of measurement error are presented here for comparative purposes.

*The authors express appreciation to L. K. Hammet and R. Weinberg for their work and assistance on this material.

MATERIALS AND METHODS

Sample of children

The data for this chapter stemmed from blind duplicate (McMahan and Strong, 1965; McMahan, 1967) aliquots of blood drawn from (reportedly fasting) children selected strictly at random during the period September 1973 through May 1974; usually four children were selected during each "screening" day from approximately 40 children being examined. The age, race, and sex distribution for the children from whom the duplicate blood specimens were drawn is presented in Table 4–1. During venipuncture, two tubes of blood were drawn from each of four children and sent to the SCOR-A laboratory along with specimens from the other children examined that day. The two tubes were labelled as follows: one with the name and identification number of the child, the other with a fictitious name and a corresponding unique identification number. Assignment of the fictitious name and number was randomized to "first tube" or "second tube" of blood drawn for each individual from whom duplicates were obtained.

Limitations

According to the protocol,* generalizations from this study refer to children from Ward 4 who meet specified conditions. Explicitly, blind duplicate aliquots of blood should be drawn only from fasting children, children from Ward 4, and children not designated as "rescreenee." The 432 pairs of blind duplicate samples analyzed in this report did not necessarily meet all the protocol restrictions. Nonetheless, the evaluation of measurement error is not affected.

Biochemical methods

β- plus pre-β-lipoprotein index. Quantiation (Srinivasan et al., 1970a; Srinivasan et al., 1970b; Berenson et al., 1972a; Berenson et al., 1972b) (referred to as an index) of a given serum was determined by a turbidimetric method as outlined in Chapter 3.

Serum total cholesterol and triglyceride. These were determined

*Detailed protocols, L.S.U. Specialized Center of Research–Arteriosclerosis

Table 4–1. Number of children providing blood samples for blind duplicate determinations of selected serum lipids and hemoglobin, by age, color, and sex, Bogalusa school children, September 1973–May 1974

Age last birthday	White			Nonwhite			Total		
	Boys	Girls	Both sexes	Boys	Girls	Both sexes	Boys	Girls	Both sexes
5	6	12	18	6	2	8	12	14	26
6	12	10	22	9	4	13	21	14	35
7	9	14	23	4	6	10	13	20	33
8	15	17	32	3	—	3	18	17	35
9	14	18	32	13	4	17	27	22	49
10	18	8	26	13	6	19	31	14	45
11	11	15	26	10	9	19	21	24	45
12	19	15	34	8	6	14	27	21	48
13	22	10	32	9	4	13	31	14	45
14	19	8	27	13	7	20	32	15	47
15	7	4	11	8	5	13	15	9	24
All ages	152	131	283	96	53	149	248	184	432

simultaneously in a Technicon AutoAnalyzer II (Technicon Instruments Corp., Tarrytown, N.Y.) according to the protocol developed by Lipid Research Clinics (1974) in collaboration with the U.S. Center for Disease Control (CDC) in Atlanta (Abell et al., 1952) and outlined in Chapter 3.

Densitometric ratios of β- and pre-β-lipoproteins. The relative proportions of β- and pre-β-lipoproteins were determined in terms of their percentages of dye staining after electrophoretic separation (Noble, 1968; Cawley, 1969; Arquembourg et al., 1970). Further amplification of the methodology is outlined in Chapter 3.

Hemoglobin. Hemoglobin was determined as cyanmethemoglobin using Hycel Diagnostic Reagent Kit (Hycel, Inc., Houston, Tex.). Whole blood (0.02 ml) was mixed with 5 ml of cyanide-ferricyanide solution using a DADE dilutor (Division American Hospital Supply Corp., Miami) and read at 540 mμ against the cyanide-ferricyanide solution as blank.

Statistical methods

In the routine monitoring of the performance of the SCOR-A laboratory, for each variable the following statistics were computed from pairs of blind duplicates: the arithmetic mean, the variance for measurement error, the standard deviation for measurement error, the coefficient of variation for measurement error (for definitions and worked examples, see Appendix 4A following this chapter), and the intraclass correlation coefficient between the laboratory-reported results of blind duplicates (for technical details, see Appendix 4B, Section 1).

RESULTS

Selected statistics for measurement error of six variables are presented in Table 4–2, namely, the variance, the standard deviation, and the coefficient of variation; in addition, the mean and the intraclass correlation coefficient are presented. Other serum variables, such as α-lipoprotein cholesterol, β-lipoprotein, pre-β-lipoprotein, and α-lipoprotein, were obtained through calculation; hence, laboratory measurement error is not presented for those variables. Note that each of those variables "contains" at least the laboratory measurement error in each of its component parts.

Interval estimates of the coefficient of variation for measurement error

The observed coefficients of variation for measurement error, cv_{me}, (see Table 4–2) ranged from 3.7 to 16.6%. If the electrophoresis-pre-β variable (which compliments electrophoresis-β) is omitted, then the range is 3.7 to 13.3%.

When we use the size of the coefficient of variation for measurement error as the criterion of how precisely we can measure, and if we delay consideration of the cv_{me} for electrophoresis-β, and electrophoresis-pre-β, inspection of the remaining four confidence intervals suggests that we take action as if we measured triglyceride poorest; as if we measured β- plus pre-β-lipoprotein index and total cholesterol equally (about medium); and as if we measured hemoglobin best.

Data were analyzed in intervals of calendar months from September 1973 through May 1974. Approximate 95% confidence intervals on the coefficient of variation for data collected in each month indicated fluctuation of magnitude of measurement error for a specified lipid from month to month, irrespective of fluctuation of the mean for

Table 4–2. Selected statistics on measurement error and the intraclass correlation coefficient

Serum variable	Number of pairs of blind duplicates	Measurement error				Intraclass correlation coefficient
		Mean	Variance	Standard deviation	Coefficient of variation (and ≈95% confidence limits[1] (percent)	
β + pre-β lipoprotein index (optical density units)	432	0.20	0.0001	0.01	5.2(4.85, 5.55)	0.96
Triglyceride (mg/dl)	431	72.87	93.2355	9.66	13.3(12.40, 14.20)	0.93
Total cholesterol (mg/100 dl)	431	166.45	83.5940	9.14	5.5(5.13, 5.87)	0.90
Electrophoresis β lipoproteins (percentage)	431	81.80	9.1914	3.03	3.7(3.45, 3.95)	0.91
Electrophoresis pre-β lipoproteins (percentage)	431	18.19	9.1531	3.03	16.6(15.46, 17.74)	0.91
Hemoglobin (g/dl)	426	12.75	0.2704	0.52	4.1(3.82, 4.38)	0.79

[1]Computations were made before the standard deviation and mean were rounded. See Appendix A, Section 2, for computational details.

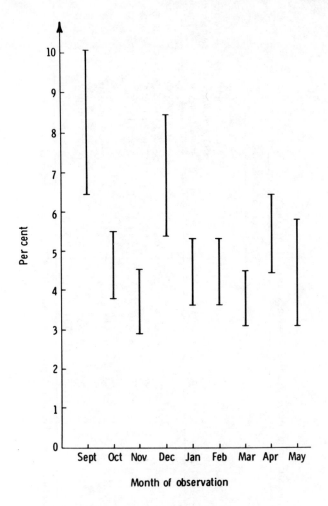

Figure 4–1. Approximate 95% confidence limits on coefficient of variation for measurement error for β- + pre-β-lipoprotein index by mouth.

some lipids. The fluctuations can be seen in Figures 4–1, 4–2, and 4–3 for β- plus pre-β-lipoprotein index, triglyceride, and total cholesterol.

For any given compound, the number of samples per month varied and was obviously small. If s for measurement error remained constant from month to month, changes in $\bar{x}$ would alter the observed cv_{me}; if s changed from month to month and $\bar{x}$ remained constant,

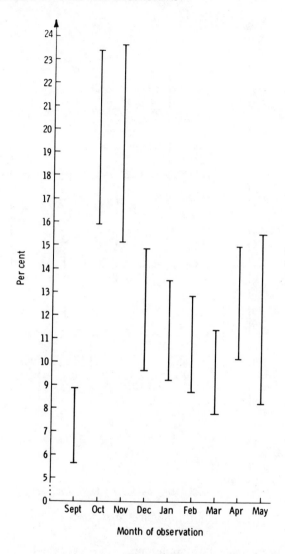

Figure 4–2. Approximate 95% confidence limits on coefficient of variation for measurement error for triglyceride by month.

likewise the cv_{me} would be altered. Examination of $\bar{x}$, s, and cv_{me} indicated that both $\bar{x}$ and s varied from month to month for each variable. In short, the variation of the cv_{me} from month to month for each variable reflects variation in relative performances of the lipid

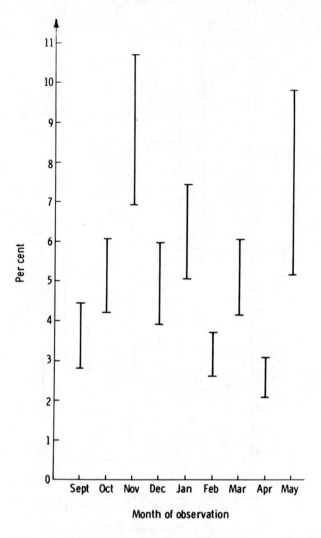

Figure 4–3. Approximate 95% confidence limits on coefficient of variation for measurement error for serum total cholesterol by month.

laboratory from time to time. As additional data are collected, these phenomena can be examined in depth. In the meantime, the SCOR-A laboratory shall continue the practice of obtaining blind duplicate measurements on at least a sample of the children undergoing screening.

Intraclass correlation coefficients

Observed intraclass correlation coefficients are presented in Table 4–2 in order to indicate the degree of agreement between duplicates relative to the inherent variability among measurements for the children. They ranged from 0.79 to 0.96. Only for hemoglobin, a service variable, was the r_I smaller than 0.90. Approximate 95% confidence intervals for these variables are presented in Table 4–3. From these confidence intervals, we conclude (with 95% confidence) that the percentage variability of true measurements that is accounted for by (included in) the variability of reported measurements is at least 95% for the variable β- plus pre-β-lipoprotein index, 92% for the variable triglyceride, 88% for total cholesterol, and 89% for electrophoresis β- plus pre-β-lipoproteins. For the service variable hemoglobin, however, this percentage was 75. The null hypothesis for equality of intraclass correlation coefficients for all five variables was rejected as well as the null hypothesis concerning the group of four research variables. Nevertheless, the overall estimate of intraclass correlation coefficient for these four variables was found to be 0.93. Thus, for research variables, reported measurements could be considered to be carrying more than 90% of the true variability of children. Summing up, if we use the intraclass correlation coefficient as our criterion, we would hypothesize as follows: we measured the β- plus pre-β-lipoprotein index better than any of the other variables examined; we measured about equally well triglyceride, total cholesterol, electrophoresis-β-lipoproteins, and electrophoresis-pre-β-lipoproteins; and we measured hemoglobin poorest.

Table 4-3. Approximate 95% confidence intervals for intraclass correlation coefficients

Serum variable	$r_{I(\ell)}$	Observed r_I	Approximate 95% confidence interval (C.I.)
β+ pre-β lipoprotein index	$r_{I(1)}$	0.96	$0.95 \leq \rho_{I(1)} \leq 0.97$
Triglyceride	$r_{I(2)}$	0.93	$0.92 \leq \rho_{I(2)} \leq 0.94$
Total cholesterol	$r_{I(3)}$	0.90	$0.88 \leq \rho_{I(3)} \leq 0.92$
Electrophoresis β-lipoproteins	$r_{I(4a)}$		
Electrophoresis pre-β lipo- proteins	$r_{I(4b)}$	0.91	$0.89 \leq \rho_{I(4)} \leq 0.92$
Hemoglobin	$r_{I(5)}$	0.79	$0.75 \leq \rho_{I(5)} \leq 0.82$

Comparison of the coefficient of variation for measurement error with the intraclass correlation coefficient confirms the fact that for variables in which there is great similarity among subjects, laboratory error is "more important" than it is for variables where subjects are vastly different from one another. Hemoglobin level, for example, has a relatively narrow range of values. The coefficient of variation for laboratory measurement error in hemoglobin was small; yet the r_I indicates that variability within blind duplicates was large relative to the amount of variability among subjects. Conversely, the r_I's for the serum lipids indicate that variability within blind duplicates was small relative to the amount of variability observed among subjects.

DISCUSSION

Consider color at two levels, sex at two levels, and age at eleven levels. For convenience, given 75 children in each color-sex-age classification (75 children in each of the 44 cells of such a table), there would be 3,300 children. Suppose that within each of the 44 cells, it was desired to follow for five years the four children with the highest lipid levels (those above the 95th percentile (P_{95}) and the four children with the lowest lipid level (P_5 and below). Assume none were lost to follow-up.

The questions are as follows: Do the observed levels of precision of measurement permit satisfactory follow-up of individuals over long periods of time, sometimes loosely referred to as "testing for tracking"? That is, can high values and low values be measured with similar precision (McMahan, 1970) and is that precision fine enough to test for tracking? Are individuals with high values of cholesterol classified as having high values, low values, or intermediate values five years later? Have the true ranks remained unchanged? In short, how much do extreme values regress toward the mean (Gardner and Heady, 1973)?

A highly technical approach for this purpose involves the relationship of "high-value percentile" P_{95}, "low-value percentile" P_5, and interpercentile range $P_{95}-P_5$; the measurement error involved is beyond the scope of this publication. We shall discuss, however, the impact of measurement error on "testing for tracking" by two examples.

Data from Appendix 4C (where subclassification by color, sex, and age has been disregarded for convenience) provide a basis for discussion of planning factors. For convenience, in Appendix 4C and in the remainder of this discussion, "high" values were defined to be those above the 92.5 percentile and "low" values were those values at the 7.5 percentile or lower (as contrasted with 95th and 5th percentiles).

Example 1: triglycerides

The standard deviation for measurement error (s) for "high" triglyceride values was about 11. The approximate 95% confidence interval for an individual observation is $x \pm 2s$, or $x \pm 2(11)$, or $x \pm 22$. For a reported value of 157 mg/dl for an individual child, call it C_1, we shall take action as if the true value for C_1 is between 135 and 179. Furthermore, the s for measurement error for "low" values was about 9; thus, for a reported observation on a second child C_2 of 36 mg/dl, the true value is probably in the interval 18 to 54. Clearly, the intervals do not overlap; we shall take action as if the triglyceride levels of these two children (C_1 and C_2) are really different, and as if the triglyceride level of child C_1 is really higher than that of a child in the "middle 85%" of children.

Example 2: serum total cholesterol

The standard deviation for measurement error for high total cholesterol values was about 18; the s for low cholesterol values was about 6. For a reported value of 228 mg/dl, the true value is probably in the interval 192 to 264; for a reported "low" value of 122, the true value is probably in the interval 110 to 134. The intervals do not overlap. In fact, Appendix Table 4A–1 shows that these intervals do not overlap the interval computed using a reported value of 166 mg/dl, which is the overall mean for 431 pairs of blind duplicate cholesterol values, and the corresponding s for measurement error.

COMMENT

Clearly, if the serum lipids are measured with· the precision demonstrated to date, and if the children do not change relative positions radically over five years, one might at least conclude that the "high-highs" remain "high"—if indeed that is the case.

The importance of knowing laboratory precision, reproducibility, and validity of analyses with respect to biological variation is obvious. The reproducibility of the laboratory data when used for diagnosis, and even more so when interpreted with respect to a treatment that alters the laboratory values being measured, is critical. Most disease processes occur over time; certainly that is true with coronary artery disease. In the study of risk factors and atherosclerosis, unfortunately, available information and resultant interpretation of laboratory data are mostly based on one point in time. Clearly important is the need to observe the natural history or risk factors over time with the natural history of anatomic changes of atherosclerosis. Interpretation cannot go beyond limitations of laboratory data, and the ability to conduct epidemiologic studies of coronary artery disease, for example in the use of drugs or diet, depends upon the time-performance of the laboratory. Blind duplicates in such investigations are essential. This study is intended to be a model of field laboratory assessment which could be adapted for other investigations.

SUMMARY

Estimates of laboratory measurement error and intraclass correlation coefficients are presented for reported values of selected serum lipid variables in Bogalusa school children. The estimates were obtained from values reported on blind duplicate aliquots of sera from 432 children. The coefficients of variation for measurement error of serum lipids ranged from 3.7% to 16.6%. The overall estimate of the intraclass correlation coefficient for serum lipid variables was 0.93; thus, reported measurements could be considered as carrying more than 90% of the (true) variability among children. These observed levels of precision of measurement would permit satisfactory follow-up of individuals with high and low levels of serum lipids over long periods of time. Such long-term tracking is a fundamental aspect of the study of relationships of hypothesized risk factors and the early natural history of arteriosclerosis, coronary artery disease, and essential hypertension.

APPENDIX 4A

Measurement error and its computation

MEASUREMENT ERROR
Measurement error has been used here to describe the failure of blind duplicate measurements by the same laboratory and the same analytical technique

on identical blood samples (blind duplicates) to yield identical results. If T is true measurement for a child and X is its reported measurement, then we may write $X = T + e$, where e is the measurement error committed. For a given laboratory or a given analytical technique, there is a possibility that reported results consistently overestimate or underestimate the true measurement (i.e., are biased) and the average of reported results differs by an amount, say B from the average of true measurements. In this situation we write $X = T + B + E$, where $e = B + E$, E being measurement error for the given laboratory or the given analytical technique. Average value of E in the population is now zero, but the variance of E in the population is the same as that of the variance of e—the actual error committed. We use variance or standard deviation (or coefficient of variation) to measure variability of error committed as it can be estimated internally from the laboratory performance without the knowledge concerning B. The measurement error E is assumed to be independent of the true value T. This gives us

$$\sigma_x^2 = \sigma_p^2 + \sigma_{me}^2$$

where σ_x^2 is the variance of reported measurements X in the population, and σ_p^2 is the variance of true values T in the population, and σ_{me}^2 is the variance of E in the population.

There follows a description of definitions and computational procedures for estimates of variance, standard deviation, and coefficient of variation of the measurement error. For convenience, definitions are made in terms of mg/dl of total serum cholesterol in the subsequent paragraphs.

ARITHMETIC MEAN
Let x_j be the amount of cholesterol as measured for one tube of serum. The mean for n tubes would be

$$\bar{x} = \frac{\sum_{j=1}^{n} x_j}{n}$$

for the special case of two tubes,

$$\bar{x} = \frac{\sum_{j=1}^{2} x_j}{2}$$

alternatively, $\bar{x} = \frac{x_1 + x_2}{2}$ mg/dl.

VARIANCE FOR MEASUREMENT ERROR, s^2
Let x_1 = measurement (amount of cholesterol) on one tube, say, the first tube of a pair of blind duplicates; let x_2 = measurement on the other tube, say, the

second tube of the pair. Then the variance for measurement error for one pair of tubes is defined as follows:

$$s^2 = \frac{\text{sum of squares}}{\text{degrees of freedom}} = \frac{ss}{df}$$

$$s^2 = \frac{\sum\limits_{j=1}^{n}(x_j - \bar{x})^2}{n - 1}, j = 1, \ldots, n$$

or $$s^2 = \frac{(x_1 - \bar{x})^2 + (x_2 - \bar{x})^2}{2 - 1} \text{ for the case } n = 2$$

clearly, s^2 is in square units and is based on 1 degree of freedom (df). It is zero when $x_1 = x_2$, and increases when the difference between x_1 and x_2 increases.

For multiple sets (k pairs of tubes) of blind duplicates,

$$s^2 = \frac{\sum\limits_{i=1}^{k}\sum\limits_{j=1}^{n}(x_{ij} - \bar{x}_i)^2}{k(n - 1)} \tag{A1}$$

where x_{ij} is the jth observation (measurement) within the ith pair, $j = 1, \ldots, $ n, here obviously $n = 2$ for blind duplicates; $\bar{x}_i$ is the mean (of the $n = 2$ observations) for the ith pair, $i = 1, 2, \ldots, k$ pairs; and $df = K(n - 1) = (kn - k)$.

STANDARD DEVIATION FOR MEASUREMENT ERROR

The standard deviation for measurement error s is the positive square root of the variance. Symbolically,

$$s = \sqrt{s^2} = \sqrt{\frac{\sum\limits_{i=1}^{k}\sum\limits_{j=1}^{n}(x_{ij} - \bar{x}_i)^2}{k(n - 1)}} \tag{A2}$$

The standard deviation is in terms of the original units of measurement; for total cholesterol, s is in mg/dl.

INTERVAL ESTIMATES

The standard deviation for measurement error can be used to obtain an interval estimate of the true value (as compared to the reported value, a point estimate) of the specified variable for a given child. For example, if a single measurement is made for a child, the interval estimate below is expected to "bracket" the true value for that child with a probability of about 0.95:

(reported value) ± [(approximately 2) × (s for measurement error)].

Table 4A–1. Approximate 95% confidence intervals for measurements of selected serum lipids and hemoglobin

Serum variable	Reported value for one reading on a child	True value is probably in the interval	
		Lower limit	Upper limit
β + pre-β-lipoprotein index (optical density units)	0.20	0.18	0.22
Triglyceride (mg/dl)	73	53.68	92.32
Total cholesterol (mg/dl)	166	147.72	184.28
Electrophoresis β-lipoproteins (percentage)	82	75.94	88.06
Electrophoresis pre-β-lipoproteins (percentage)	18	11.94	24.06
Hemoglobin (g/dl)	13	11.96	14.04

For illustrative purposes, six examples are presented in Table 4A-1 (where data from Table 4–2 have been applied).

COEFFICIENT OF VARIATION FOR MEASUREMENT ERROR
The coefficient of variation (cv_{me}) for measurement error is defined as follows:

$$cv_{me} = \frac{s(\text{units})}{\bar{x}(\text{units})} \times 100$$

where s is the standard deviation for measurement error. Hence,

$$cv_{me} = \frac{s}{\bar{x}} \times 100 \text{ in percent}$$

Notice here that cv_{me} is not subject to units of measurement.

EXAMPLES
In order to explicity illustrate the direct computation of measures of variability between blind duplicates, the following worked examples are based on the raw reported total cholesterol values for 40 children (September 1973) presented in Table 4A–2. For child (examinee) number 1, the measurement on

Table 4A–2. Observed measurement error in blind duplicate measurements, total cholesterol (mg/dl)

Examinee	Reading 1	Reading 2	Sum	Mean	ss	Examinee	Reading 1	Reading 2	Sum	Mean	ss
1	140	134	274	137.0	18.0	21	239	230	469	234.5	40.5
2	110	105	215	107.5	12.5	22	139	142	281	140.5	4.5
3	193	197	390	195.0	8.0	23	168	170	338	169.0	2.0
4	146	146	292	146.0	0.0	24	166	162	328	164.0	8.0
5	171	186	357	178.5	112.5	25	161	166	327	163.5	12.5
6	149	151	300	150.0	2.0	26	173	173	346	173.0	0.0
7	143	137	280	140.0	18.0	27	185	193	378	189.0	32.0
8	145	165	310	155.0	200.0	28	128	139	267	133.5	60.5
9	122	121	243	121.5	0.5	29	164	168	332	166.0	8.0
10	190	182	372	186.0	32.0	30	147	147	294	147.0	0.0
11	125	131	256	128.0	18.0	31	119	119	238	119.0	0.0
12	167	173	340	170.0	18.0	32	167	175	342	171.0	32.0
13	176	181	357	178.5	12.5	33	175	145	320	160.0	450.0
14	166	170	336	168.0	8.0	34	120	122	242	121.0	2.0
15	128	125	253	126.5	4.5	35	179	179	358	179.0	0.0
16	147	140	287	143.5	24.5	36	168	175	343	171.5	24.5
17	139	141	280	140.0	2.0	37	184	188	372	186.0	8.0
18	142	148	290	145.0	18.0	38	184	194	378	189.0	50.0
19	189	181	370	185.0	32.0	39	141	140	281	140.5	0.5
20	150	144	294	147.0	18.0	40	148	144	292	146.0	8.0
						Total			12622	157.77	1302.0
								$df = 40$			

one tube of serum was 140; on the other tube it was 134. The sum of squares (*ss*) associated with the first pair of blind duplicates is computed as follows:

$$(140 - 137)^2 + (134 - 137)^2$$
$$= (3)^2 + (-3)^2 = 18 \,(mg/dl)^2$$

For those who prefer a computing formula, the *ss* associated with a pair of blind duplicates can be obtained as follows:

$$ss = \frac{(x_1 - x_2)^2}{2}$$

Here

$$ss = \frac{(140 - 134)^2}{2} = 18$$

the same result as was obtained using the defining formula. Note that there is one degree of freedom (*df*) for each pair of blind duplicates.

Applying Eq. (A2) to the duplicate readings of Table 4A–2,

the standard deviation for measurement error $s = \sqrt{\dfrac{\displaystyle\sum_{i=1}^{40}\sum_{j=1}^{2}(x_{ij} - \bar{x}_i)^2}{40(2 - 1)}}$

(where $j = 1, 2$; and $i = 1, 2, \ldots, 40$):

$$s = \sqrt{\frac{1302}{40}}$$

$$s = 5.71 \,mg/dl$$

The coefficient of variation for measurement error,

$$cv_{me} = \frac{5.71}{157.77} \times 100$$

$$cv_{me} = 3.6\%$$

Confidence limits for the coefficient of variation

The coefficient of variation for measurement error for the ℓth lipid is denoted $cv_{me(\ell)}$.

Let

$$\hat{C}_\ell = \frac{cv_{me(\ell)}}{100}$$

which is an estimate of the true proportion that the standard deviation is of the mean (σ_{me}/μ). Approximate 95% confidence limits (Hald, 1952) for the true coefficient of variation for measurement error based on the estimate $\hat{C}_\ell$ are given by the following:

$$\hat{C}_\ell \left[1 \pm 1.96 \sqrt{\frac{1 + 2\hat{C}_\ell^{\,2}}{2(k-1)}} \right]$$

Applying this equation to the data of Table 4A-2 on 40 pairs of blind duplicate readings of total serum cholesterol ($\ell = 3$),

$$\hat{C}_3 = 5.71/157.77 = 0.0362$$
$$\hat{C}_3^2 = 0.00131044$$
$$k_3 = 40$$

$$\text{C.L. } (C_3) = 0.0362 \left[1 \pm 1.96 \sqrt{\frac{1 + 2(0.00131044)}{2(39)}} \right]$$

$$= 0.0362 \left[1 \pm 1.96 \sqrt{\frac{1.0026}{78}} \right]$$

$$= 0.0362[1 \pm 1.96\sqrt{0.012854}]$$
$$= 0.0362[1 \pm 1.96(0.113)]$$
$$= 0.0362[1 \pm 0.2215]$$
$$= 0.0362[0.7785, 1.2215]$$
$$\text{C.L. } (C_3) = (0.0282, 0.0442)$$

Hence, the confidence limits (with coefficient 0.95) on the true coefficient of variation for measurement error for $\ell = 3$ = cholesterol are 2.82% and 4.42%.

APPENDIX 4B

Intraclass correlation coefficient and its computation

The overall agreement among independent determinations (blind duplicates in the present case) relative to inherent variability of children can be indicated by computing the intraclass correlation coefficient.

The population intraclass correlation coefficient ρ_I is defined as follows:

$$\rho_I = \frac{\sigma_p^2}{\sigma_{me}^2 + \sigma_p^2} \tag{B1}$$

where σ_p^2 is the true component of variance among children (Table 4B-1) and σ_{me}^2 is the true variance for measurement error (Table 4B-1). Note that for $n = 2$,

$$\rho_I = \frac{\text{cov }(x_1, x_2)}{\sqrt{(\text{var } x_1)(\text{var } x_2)}}$$

Table 4B–1. Skeleton analysis of variance (ANOVA) for use in calculating the intraclass correlation coefficient

Source of variation	Degrees of freedom	Sum of squares	Mean square		Expected mean square
(1)	(2)	(3)	(4)	(5)	(6)
Mean	1	$\left(\sum\limits_{i=1}^{k}\sum\limits_{j=1}^{n_i}x_{ij}\right)^2 \Big/ \sum\limits_{i=1}^{k}n_i$			
Among children	$k-1$	$\sum\limits_{i=1}^{k}n_i(\bar{x}_i - \bar{x})^2$	MS_p	$s^2 + ns_p^2$	$\sigma_{me}^2 + n\sigma_p^2$
Within (pairs of) blind duplicates	$k(n-1)$	$\sum\limits_{i=1}^{k}\sum\limits_{j=1}^{n_i}(x_{ij} - \bar{x}_i)^2$	MS_w	s^2	σ_{me}^2
Total	kn	Σx_{ij}^2			

Inspection of Eq. (B1) clearly indicates that ρ_I is the proportion of variance of true measurements in the population as compared to variance of laboratory-reported measurements for the population. Variance components σ_p^2 and σ_{me}^2 are usually positive and their least possible (but improbable) value is zero. Clearly, $\rho_I = 1$ when $\sigma_{me}^2 = 0$, i.e., when for every child of the population, the blind duplicate results agree completely. Conversely when $\rho_I = 1$, $\sigma_{me}^2 = 0$ and blind duplicate results have to agree completely. Notice that $1 - \rho_I = \sigma_{me}^2/(\sigma_{me}^2 + \sigma_p^2)$, i.e., $1 - \rho_I$ is the proportion of variance for measurement error as compared to the variance of laboratory-reported values. Also $(1 - \rho_I)/\rho_I = \sigma_{me}^2/\sigma_p^2$. Thus, while the estimates of measurement error discussed in Appendix 4A (i.e., variance for measurement error, standard deviation for measurement error, and cv_{me}) do not themselves relate to true inherent variability among children, the intraclass correlation coefficient does so besides being free from units of measurement for the variables.

In this problem, in order to obtain an estimate of ρ_I, first consider the dummy analysis of variance table (Table 4B–1). A sample estimate of ρ_I is provided by the following computing formula:

$$r_I = \frac{MS_p - MS_w}{MS_p + (n-1)MS_w} \tag{B2}$$

where

$$MS_p = \text{mean square among groups (among children)}$$
$$= \hat{\sigma}_{me}^2 + n\hat{\sigma}_p^2$$

and

$$MS_w = \text{mean square within groups (within pairs of blind duplicates)}$$
$$= \sigma_{me}^2$$

Clearly, in Table 4B–1, $MS_w = s^2$; moreover, the s^2 of Table 4B–1 is identical to an s^2 computed by using Eq. (A1).

EXAMPLE

To illustrate the computations of the sample intraclass correlation coefficient, r_I, it is convenient to use analysis of variance techniques. Again making use of the data on total cholesterol for September, the analysis of variance is shown in Table 4B–2. The s_p^2 of column 4 is computed from column 5, as follows:

$$s^2 + ns_p^2 = 1320.2038$$

Substituting for s^2 and n,

$$32.5500 + 2(s_p^2) = 1320.2038$$
$$2\ s_p^2 = 1287.6538$$
$$s_p^2 = 643.8269$$

The estimate of the intraclass correlation coefficient is computed as follows:

$$r_{I(3)} = \frac{643.8269}{32.5500 + 643.8269} = \frac{643.8269}{676.3769}$$
$$r_{I(3)} \approx 0.95.$$

More directly, using Eq. (B2),

$$r_{I(3)} = \frac{1320.2038 - 32.5500}{1320.2038 + (2 - 1)(32.5500)} = \frac{1287.6538}{1352.7538}$$
$$r_{I(3)} \approx 0.95 \text{ as before}$$

The computation of 95% confidence limits on $\rho_{I(\ell)}$ also can be demonstrated using data on total cholesterol for the children screened in September 1973.

Fisher (1954) suggests the transformation

$$z_\ell = \tfrac{1}{2}ln\ \frac{1 + (n - 1)r_{I(\ell)}}{1 - r_{I(\ell)}} \tag{B3}$$

and has shown for the case $n = 2$ that z_ℓ is approximately normally distributed with mean μ_ℓ and variance

$$\sigma_{z_\ell}^2 = \frac{1}{k_\ell - 3}$$

Dixon and Massey (1969) obtain a confidence interval for $\rho_{I(\ell)}$ by using z_ℓ. In this example, $\ell = 3$ and $r_3 = 0.95$; hence,

$$z_3 = \tfrac{1}{2}ln\ \frac{1 + 1(0.95)}{1 - (0.95)}$$
$$z_3 \approx 1.83$$
$$\hat{\sigma}_{z_3} = 1/\sqrt{k_3 - 3} = 1/\sqrt{40 - 3} = 1/6.082763$$
$$\hat{\sigma}_{z_3} \approx 0.164$$

Table 4B-2. Analysis of variance for calculating the intraclass correlation coefficient for total serum cholesterol

Source of variation (1)	Degrees of freedom (2)	Sum of squares (3)	(4)	Mean square (5)
Mean	1	1,991,436	1,991,436	. . .
Among children	39	51,488	1,320.2038	$s^2 + ns_p^2 = 32.5500$ $+ 2(643.8269)$
Within pairs of blind duplicates	40	1,302	32.5500	$s^2 = 32.5500$
Total	80	2,044,226	. . .	. . .

Let z be an estimate of the parameter ζ (zeta), then

$$95\% \text{ C.L. } (\zeta_3) = z_{z_3} \pm 1.96 \; \hat{\sigma}_{z_3}$$
$$= 1.83 \pm 1.96(0.164)$$
$$95\% \text{ C.L. } (\zeta_3) = (1.51, 2.15)$$

and noting that

$$r_\ell = \tanh z_\ell$$
$$95\% \text{ C.L. } (\rho_{I(3)}) = (\tanh 1.51, \tanh 2.15)$$
$$= (0.91, 0.97)$$

Thus, for September it is estimated that

$$(0.91 \leq \rho_{I(3)} \leq 0.97)$$

Comparison of intraclass correlation coefficients

Let $x_{ij\ell}$ denote the jth measurement made on the ith child for the ℓth lipid or hemoglobin, where $i = 1, 2, \ldots, k_\ell$; $j = 1, 2, \ldots, n$; $\ell = 1, 2, \ldots, L$.

Let $r_{I(\ell)}$ represent the ANOVA estimate of the intraclass correlation coefficient $\rho_{I(\ell)}$ for the ℓth lipid (or hemoglobin) based upon n measurements made on each of k_ℓ children [see Eq. (B2)].

Fisher tests the hypothesis that two intraclass correlations are equal. Ostle (1963) gives an example (using the product-moment correlation coefficient) for testing the hypothesis that

$$\rho_{(1)} = \rho_{(2)} = \ldots = \rho_{(L)}$$

under the assumption that the L sets of measurements represent L independent samples. (Clearly, the same procedure is applicable to the intraclass correlation coefficient because z_ℓ is approximately normally distributed when $n = 2$.)

Although the serum lipids are intercorrelated, the estimates of $\rho_{I(\ell)}$ can be used for an approximate test using these data. For this test, let $\ell = 1$ correspond to β + pre-β lipoprotein index, $\ell = 2 \rightarrow$ triglyceride, $\ell = 3 \rightarrow$ total cholesterol, $\ell = 4$ represent either electrophoresis β or pre-β, $\ell = 5 \rightarrow$ hemoglobin.

We can make use of the Ostle procedure as follows: Using Fisher's transformation [Eq. (B3)], we have

$$\frac{z_\ell - \mu_\ell}{\sigma_{z_\ell}}$$

approximately normally distributed with mean 0 and variance 1. Consequently,

$$\sum_{\ell=1}^{L} \left(\frac{z_\ell - \mu_\ell}{\sigma_{z_\ell}} \right)^2$$

can be approximated by a chi-square distribution with L degrees of freedom. If we estimate μ_ℓ by taking a weighted average of the L z-values (call it $\hat{\mu}$), we lose one degree of freedom. With $L = 5$ in our example, we have a test statistic.

$$\chi_c^2 = \sum_{\ell=1}^{5} (k_\ell - 3) (z_\ell - \hat{\mu})^2$$

[where the subscript c on χ^2 indicates computed value], approximately distributed as χ^2 with $4\,df$.

In calculating $\hat{\mu}$, use as weights (in the weighted average) the reciprocals of the variances of z_ℓ. Thus

$$\hat{\mu} = \frac{\sum_{\ell=1}^{5} (k_\ell - 3)\, z_\ell}{\sum_{\ell=1}^{5} (k_\ell - 3)}$$

Hence,

$$\chi_c^2 = \sum_{\ell=1}^{5} (k_\ell - 3)\, z_\ell^2 - \hat{\mu} \sum_{\ell=1}^{5} (k_\ell - 3)\, z_\ell$$

and χ_c^2 is approximately distributed as χ^2 with $4\,df$.

Calculations for testing the hypothesis that all five true intraclass correlation coefficients (based on data for September through May) are equal are shown in Table 4B–3; we take action as though at least two of the $\rho_{(I)}$'s are not equal.

Table 4B–3. Calculations for testing the hypothesis that
$\rho_{I(1)} = \rho_{I(2)} = \cdots = \rho_{I(5)}$

ℓ	k_ℓ	$k_\ell - 3$	r_ℓ	z_ℓ	$(k_\ell - 3)z_\ell$	$(k_\ell - 3)z_\ell^2$
1	432	429	0.96	1.95	836.55	1631.27
2	431	428	0.93	1.66	710.48	1179.40
3	431	428	0.90	1.47	629.16	924.87
4	431	428	0.91	1.53	654.84	1001.91
5	426	423	0.79	1.07	452.61	484.29
Total	2151	2136			3283.64	5221.74

$\hat{\mu} = \dfrac{3283.64}{2136} = 1.54$

$\chi_c^2 = 5221.74 - 1.54(3283.64) = 164.93$

$\chi_{\alpha,\,\nu}^2 = \chi_{0.05,\,4} = 9.49$

Therefore, we reject

$H_0\colon \rho_{I(1)} = \rho_{I(2)} = \ldots = \rho_{I(5)}.$

At this stage it seems desirable to test the hypothesis that $\rho_{I(3)} = \rho_{I(5)}$ and perhaps also that $\rho_{I(3)} = \rho_{I(4)}$. Apparently the Ostle procedure could be used in either case taking $L = 2$ and using $1 df$. However, the Dixon-Massey procedure is simpler: with $\ell = 3$, $r_3 = 0.90$, $z_3 = 1.47$, $k_3 - 3 = 428$, $\hat{\sigma}_{z_3} = \dfrac{1}{\sqrt{k_3 - 3}} =$

$\dfrac{1}{\sqrt{428}} = 0.048$.

The 95% confidence interval (C.I.) for

$$\tfrac{1}{2} \ln \frac{1 + \rho_{I(3)}}{1 - \rho_{I(3)}} \text{ is } z_{(3)} \pm 1.96\, \hat{\sigma}_{z_3}$$
$$1.47 \pm 1.96\,(0.048)$$
$$95\% \text{ C.I.} = (1.376,\ 1.564)$$

Noting that $r_\ell = \tanh z_\ell$, we have for our confidence interval on $\rho_{I(3)}$ the interval $(\tanh 1.376, \tanh 1.564)$. According to Selby (1970) the 95% confidence interval is $0.88 \le \rho_{I(3)} \le 0.92$.

The C.I. for $\rho_{I(4)}$ overlaps the C.I. for $\rho_{I(3)}$ and the C.I. for $\rho_{I(5)}$ does not overlap the C.I. for $\rho_{I(3)}$. Obviously, the use of confidence intervals is merely an approximation; nevertheless, we shall take action as if $\rho_{I(3)} = \rho_{I(5)}$, $\rho_{I(4)} = \rho_{I(5)}$, and as if $\rho_{I(3)} = \rho_{I(4)}$.

APPENDIX 4C

High values versus low values as planning factors for selection of children for long-term follow-up

For this analysis, age, color, and sex were disregarded. The initial step was to inspect the original value reported for a child; the associated blind duplicate was disregarded. These original sample values were ranked from high to low. The 30 high values were selected for analysis. In cases where rank number 30 involved tied values, values were eliminated strictly at random as required. Data on measurement error reported in Table 4C–1 were computed by using the blind duplicate associated with each original value. These 30 pairs of values constituted the "high group." The "low group" was selected in a similar manner, where obviously the selection was based on values of low rank.

We recognize that we are dealing with "censored" data; nevertheless, inspection of Table 4C–1 suggests that it may not be advantageous to measure electrophoresis-pre-β-lipoproteins in the follow-up studies of children selected in terms of high and low values. This is related to limitations of the methodology at extremely low values.

Table 4C–1. Selected statistics, measurement error, and the intraclass correlation coefficient for selected serum variables, for 30 high and 30 low original values[1]

Variable		Number of pairs	Mean (of original values only)	Range (of original values only)	Measurement error			Intraclass correlation coefficient
					Variance	Standard deviation	Coefficient of variation	
β + pre-β lipoprotein index	High	30	0.33	0.28–0.51	0.0001	0.01	3.1	0.97
	Low	30	0.12	0.09–0.13	0.0002	0.01	11.8	0.30
Triglyceride	High	30	160.33	123–506	120.2167	10.96	7.0	0.98
	Low	30	33.60	21–39	84.2000	9.18	25.4	0.10
Total cholesterol	High	30	232.67	212–313	320.3665	17.90	7.9	0.57
	Low	30	120.33	98–128	32.6333	5.71	4.7	0.60
Electro-β lipoprotein	High	30	97.07	96–99	5.0333	2.24	2.3	–0.01
	Low	30	59.47	48–65	16.3333	4.04	6.7	0.59
Electro-pre-β lipoprotein	High	30	40.53	35–52	16.6667	4.08	10.4	0.59
	Low	30	2.93	1–4	5.0333	2.24	65.3	–0.01
Hemoglobin	High	30	15.18	14.4–17.5	0.6473	0.80	5.4	0.24
	Low	30	10.70	9.7–11.0	0.4823	0.69	6.3	0.17

[1]High and low values selected from a random sample of approximately 430 children. Measurement error obviously computed using original and duplicate values.

5. Approaches to studying instruments for blood pressure measurements in children

The important role of mass surveys in detecting individuals with hypertension has stimulated an interest in improving techniques and instruments for measuring indirect blood pressure. As new technology is applied (U.S. Dept. of H.E.W., 1976a), new insights are gained into the pathophysiology of blood pressure control (Guyton et al., 1974), furthering the need for improved methods that will obtain valid and reliable indirect measurements. Although automatic instruments could reduce such factors as examiner fatigue and observer bias in measuring blood pressure, a recent report suggests (Labarthe et al., 1973) that the available instruments are not yet adequate for use in epidemiologic studies. Our studies do not support this conclusion.

In preparing for an extensive survey of blood pressure in children, we investigated the currently available automatic blood pressure instruments for measurement reliability. The mercury sphygmomanometer was considered the general reference instrument since it is so widely used by physicians; however, several questions were posed: (1) Are there differences among commonly used instruments that are comparable to the standard mercury sphygmomanometer? (2) Do examiners using the same instruments on the same subjects obtain different measurements? (3) Which instruments would be most satisfactory for studying children, especially in a large survey? (4) In a complete field setting, will the measurements be similar to those obtained under a rigidly controlled statistical design? (5) Can the graphic recordings of automatic measuring devices be interpreted without reader bias? (6) Can differences among equally trained readers be explained?

GENERAL METHODS AND INSTRUMENTS

In these studies a number of instruments were used in several experimental designs (Table 5–1). We used as many automatic instruments as became available. A recently published catalog of all available automatic instruments (U.S. Dept. of H.E.W., 1976a) fully describes the instruments.

Arteriosonde 1216. The Arteriosonde registers phonosound Korotoff signals detected by an ultrasonically produced Doppler principle. Systolic and diastolic pressures are registered directly on vertical mercury columns when the falling mercury automatically stops at these levels (Hochberg and Saltzman, 1971; Hoffman-LaRoche, unpublished).

Bonn (Sela Electronics Co.). This instrument converts Korotoff sounds into visual or sonic signals but does not produce a permanent record. The transducer is a phonosound microphone.

Kass-Zinner (Boston) Automatic Recorder. Korotoff sounds, detected by phonosound microphone, are recorded on electrocardiographic paper moving with constant speed. As in the Narco Physiograph, these sounds are superimposed on the cuff pressure curve, which is calibrated by reference standard square waves (Boston City Hospital, unpublished).

Mercury Sphygmomanometer (Baumanometer). We used a portable model of a standard mercury sphygmomanometer (The Clinical Measurement of Blood Pressure, 1969). While standard cuff bladder sizes were used (child, adult, obese), we selected a size according to a rigid protocol for each child based on his arm size, using as large a bladder width as possible without obstructing the stethoscope with the elbow skin crease (Voors, 1975).

Table 5–1. Criteria for selection among representative, currently available automatic sphygmomanometric devices

Physical principle of gauging arterial sounds	Baumanometer — Audible (phono-sound)	Arteriosonde 1216 — Doppler (ultrasound)	Physiometrics[1] (USM–105) — Low frequency (infrasonde)	Physiograph — Audible (phono-sound)	Bonn — Audible light flashing[2]	Boston automatic (Kass-Zinner) — Audible (phono-sound)
Detailed permanent record	No	Available	Yes	Yes	No	Yes
Diagnostic reading capabilities, phase	4,5	4	4	4,5	4,5	4.5[3]
Ease of interim calibration	+	–	+	+	+	+
Portability, sturdiness	+	+	+	+	+	–
Ease of maintenance, exchangeability of parts	+	–	+	+	–	–
Ease of operating and trouble-shooting	+	–	+	–	–	–
Can errors made during the operation be detected later by the permanent record?	No	No	Yes	Yes	No	Yes
Approximate cost in U.S. dollars	50	3,000	1,000	1,000	Not available	Not available
Ease of reading record within 5 mm Hg	–	±	+	–	–	—[3]

[1]Subsequent modifications have been made with new series of instruments.
[2]Several instruments of similar design are available.
[3]Difficulty with fourth and fifth phase

Narco Physiograph. The instrument records (by phonosound micro-phone) Korotkoff sounds superimposed on the cuff pressure curve, written on a record moving with constant speed, and calibrated by re-ference standard square waves. Particular skills (Fernandez and Robinson, 1971) are needed in calibrating the record and handling the instrument.

*Physiometrics Recorder.** The Physiometrics instrument records on a small precalibrated paper disk rotated on an aneroid manometer in open communication with an oversized rubber cuff bladder. This bladder contains an infrasonic transducer that detects low-pitched vibrations (Sphygmetrics, Inc.). Biophysical measurements have suggested that the low-frequency observations may be more valid than those produced by a Doppler system.

Random-zero (Hawksley). This device is similar to the mercury sphygmomanometer, but has in addition a pressure-changing device between manometer column and mercury reservoir, that allows the examiner to obtain "blind" readings from the examinee and avoids bias of readings by observers (Wright and Dore, 1970; Hawksley/Gelman, unpublished).

STUDY APPROACHES, DESIGNS, AND OBSERVATIONS

Single-investigator studies

Twice during this preliminary testing period one investigator studied various blood-pressure measuring devices. In conducting the study session, the order of use of instruments was randomized. In one series, thirteen subjects were observed on each of three instruments—sphygmomanometer, Physiometrics, and Arteriosonde. A similar series was conducted on twelve subjects with these three instruments (the Arteriosonde instrument was replaced because it produced low readings in some of the preliminary studies) plus a Zero Muddler. Dif-ferences between means, each based on the average of three readings per instrument, were tested. Although in both studies the mean sys-tolic reading for the sphygmomanometer was highest, none of the dif-

*Physiometrics USM-105 recorder was used in the entire program. Subsequent testing of Physiometrics SR-2 indicated slight differences in diastolic readings in children.

ferences among the means were significant. Similarly, the mean diastolic readings for each instrument did not differ significantly, although the mean readings on the Arteriosonde were lower.

The readings from the Physiometrics, Arteriosonde, and Zero Muddler were compared to that of the sphygmomanometer. In all cases the correlation coefficients were very high, 0.86–0.95. This was to be expected since there was a wide range in blood pressures of the subjects, and one investigator took all readings in a nonblind manner. This approach does provide a rapid and subjective evaluation of available instruments for a research survey of blood pressure.

Graeco-Latin Square design

This design utilized three-factor blocking and randomization of all treatments for each replication of an experiment. Implementation of this design required n examiners to measure the blood pressure of n examinees with n instruments during n time periods. During the course of a year-long testing period, four implementations of such designs incorporated four unique combinations of examiners, instruments, and examinees. Each study was conducted with specific protocols that included standards for cuff selection and methods of taking and recording blood pressure. When possible, first-, fourth-, and fifth-phase Korotkoff sounds or their equivalents were obtained. Since not all instruments allowed fifth-phase measurements, the term "diastolic" will generally refer to the fourth phase. The following studies and observations are briefly presented as examples of the use of this design under various conditions.

1. FIVE SIMILAR INSTRUMENTS
A study was conducted using five mercury sphygmomanometers. Since this was the initial experiment to train examiners to use this instrument and this statistical design, five adults instead of children were used as examinees. It was thus possible to compare five similar instruments in a highly controlled situation. Three physicians and two medical students were used as examiners. Preliminary sessions were conducted to organize and train staff in the flow of personnel and the recording of observations. Three readings were obtained at each station by each observer. The entire experiment was replicated twice.

The hypothesis that the mean readings from each instrument were the same was rejected ($p < 0.01$) for both the systolic and diastolic readings. The means of readings from the two replications ranged from 123.8 to 131.8 mm Hg systolic and 85.1 to 93.9 mm Hg diastolic. Specifically, two of the instruments appeared to give lower readings than the other three. The null hypothesis of no difference among examiners was rejected ($p < 0.01$) for systolic and diastolic readings. The means for the five examiners ranged from 122.4 to 130.1 mm Hg systolic and 84.7 to 94.8 mm Hg diastolic.

Since multiple readings were taken at each of the stations during each time period, the precision (measurement error) of each of the sphygmomanometers could be compared. This is a pseudoprecision since multiple readings on each sphygmomanometer could not be obtained in a blind manner. The standard deviations for a pseudomeasurement error for each of the five instruments showed no statistically significant differences ($p > 0.05$). This was not unexpected since the three readings at each station were nonblind. For the most part, there were similar findings for pseudoprecision among examiners and examinees, except for systolic pressure. Such a study is not difficult to conduct when the examiners are familiar with the instruments and the instruments are functional. In addition, subtle differences among instruments and among examiners can be detected in an unbiased manner. These differences may be due to such factors as parallax or inadequate levels of mercury in the reservoirs of the sphygmomanometers. These factors were considered and rectified in future studies by raising the sphygmomanometers to eye level, by adding an additional light source, and by adding mercury to the reservoirs to equalize the instruments. This experiment was a prepilot study in that there are many sources of variability in blood pressure readings. Future protocols take these factors into consideration.

A complete analysis of the data of this experiment is available as an unpublished report.

2. FIVE DIFFERENT INSTRUMENTS

Further studies were conducted to compare five different instruments (Physiograph, Physiometrics, Kass-Zinner, mercury sphygmomanometer, and Bonn) in a 5×5 Graeco-Latin Square design. Physicians and children served as examiners and examinees, respectively. Two replications of the experiment were conducted for each of three different age groups (6-, 10-, and 14-year-olds). The first three instruments were automatic recorders yielding permanent records. Three readers, not acting as examiners and independent of each other, read these records. Because of the difficulty that arose in training examiners and readers for each instrument and because of instrument malfunction during the course of the experiment, no detailed analysis of the data was warranted. The observations indicated the need to conduct a design of this type with equipment and personnel operating satisfactorily.

3. FIELD STUDY

Third-grade children, 8–10 years of age, participated in a 4×4 Graeco-Latin Square design aimed at testing the performance and practicability of two promising automatic instruments under actual field conditions in Franklinton, Louisiana. Registered nurses, well-trained according to a specific protocol, observed blood pressures of children with the mercury sphygmomanometer and the two automatic instruments. The experiment was conducted four times, twice for each sex with different children used in each replication.

The hypothesis that the four instruments—an Arteriosonde, a Physiometrics, and two mercury sphygmomanometers—measured the same on the average was rejected for both systolic ($p < .05$) and diastolic ($p < .01$) readings by using an analysis of variance for a Graeco-Latin Square design; however, multiple comparison tests between pairs of instruments failed to reject the hypothesis that the systolic means were the same. Diastolic readings on the Arteriosonde ($\bar{x} = 54.2$ mm) were significantly lower than the diastolic readings on the Physiometrics ($\bar{x} = 62.7$ mm) and each of the sphygmomanometers ($\bar{x} = 60.5$ mm, $\bar{x} = 62.0$ mm), each at the 0.01 level. The hypothesis that the four examiners measured identically and the hypothesis of equal mean pressure for the four time periods were not rejected. The studies were effective in the testing of instruments capable of obtaining reproducible blood pressures in children under survey conditions, and they allowed comparison of measurements characteristic for each instrument.

4. FOUR DIFFERENT INSTRUMENTS

The fourth series of Graeco-Latin Square design studies was conducted to test the mercury sphygmomanometer, Arteriosonde, Physiometrics, and Zero Muddler. The latter two instruments give blind measurements, thus allowing the evaluation of precision among the examiners. Trained physicians replicated the experiment four times on adult subjects.

The only differences for systolic pressures indicated significant by the Newman-Keuls test were those obtained by the Physiometrics, which gave significantly lower readings than the Arteriosonde (a second instrument was obtained because of low readings produced earlier). Similarly, for diastolic readings the Physiometrics was lower than the other three instruments. This was partly due to inexperience in reading the recordings, particularly the diastolic. There appeared to be no significant differences among the four examiners. This study allowed comparisons of the levels of indirect blood pressure measurements on certain properly working instruments to blind mercury sphygmomanometric readings.

Field studies

The final test for any blood pressure measuring device must be its use in the field by those observers who will do the recordings. The reproducibility of observations in the field and agreement with reference methods are obviously important in conducting epidemiologic studies.

First Franklinton field study. In an examiner training session, and as part of a prepilot study to develop a fixed protocol for obtaining blood pressure measurements in children, some 215 school children were examined in Franklinton in April of 1973. Each child was placed in random waiting order and measured three times in sequence with each of two mercury sphygmomanometers and with one of the two automatic instruments (Physiometrics or Arteriosonde). The order in which these instruments were applied was determined by randomization for each child separately. The objective of this study was to compare each automatic instrument to the reference technique on a large sample in a field setting.

Means (± one standard deviation) for both systolic and diastolic readings are given in Table 5–2. The mean readings are shown for first mercury station visited, second mercury station visited, and automatic instrument.

For those children examined on two mercury sphygmomanometers

Table 5–2. Means (±1 standard deviation) and product moment correlation coefficient between means of three readings on each of three instruments, Franklinton, April 1973

N = 99	Systolic			Diastolic		
	Baum 1	Baum 2	Physiometrics	Baum 1	Baum 2	Physiometrics
	105.0	101.5	100.5	72.7	68.5	63.1
	(± 10.0)	(± 11.0)	(± 9.6)	(± 8.6)	(± 9.4)	(± 6.2)
Baum 1		0.81	0.70		0.64	0.41
Baum 2			0.66			0.35

N = 114	Systolic			Diastolic		
	Baum 1	Baum 2	Arteriosonde	Baum 1	Baum 2	Arteriosonde
	104.3	101.0	97.4	74.0	68.8	58.8
	(± 12.2)	(± 12.1)	(± 13.1)	(± 9.3)	(± 9.5)	(± 8.2)
Baum 1		0.81	0.79		0.57	0.54
Baum 2			0.79			0.56

and the Physiometrics, the mean systolic readings at the first mercury station visited were greater than those at the second mercury station or on the Physiometrics ($p < 0.01$). The mean diastolic readings for each of the three stations differed ($p < 0.01$). Although these differences are statistically significant, they are small. The readings from the Arteriosonde were somewhat lower. These observations suggested that the automatic instruments can obtain reliable blood pressure measurements in the field, equivalent to those measured by the mercury sphygmomanometer.

Second Franklington field study. Thirty-seven children were examined in May of 1973 in Franklinton to compare examiners and to test replicability with the same examiner. The children were randomly assigned to one of two teams. A team consisted of three examiners at three mercury sphygmomanometer stations. Because each examiner remained at the same station over the duration of the two-day study, differences among examiners rather than instruments were the prime focus of the study. For each team the examiner at one station had both systolic and diastolic readings lower than either of the examiners at the other stations. In most cases, these differences were statistically significant.

In addition, seventeen of the children were rescreened; that is, they were examined a second time in the same order on the same instruments by the same examiner. To obtain an unbiased sample, the random drawing of the sample of children for rescreening was not revealed until all children had been screened initially. Although the sample was small, it did appear that the diastolic rescreenee readings for one examiner were higher than the original readings. Although a true measurement error could not be calculated (due to time delay in obtaining rescreenee blood pressure) the variability of each individual examiner was calculated. For five examiners there appeared to be little variability in replicability. However, one of the examiners had a greater variability than the other five for diastolic readings. Such observations can help determine the need for further training of examiners. The method of rescreening is a valuable research tool for studies attempting to obtain reliable blood pressure measurements in an epidemiologic survey.

Replicability within and among readers of automatic blood pressure records

After the series of studies described above, the Physiometrics automatic recorder was selected for indirect measurement of blood pressure in addition to the mercury sphygmomanometer. A major reason for selecting the former instrument was its provision of a permanent record in the form of a graph on a paper disk. The difficulty with the instrument may not be its lack of recording reliability, but the interpretation of its permanent records, especially for diastolic readings. In order to evaluate readings of these disks, a study was conducted in July of 1975 to evaluate reproducibility of readings. Specifically, the experiment was designed to measure the degree of agreement among four readers and the reproducibility of each reader. Since three disks are made for each subject observed, a second purpose of the experiment was to estimate the pseudo-measurement error of the instrument, with the assumption that the blood pressure was not altered during the 3 to 4 min required to obtain three readings.

Three disks from each of 112 subjects (randomly selected from children, age 5–14 years, examined from September of 1973 through May of 1974) constituted the sample for this study. The 336 disks were divided randomly into four disk packs (A, B, C, and D) so that no two disks from the same subject appeared in the same pack. A 4 × 4 Graeco-Latin Square design was employed to compare readers (numbered 1, 2, 3, 4), recorders (who gave the disks in random order to the reader and recorded each reading), time periods, and disk packs. A fifth time period was added at the end of the experiment in which one of the first time periods was repeated. The disks were given new random identifying numbers before this fifth period. Each of the four readers were trained in reading the disks according to a standardized protocol. Table 5–3 contains the mean systolic and diastolic readings for each of the four readers, recorders, time periods, and disk packs. None of the pairwise differences among the readers, recorders, and time periods were significant at the 0.05 level. The systolic readings for disk pack D were lower ($p < 0.05$) than the readings for the other three disk packs, while the diastolic readings for disk pack D were lower ($p < 0.05$) than the readings for disc pack A and disc pack C. Each mean is based on 336 observations.

Estimates of pseudomeasurement error by reader for both systolic

Table 5–3. Mean systolic and diastolic blood pressure readings for four readers, four recorders, four time periods, and four disk packs, Physiometrics disk experiment, July 1975.

	Reader			
	1	2	3	4
Systolic N = 336	100.5	100.5	100.4	100.9
Diastolic N = 336	62.8	62.7	63.1	63.6

	Recorder			
	a	b	c	d
Systolic N = 336	100.7	100.6	100.5	100.6
Diastolic N = 336	62.9	63.2	63.2	62.8

	Time period			
	I	II	III	IV
Systolic N = 336	100.4	100.7	100.7	100.6
Diastolic N = 336	63.3	63.0	62.9	62.9

	Disk pack			
	A	B	C	D
Systolic N = 336	102.1[1]	101.1[1]	100.5[1]	98.6
Diastolic N = 336	63.9[1]	62.6	63.9[1]	61.8

[1]Mean for disk pack greater than mean for disk pack D ($p < .05$)

and diastolic readings are given in Table 5–4. The standard deviations for pseudomeasurement error for both systolic and diastolic readings were about the same for each reader; however, the coefficient of variation for this pseudomeasurement error was greater for diastolic readings due to their smaller magnitude. For each reader the first systolic reading was higher than the second ($p < 0.05$, except for reader 2, with $p < 0.01$) and third reading ($p < 0.01$). No significant differences among the three diastolic readings were found. These observations can be interpreted to mean that the standard deviation corresponding to the replicability variance of any reading is on the average between 4 and 5 mm Hg for both systolic and diastolic, respectively, due to either measurement aberration or short-term subject variability, or both.

Table 5–5 gives the mean systolic and diastolic readings for the first and fifth time periods in which 84 disks were reread by each examiner. The mean differences were significant for reader 4, for

Table 5–4. Standard deviation(s) and coefficient of variation (CV) for pseudo-measurement error about three consecutive systolic and diastolic blood pressure readings for 112 children by each of four readers, Physiometrics disk experiment, July 1975

Reader	Number of children	Mean pressure at time			Significance level	Pseudo-measurement error	
		1	2	3		s	CV
Systolic blood pressure (mm Hg)							
1	112	101.7	100.3	99.6	$p < 0.002$	4.51	4.49
2	112	101.6	100.2	99.7	$p < 0.004$	4.32	4.29
3	112	101.4	100.2	99.6	$p < 0.003$	4.08	4.06
4	112	102.0	100.6	100.0	$p < 0.003$	4.44	4.40
Diastolic blood pressure (mm Hg)							
1	112	63.1	62.9	62.6	$p < 0.69$	4.41	7.01
2	112	62.6	62.8	62.5	$p < 0.91$	4.59	7.33
3	112	62.8	63.2	63.2	$p < 0.76$	4.52	7.17
4	112	64.2	63.4	63.0	$p < 0.10$	4.26	6.71

Table 5–5. Means, difference in means, standard deviation(s) for measurement error, and coefficient of variation (CV) for measurement error for systolic and diastolic blood pressure for 336 disks read twice (84 by each reader), Physiometrics disk experiment, July 1975

Reader	N	Mean		Difference $\bar{d}$	Measurement error	
		Time 1	Time 5		s	CV
Systolic blood pressure						
1	84	101.7	101.6	0.12	1.52	1.50
2	84	100.8	100.8	0.01	0.83	0.83
3	84	100.1	100.2	−0.13	0.79	0.79
4	84	98.9	99.5	−0.56[2]	1.24	1.25
Diastolic blood pressure						
1	84	63.9	63.1	0.83	2.93	4.61
2	84	62.5	61.7	0.81[1]	2.35	3.78
3	84	64.5	63.9	0.58	2.45	3.81
4	84	62.3	63.8	−1.47[3]	2.81	4.45

[1]$p < 0.01$
[2]$p < 0.05$
[3]$p < 0.001$

whom the second systolic reading was higher ($p < 0.001$). The first diastolic reading was higher for reader 2 ($p < 0.05$). The measurement error for the two readings was about twice as great for diastolic as for systolic readings, indicating the difficulty in assessing the diastolic measurement. The differences in readings, although significant, are rather small and are a measure of the reproducibility of reading the disks after training and adhering to a protocol. The observations suggest that this automatic instrument can be reliably used in a large survey, and resting indirect blood pressure measurements on children can be reproduced.

COMMENT

The two major techniques we used to assess instruments for obtaining indirect blood pressure measurements on children, the Graeco-Latin Square design and field studies, tend to complement each other. The Graeco-Latin Square design provides a method for eliminating bias and the effect of levels of blood pressure on the instruments and the performance of the observers. Unfortunately, thorough training of all participants and proper functioning of all instruments are necessary for its use. Studies done in the field not only evaluate the conditions under which a survey is to be conducted, but can also help detect subtle differences occurring only through many observations.

The technical problems of instruments cannot be overemphasized. Differences between mercury sphygmomanometers can arise not only from parallax in reading instruments, but also from under- and over-filling the mercury reservoirs of the instrument. The initial inability to cope with some of the mechanical aspects of the newly tried automatic devices and inefficient calibration of such devices (even at the factory) can cause differences in readings between instruments of the same type, as was observed with the Arteriosonde 1216.

Biologic variations of blood pressure in any one child cause difficulty in obtaining reproducible blood pressures and in evaluating the reproducibility of an individual examiner; however, use of the several approaches outlined here and extensive training programs preceding these studies (training with tapes, film, split stethoscope, and the technique of rescreening and reexamining the same subject) can reveal problems encountered by a specific examiner. Those who consistently differ from the other examiners when examining the same children under similar conditions can be identified and either given additional training or shifted to other assignments. This examiner surveillance was repeated periodically, each time followed by appropriate adjustments.

These studies further illustrate the potential of an epidemiologic program to detect small differences and subtle biologic effects in blood pressure, i.e., racial differences and examiner-examinee interaction. Automatic recording instruments that can produce permanent records have the advantage of evaluating replicability of record reading. Another advantage, since the recording process does not involve examiner judgement, is that such instruments allow the study of the influence of the examiner as a person on the blood pressure of the examinee, which is difficult to evaluate with a mercury sphygmomanometer. For these reasons we chose the Physiometrics recorder to complement observations recorded by the mercury sphygmomanometer. The oversize cuff, the ability to detect fourth-phase Korotkoff sounds, and the ease in operation and maintenance of the machine made it a suitable addition to the study. A comparison of the results of the two instruments in an epidemiologic survey are presented elsewhere (Chapter 16 and Voors et al., 1976). The use of this instrument led to the detection of higher levels in black children and cuff artifacts in indirect blood pressure measurements by the mercury sphygmomanometer in young children (Chapter 16 and Voors et al., 1976; Golden et al., 1974).

In the past few years, many new instruments have been introduced which measure indirect blood pressure and can produce values equiv-

Table 5–6. Potential sources of error in blood pressure surveys

Variable	Validity testing	Replicability testing
Instrument	Graeco-Latin squares	Rescreening
Overall effect	Daily calibration	
Cuff size		
Sound transducer		
Pressure indexing		
Examiner	Multiple regression	Rescreening
Overall effect	Split stethoscopes	Rereading of permanent
Interpretation of sound	Audiometry	records
signals	Graeco-Latin squares	
Interaction with		
subjects		
Field	Field studies	Rescreening
Overall effect	Graeco-Latin squares	

alent to those obtained by listening for Korotkoff sounds. The low-frequency sound transducer of the Physiometrics may have an advantage over the recording via transducer filters concentrating on higher-pitched components (Golden et al., 1974). Table 5–6 summarizes the contingencies on the strategy of designing and monitoring on ongoing blood pressure study. Tests should be conducted often and should be both sensitive and specific enough to reduce the probability of false results. These tests should begin at the inception of the study and should end only when the last report of the results is complete. These studies are intended to aid in evaluations of instruments, which should always be tested extensively before widespread use. (See Chapter 14 for more detail regarding methods to decrease measurement error in blood pressure readings.)

For clinical purposes, the mercury sphygmomanometer remains an excellent and useful instrument in measurement of blood pressure in children around five years of age and older. For younger children and infants, other instruments are required, as discussed in Chapter 15. The automatic instruments do contribute to studies on a large population and can complement observations obtained with the mercury sphygmomanometer.

SUMMARY

To obtain accurate measurements of blood pressure in children, we conducted several studies to monitor the validity and replicability of instruments, methods, and observers in measuring indirect blood pressure. These studies included Graeco-Latin Square designs, examination of children in a field setting, and assessments of the replicability of reading automatically recorded blood pressures. We computed biases and, where possible, eliminated them in the ensuing studies.

One automatic instrument, the Physiometrics recorder, was used in conducting epidemiologic studies where it complemented the measurements by the commonly used mercury sphygmomanometer.

Although direct arterial pressure measurements are desirable to assess validity of levels obtained with instruments and indirect measurements, these are not practical for routine observations or for epidemiologic studies of children. Future studies are needed to evaluate methods for measuring moment-to-moment changes of blood pressure in a given individual.

6. A comparison of fourth and fifth Korotkoff phases of blood pressure in school-age children

There is no uniform agreement in reporting·diastolic blood pressure as fourth or fifth Korotkoff phases. This is especially true for children, in whom there have been fewer reliable blood pressure studies. A prominent textbook on the measurement of blood pressure states: ". . . whether the onset of Phase 4 or Phase 5 should be used . . . is, in most instances, an argument over a few millimeters of mercury . . . Our practice is to note both diastolic pressures. If only one value is to be recorded, we employ the onset of Phase 5" (Burch and de Pasquale, 1962). The latest recommendation of the Committee on Postgraduate Education of the American Heart Association (Kirkendall et al. 1967) is to record fourth and fifth Korotkoff phases, the fourth being the best index of diastolic pressure. The difference noted between the fourth and fifth phase is 7–10 mm Hg. In a literature review, Geddes (1970) seems to agree with this recommendation.

In children, the difference between fourth and fifth phases was found to be 5 mm Hg by Johnson et al. (1965), but much larger, namely 17 mm Hg., by Moss and Adams (1962). Londe and Goldring (1976), in giving guidelines for blood pressure evaluation in children, used fifth phase because: " . . . we were more certain of this end point than of others." It is clear that further studies are needed to make a selection of Korotkoff phase so that it is most easily reproduced by indirect blood pressure measurements.

This chapter describes fourth and fifth phase measurements with the use of mercury sphygmomanometry on 3,524 children, ages 5–14 years.

GENERAL METHODS

Instruments

During the school year 1973–74, indirect blood pressures were obtained on the children 5–14 years of age by using the mercury sphygmomanometer and by the Physiometrics automatic blood pressure recorder. Selection of the bladder sizes for the Baumanometer cuff was based on arm measurement criteria recommended by Karvonen et al. (1964), Simpson et al. (1965), and King (1967), but with the restriction that commonly available bladders be used and that shorter arms require a narrower cuff in order to leave room for the stethoscope at the elbow skin crease.

Observer training

The measurements were taken by eight carefully trained and monitored observers. All blood pressure observers (registered and licensed practical nurses) were selected after an intense training period and a clearance for hearing by audiometry testing. After intitial testing they were retested at regular intervals (four times) during the nine months of screening. Several materials were used for training and testing: 1. tape recordings; 2. the sound film, "Practice in Blood Pressure Reading" (National Medical Audiovisual Center at the Center for Disease Control, Atlanta); and 3. a cuff with a Y-shaped tube leading to two Baumanometers combined with a stethoscope with Y-shaped tubes leading to two sets of earpieces. These materials enabled blind measurements by two observers on the same subject simultaneously. As criteria for passing these tests, preestablished relative tolerance limits were used and observers were replaced if they consistently reported different values relative to the other observers.

Blood pressure measurement

The children were encouraged to void before the blood pressures were measured. Volunteer workers then guided them through a designated random sequence for examination. For each child the blood pressure was determined by three trained observers in a rigid random order, each observer independently measuring three consecutive blood pressures per child. Two of these observers each used a well-illuminated mercury sphygmomanometer placed at eye level, and the third a Physiometrics recorder; each instrument was assigned randomly on a daily basis to an observer. An instrument and an observer formed a "station." Under quiet conditions in a screened-off corner, observers recorded the first and fourth Korotkoff phases to determine the right-arm blood pressure while each child was seated. The fifth phase was also recorded with sphygmomanometer readings. Care was taken to cover the brachial artery with the center of the rubber bladder. Blood pressures were recorded as the last procedure of the examination process that took $1^{1}/_{2}$ to 2 hr. At the end of each examination day, in which 30–40 children were examined, a random sample of four children (slightly more than 10%) were reexamined. This enabled us to assess the replicability of measurements by an observer after about one hour.

GENERAL OBSERVATIONS

Observations of diastolic pressures

The distribution of the fifth-phase measurements in all children is given in Table 6–1. In 5.7% of the readings disappearance of the Korotkoff sound was not perceived by the observers. In another 0.9% this disappearance was heard at a cuff pressure of less than 20 mm Hg. In order to increase the empirical biologic validity of the results these readings were eliminated. This frequency distribution was bimodal, and the elimination of all fifth-phase observations below 20 mm Hg seemed to yield an approximate Gaussian distribution of the remaining values. For these reasons, at this point all children having fifth-phase measurements less than 20 mm Hg were excluded from the study data. Thus, 2,884 children remained in the study population.

Table 6–1. Diastolic (fifth-phase) blood pressure measurements on Baumanometer for 3,524 children, 5–14 years of age, before and after exclusion of children with at least one fifth phase measurement less than 20 mm

Fifth-phase blood pressure (mm Hg)	Before exclusion		After exclusion	
	n	%	n	%
0	1,208	(5.7)	0	(0)
1–19	194	(0.9)	0	(0)
20–39	4,634	(22.0)	3,667	(21.2)
40–59	11,446	(54.3)	10,207	(59.0)
60–79	3,573	(16.9)	3,387	(19.6)
80[1]	43	(0.2)	43	(0.2)
Total	21,098[1]	(100.0)	17,304	(100.0)

[1]Each of 3,524 children was measured six times; 46 missing values were excluded from above totals.

Figure 6–1. Diastolic fourth and fifth phase blood pressures (mean ±2 S.E.) by mercury sphygmomanometer in children ages 5–14 years; N = 2,884. Children with fifth-phase measurements below 20 mm Hg were omitted.

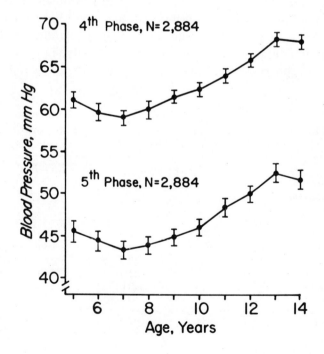

Mean ($\pm$ 2 S.E.) resulting blood pressures by age for the fourth and fifth phases are given in Figure 6–1. The average difference is 16 mm Hg. The yearly ranges approximated 40 mm Hg for the fourth, and 40–55 mm Hg for the fifth phase. The distributions of the fourth phase measurements approximated Gaussian curves.

Replicability between stations

The distribution of absolute differences between the means of two stations is given in Table 6–2 for fourth and fifth phases. We found that this distribution is not affected by race, sex, or by level of individual mean fourth phase blood pressure (chi-square test). Absolute differences were on the average larger for the fifth phase than for the fourth. (Mean absolute differences were 9.8 and 6.5 mm Hg, respectively; the distribution was evaluated by chi-square test, resulting in statistical significance — $p < 0.0001$.)

Determinants of variability

Multiple regression analysis was applied to the mean of six blood pressure readings made per individual, and controlled for all measured biologic determinants (age, body height, weight, maturation, etc.) on which the blood pressure had a statistically significant partial regression (Table 6–3). Significant coefficients of regression that were

Table 6–2. Absolute differences between means for two Baumanometer stations of fourth and fifth-phase blood pressures measured approximately 5 min apart by different observers in 2,884 children, 5–14 years of age

Absolute difference in blood pressure between stations (mm Hg)	Fourth phase		Fifth phase	
	n	%	n	%
0.0–0.9	303	10.5	195	6.8
1.0–4.9	1,073	37.2	684	23.7
5.0–9.9	829	28.7	748	25.9
10.0–19.9	617	21.4	939	32.6
20.0–29.9	59	2.0	277	9.6
30.0 +	3	0.1	41	1.4
Total	2,884	99.9	2,884	100.0

Table 6–3. Stepwise multiple linear regression for fourth and fifth-phase blood pressure on Baumanometer in 2,884 children, 5–14 years of age[1]

Source	Fourth phase		Fifth phase	
	Regression coefficient	Partial correlation coefficient	Regression coefficient	Partial correlation coefficient
Intercept	6.86		9.78	
Right upper-arm circumference[2]	32.90[a]	0.28[a]	23.56[a]	0.16[a]
Maturation	0.55[a]	0.17[a]	0.73[a]	0.18[a]
Hemoglobin	0.56[a]	0.09[a]	0.52[b]	0.07[b]
Black race	0.86[c]	0.06[c]	—	—
Observer 1	1.44[a]	0.08[a]	− 1.21[c]	−0.05[c]
2	—	—	—	—
3	2.95[a]	0.12[a]	1.76[c]	0.05[c]
4	2.73[a]	0.18[a]	—	—
5	—	—	− 2.36[a]	−0.09[a]
6	—	—	− 5.97[a]	−0.30[a]
7	2.23[a]	0.15[a]	—	—
8	—	—	—	—

Multiple correlation coefficient squared is 0.30 (4th phase) and 0.26 (5th phase)

[1]118 out of 2,884 children were not analyzed due to missing data
[2]Log_{10}
[a]$p < 0.0001$
[b]$p < 0.001$
[c]$p < 0.01$

due to the individual observers measuring blood pressure ranged from 1.44 to 2.95 mm Hg for Phase 4 and from −1.21 to −5.97 mm Hg for Phase 5. The true effects on the three measurements made are twice as large as the regression coefficients given for individual observers because the dependent variable represented six measurements: three by one observer and three by another. Therefore, the maximum absolute size of any significant observer effect was higher for the fifth phase than for the fourth phase.

Examination-reexamination comparison

Comparing the first examination with the reexamination (Table 6–4), we found for each station that the absolute differences of the mean pressure between examination and reexamination of a child were much larger for the fifth than for the fourth phase. (Mean absolute differences were 7.1 and 5.0 for fifth and fourth phases, respectively; the

Table 6–4. Absolute differences between means for two Baumanometer
stations of fourth and fifth phase blood pressure measured approximately
one hour apart by the same observer in 268 children, 5–14 years of age

Absolute difference in blood pressure between stations (mm Hg)	Fourth phase		Fifth phase	
	n	%	n	%
0.0–0.9	89	16.6	64	11.9
1.0–4.9	226	42.2	182	34.0
5.0–9.9	153	28.5	132	24.6
10.0–19.9	65	12.1	137	25.6
20.0–29.9	3	0.6	19	3.5
30.0+	0	0.0	2	0.4
Total	536	100.0	536	100.0

distribution of the data was evaluated by chi-square test, resulting in
statistical significance—$p < 0.0005$.)

Statistical tests

Some statistical tests for the results given above are presented in
Table 6–5. In general, the difference between first and second station
was positive (at the station of first measurement the pressure was
higher) but small in size. Standard deviations of these differences, on
the other hand, were quite large. When F-tests of differences between
the squared deviations of fourth and fifth phases were applied, all
turned out to be statistically highly significant ($p < 0.0001$).

COMMENT

Korotkoff sounds in the informative spectrum band (being 10–80 Hz
according to Golden et al. (1974), are likely to be generated by relaxa-
tion oscillation (Ur and Gordon, 1970) and therefore to decrease in
frequency with a decrease in diastolic blood pressure (Whitcher, 1969;
Maurer and Noordergraaf, 1976). Clearly, the lower end of this band is
not audible by the human ear. We surmise that if the diastolic pressure
is correspondingly low (as in young children), the human ear sometimes misses the informative change in amplitude but remains tuned
to the higher frequencies which are informative only for adults with

Table 6–5. Measures of variability in fourth and fifth-phase blood pressures in children 5–14 years of age[1]

Description		Fourth phase	Fifth phase
		mm Hg	
Replicability between stations			
Difference (mean ± S.D.) between mean pressures for two Baumanometer stations		0.15 ± 8.25 (N = 2884)	0.25 ±12.28 (N = 2884)
Examination-reexamination Difference			
(mean ± S.D.) between mean pressures for two examining and reexamining Baumanometer stations	first station	−0.44 ± 6.62 (N = 268)	−0.85 ± 9.20 (N = 268)
	second station	−0.96 ± 6.26 (N = 268)	−1.89 ± 9.05 (N = 268)

[1]F-tests of differences of the squared standard deviations between the fourth and fifth phases resulted in high significance ($p < 0.001$).

their higher diastolic pressures. Apparently our observer training, which emphasized the change in pitch at the fourth Korotkoff phase, succeeded in enabling the observers to identify this phase in each child, but was unable to sensitize their ears for the change in amplitude at the lower frequency of the fifth phase in some children.

We conclude that in the examination of children the Korotkoff Phase 4 is likely to give a more reliable measure of indirect diastolic blood pressure than Phase 5. This conclusion cannot be extrapolated to the screening of adults for hypertension by paramedical personnel because in adults Phase 5 may offer the distinct advantage of requiring less intensive training.

Our data do not reflect on the validity of the measurements as applied to intra-arterial pressure.

SUMMARY

Six blood pressures were taken on 3,524 children by trained observers using mercury sphygmomanometers in a rigid, randomized design. At the end of each examination day, a random sample of children was reexamined by the same observers. Both Korotkoff fourth and fifth phases were recorded, and measurement reliability was systematically maintained. Six percent of the fifth-phase pressures were 0 mm Hg. After elimination of the children with recorded fifth phases under 20 mm Hg, the difference between age-specific mean fourth and fifth phase pressures was 16 mm Hg. The standard deviation of the mean difference between station pressures was 8.1 mm Hg for fourth, and 12.3 mm Hg for fifth phase, the latter significantly larger than the former. Likewise, the standard deviation of the mean difference (keeping the same examiner) between examined and reexamined pressure was 6 mm Hg for fourth, and 9 mm Hg for fifth phase, the latter again significantly larger than the former. In multiple regression analysis with fourth and fifth phase pressure as the respective dependent variables, the significant effects due to the individual examiners averaged 4.7 mm Hg for fourth and 7.5 mm Hg for fifth phase. Despite painstaking efforts, fifth-phase measurements did not seem to approach the consistency and replicability of the fourth phase measurements as an index of diastolic blood pressure in children in a survey conducted by trained observers.

7. An improved 24-hour dietary recall —a useful technique for nutritional studies of children

You have to ask children and birds how cherries and straw-
berries taste.

GOETHE

Hypercholesterolemia is generally recognized as a risk factor for coronary artery disease, but the relationship of the American diet to hyperlipoproteinemia remains controversial (Kannel et al., 1971b). Since
the influence of nutrition (like many other environmental factors) has
not been determined, improved methods are needed to evaluate precisely the food and nutrient intake of individuals being studied.

A principal objective of the Bogalusa Heart Study was to develop
methods which would assess and characterize the dietary intake of
children, yield reproducible dietary data, allow a child to serve as his
own respondent, and require only a small staff. A basic question asked
was: "Can an improved 24-hour dietary recall serve as a reliable tool
for collecting data on children?" If the method would repeat the same
results under identical conditions in a pilot sample, then the error of
measurement could be defined (Rose and Blackburn, 1968). The 24-
hour dietary recall was improved and adapted for use with school-age
children, tested for its reproducibility, and then used as the tool for
studying the composition of children's diets.

METHODS

A detailed protocol outlining both the verbal and written methods of
the 24-hour dietary recall was developed, tested, and subsequently

used to train interviewers. This protocol standardizes procedures for collecting school lunch data, for calculating recalls, and for developing interview techniques to minimize interviewer variability. The method consists of five parts: interview technique, identification of food items—qualification and quantification, school lunch measurement, food calculations, and nutrient calculations.

The 24-hour recall reflects an hour-by-hour history, beginning with the food and beverages consumed on the same day of the interview and ending with the food from the day before to complete a 24-hour period. The recall usually includes three meals plus interim snacks, all of which outline a meal pattern for each child (Fabry et al., 1966).

Interview technique

The protocol establishes a basic structure which must be used by every participating interviewer. Specifically, the interview technique follows the script of a dialogue between interviewer and child in which the interviewer explains the purpose of the inquiry and asks probing questions which elicit a seemingly complete recall. Certain questions expedite the interview and stimulate the child to remember the time and place of eating. For example, the time can be evoked by the following questions:

When did you eat or drink something?

Do you have a recess or a break in the morning or afternoon?

Did you eat anything then?

Were any of your favorite shows on TV last night? Did you have a sucker, doughnut, cookie, soft drink, or popcorn while you watched TV?

When do you usually go to bed? Did you have a bedtime snack? Did your mother fix a bedtime snack for you?

The first question asks "when" rather than "what," to prompt a child to review his day and improve his recall of between-meal snacks. The second question can be verified by the student's teacher or school schedule. Correlation of snacks with TV shows indicates the precise hour of eating.

Mentioning locations or situations which are often accompanied by eating can help a child to recall easily forgotten foods:

How do you get home after school? Do you buy anything from the candy machine or corner store before you get on the bus?

Do you have a snack when you first get home after school?

Did you go to a meeting, football game, or party last night? Did they serve refreshments?

When a child knows he has eaten a serving of food but cannot remember exactly what it was, suggesting names of similar foods usually evokes recall.

The interview technique follows detailed guidelines for recording all information at each stage of the interview on a standardized form (Fig. 7–1) which is also used for keypunching for the computer.

Identification of food items—qualification

This section of the protocol describes information to be recorded for each food, specifically: 1. The name—common and/or brand; 2. the method of preparation—homemade, commercial, ready-to-eat, fried, baked, or casserole; and 3. the physical nature—color, shape, fresh or frozen, and unit size. Each food eaten or recipe is clearly identified during the interview or verified by a phone conversation with the mother. Then foods and recipes can be assigned proper identification numbers for computerized nutritional analysis.

Since children are apt to forget many snack foods eaten during a day, gentle probing with visual aids is used to remind the interviewee of them. A Product Identification Notebook (PIN) was developed to aid in distinguishing brands, sizes, and colors of snack foods (Fig. 7–2.) Snacks were grouped into five categories according to consistency and texture and were given fun names. The creamy mixtures and liquid snacks, such as ice cream, soft drinks, and puddings, are the "soft surprises"; cookies, cakes, pies, and crackers become "baked bits"; and chocolate-covered candies, nougats, and hard candies comprise the "sugary sweets." Fresh, canned, or frozen fruits and juices are named the "fruity fragments," and snacks producing noise when eaten, for example, chips, crackers, and nuts, are called "crunchy

1 2 3 4 5 6
00000 1 RECORD NO.
7 8
01 INTERVIEW NO.
NAME JOHN DOE

LSU-SCOR
BOGALUSA HEART STUDY
24-HR. DIETARY RECALL

PAGE 1 of 2
DATE FORM COMPLETED 02 06 74 (10 11 12 13 14 15)
Mo/ Day/Yr.

Form B 14

FOOD I.D. (16–20)	FREQ. (21–23)	AMOUNT x(gm)x.x (24–27)	TYPE (28)	NO. OF DAYS	C.F.	TIME OF EATING	SOURC	NAME OF FOOD ITEM	AMOUNT: MODEL	AMOUNT: EQUIV.	AMOUNT: CALCULATION	COMMENTS
06105	1	1140	1	1	1	0700	1	Egg, fried	2 units	x 57.0	gms/unit = 114.0 gms.	in Crisco hydrog., c̄ salt + pepper
00043	1	160	1	1	1	0700	1	Bacon	2 pcs.	x 8.0	gms./pe. = 16.0 gms.	~ 7" each
00357	1	6820	1	1	1	0700	1	Orange Jc.	2B	= 22.0	x 31.0gms/f.c. = 682.0 gms.	fresh, jar, no sugar
00472	1	1120	1	1	1	0700	1	Sausage, smoked	2 pcs.	x 56.0	gms. = 112.0 gms.	~ 5" each, fried, no extra fat
00325	1	7091	1	1	1	0700	1	Milk, whole	¾V+(2x¾B)	= (.75x9.0)+(1.5x11.0)	= 23.25x30.5 = 709.1 gms.	orange carton
00649	1	560	1	1	1	0700	1	Toast	2 pcs.	x 28.0	= 56.0 gms.	Holsum
00770	1	28	1	1	1	0700	1	Margarine	½ E	.1 x	28.4 = 2.84 gms.	bowl, white package
00747	1	2	1	1	1	0700	1	Salt on egg	3 pinches	x .05	gms/pinch = .15 gm.	
00408	1	1200	3	1	1	0815	4	Japanese Plum	4	x 30.0	= 120.0 gms.	on way to school size of small ball model
00670	1	4800	3	1	1	1000	5	Chocolate Milk	2 cartons x	8 fl.oz.	x 30.0gms/fl.oz. = 480.0gms.	
00131	1	3000	3	1	1	1300	5	Coke	A	= 10.0	x 30.0gms/fl.oz. = 300.0gms.	
00139	1	72	2	1	1	1200	2	Celery stick	1 stick	= 7.15 gms.		School lunch
06351	1	536	2	1	1	1200	2	Meat, gravy	1 unit	= 53.6 gms.		"
06004	1	753	2	1	1	1200	2	Rice	1 unit	= 75.3 gms.		"
06012	1	1084	2	1	1	1200	2	Biscuit	2 units	= 54.2 gms.	x 2 = 108.4 gms.	"
00136	1	206	2	1	1	1200	2	Carrot sticks	3 sticks	= 20.6 gms.		"
00325	1	2440	2	1	1	1200	2	Milk, whole	1 carton	= 244.0 gms.		"
06315	1	533	2	1	1	1200	2	Red Beans	1 unit	= 53.3 gms.		"

Is the way you ate yesterday the way you usually eat? (39) 1 ____ Do you take a vitamin or mineral supplement? (40) 0

What type? (41) 0 ____ When do you salt your food? (42) 5 ____ What time do you usually get up? (43 44 45 46) 0 6 1 0

What time do you usually go to bed? (47 48 49 50) 2 2 0 0 Completion code (51) 1 Interviewer (52 53) 0 1 7/73

Figure 7–1. Standardized form for recording quantities and names of foods appearing in a 24-hour dietary recall.

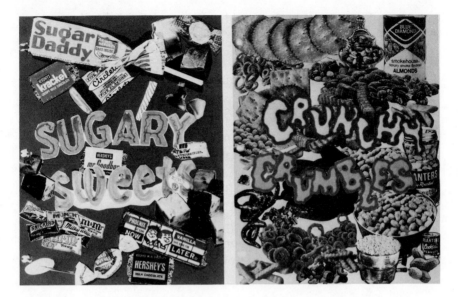

Figure 7-2. Product Identification Notebook categorizes snacks by consistency and texture.

crumbles." Each page of the PIN illustrates a snack group with pictures, product labels, or drawings of many foods. In addition, labels of local products, a color wheel, and a ruler (for specific lengths of certain foods) are included. At the close of each interview, the PIN is reviewed, page by page, to glean any other food which may have been forgotten.

On completing the recall, the interviewee is asked six questions about his sleeping and eating habits and about his use of salt. To define eating and fasting spans, the usual hours of rising and retiring are ascertained. When the respondent is asked, "Is the way you ate yesterday the way you usually eat?" the meal pattern outlined in the recall is reviewed to determine whether the times of eating and amounts of food consumed are typical. The response is coded as either "yes" or "no," and the "no" is qualified as "more" or "less" than usual. The question, "When do you salt your food?" is explored again by reviewing the recall and asking the child about his and his mother's use of the salt shaker. The interviewer assigns the salting procedure to one of seven categories that include tasting and cooking processes. The respondent is also asked whether he takes a vitamin, and if so, the frequency and brand name. Finally, the ability of the child to serve as a respondent is coded, for example, "completed satisfactorily by self."

Identification of food items—quantification

Correct quantification of foods and beverages relies on precise use of graduated food models developed by Moore and colleagues (1967) (Fig. 7–3). The models are not intended to depict any one food, but rather to assess portion size, weight, or volume without using standard household measurements, such as cups, tablespoons, or teaspoons. These models are equated for weights of specific meats and fats. Labels of various brands of margarine and butter sold in the area are shown to the child to help him identify specific types of fat used. Ordinary household beverage cups, rather than measuring cups, are used to assess volumes of other foods and drinks.

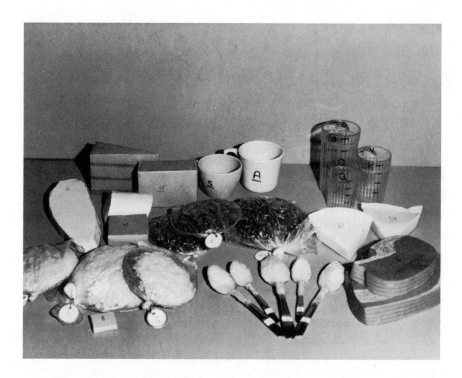

Figure 7–3. Graduated Food Models for quantification of foods.

School lunch measurement

With this technique, detailed information is obtained about the school lunch served on the day reflected in each 24-hour recall. In the cafeteria, the nutritionist uses standardized forms to record each ingredient in each recipe by weight, volume, or package unit. To determine an average unit weight, she obtains gram-weighings of a 1-cup measure of foods and three weighings of each average serving. If, for example, a child eats a whole biscuit, it would be coded as "1 unit." The average weight of a biscuit might equal 54.2 gm for that day, and this figure would appear on the child's recall. If only a portion of an item is eaten, then food models are used, and the gram-weight equivalency is calculated from the weight of a 1-cup measure of that food. By probing, any "traded" item is assessed, and since only items eaten are recorded, plate waste is indirectly quantitated.

Food calculations

A cumulative data file for converting food quantities to grams, based on $1/8$-cup weights plus actual gram-weights of units—such as candy bars and cookies—is continuously updated for accurate calculations. These data are recorded on large index cards bound in a Ready Reference Notebook for immediate use, and eventually they are placed in the computer data bank.

Each nutritionist calculates only the recalls she obtains, because she is familiar with the data. The calculations are checked by a second nutritionist, and disagreements are resolved in conference.

Nutrient calculations

The 24-hour recalls can be analyzed for 58 dietary components by the Extended Table of Nutrient Values (ETNV) (Hankins et al., 1965; Moore et al., 1974), a computer program which is comprised of over 1,600 single or basic food items and more than 1,000 composite foods or recipes derived from the single foods. A descriptive computer printout for the analysis of each recall is available. The system permits the addition of basic foods and recipes and changes of values in both when warranted.

Nine quality control programs internal to the ETNV system are applied to the data to insure consistency. For example, one program checks to be certain that, when the total fat of a food is multiplied by 0.95, the result is equivalent to the sum of saturated fatty acids, unsaturated fatty acids, and unknown fatty acids ($\pm$ 0.1%). All recipes are processed by one of three available recipe programs. The programs are based on what is known about the recipes, that is, gram-weight of all ingredients and the finished-product weight, when there is gain or loss of moisture. The third program substitutes the percentage of moisture and total solids in the final product for its final weight. An optional subprogram corrects recipes for losses of B-vitamins and ascorbic acid during cooking.

STUDIES ON A SAMPLE OF CHILDREN

The method was tested on 76 students in a pilot study in Franklinton, Louisiana. The sample met the recommendation of Young et al. (1952) that it include at least 50 persons. The group consisted of 39 girls (9 white and 30 black) and 37 boys (12 white and 25 black). Seventy-five children were 10 to 16 years old; one was 6 years old. The children were randomly selected and scheduled for one interview each; they were interviewed from Tuesday through Friday, so that a school lunch would be reflected in the recall. Interview time ranged from 30 to 40 min per child. Quiet areas were used for the interviews (the nutritionist often found herself in a bookroom, library, or behind the curtain on the auditorium stage). Only the nutritionist and the interviewee were present.

Ten of the 76 children were selected to be duplicate responders. Two trained nutritionists independently interviewed each child, covering the same 24-hour period. Half the children began with one interviewer, and the other half with the other interviewer. To prevent bias, a third nutritionist checked the duplicate recalls before computer analysis of the ETNV.

RESULTS—TEST OF REPEATABILITY

The dietary recalls of the ten duplicate responders were compared to evaluate whether the two interviewers obtained the same information. A paired t-test showed no significant difference ($p > 0.05$) between interviewers for the mean intakes computed for selected variables (Table 7–1). In addition, the coefficients of variation were relatively low (less than 20%) for all variables except total cholesterol and the

Table 7–1. Means for selected dietary variables from 24-hour dietary recalls for ten children each interviewed by two nutritionists; paired *t*-test statistics; and coefficients of variation

Variable	Means		*t*-value[1]	Coefficient of variation (%)
	interviewer 1	*interviewer 2*		
Total calories	2,342	2,225	0.68	16.9
from carbohydrate (%)	54.0	48.3	2.20	11.3
from fat (%)	34.7	38.9	1.95	13.1
from protein (%)	12.9	13.8	1.47	9.5
Total cholesterol (mg)	365	355	0.24	27.3
Polyunsaturated:saturated fatty acids ratio	0.34	0.33	0.43	15.3
Sucrose:starch ratio	1.29	1.20	0.74	20.9

[1]The *t*-test statistic has 9 degrees of freedom.

sucrose:starch ratio. As a check on the ETNV, one recall was reprocessed as a blind duplicate; identical analyses resulted.

DISCUSSION

Improved techniques for evaluating food consumption are essential in characterizing a diet which might prove to influence the risk of coronary artery disease and hypertension. With the advent of pediatric screening and risk factor programs, techniques are needed to make dietary data collection both practical and precise.

The 24-hour dietary recall is both practical and simple. Numerous studies have compared this technique with more lengthy ones and found that it saves time for both the interviewer and interviewee and is acceptable for studying a group (Young et al., 1952).

The age at which a child can serve as a valid respondent is an important criterion to determine. In Franklinton, children 10 to 12 years old were eager to talk about what they had eaten. Bosley (1947) found that children 9, 10, and 11 years old are spontaneously curious and honest and more likely to answer truthfully than older children, who tend to answer as they think they should.

The Franklinton children established rapport quickly and usually remembered brand names of the foods they had eaten. They seemed to remember eating times logically and clearly. When asked to recall a known school lunch, they were quite aware of their meals, but remembered the menu items in much simpler terms than those used by the school lunch personnel. For example, a child would recall a fruit salad with pineapple, oranges, coconut, and salad dressing, but not the name, "Polynesian pie."

Since Emmons and Hayes (1973) conclude from their experiments "that young children can provide information on their diets as accurately or more accurately than their mothers," a recall was not obtained from the mothers. Emmons and Hayes further state that with increasing age from Grade 1 to 4, a child's ability to recall a known school lunch menu improves. Using strict criteria for grading agreement, Meredith et al. (1951) interviewed students 9 to 18 years old

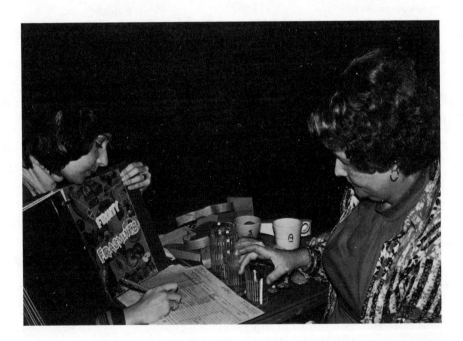

Figure 7–4. Nutritionist Rosanne Farris, R.D., helps Mrs. John Carpentar, mother of a 4-year-old participant remember the amount and kinds of foods her son has eaten over a 24-hour period. Food models and the product identification notebook being held are essential in efforts to quantitate diets and snack foods.

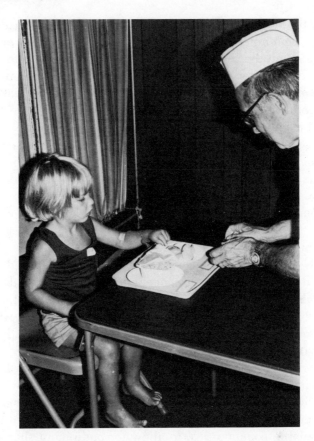

Figure 7–5. As part of an unpublished dietary study on an infant cohort (Frank, 1979a), 4-year-old George Bertoniere, Jr., is offered a choice of foods by a staff member. The choices may help nutritionists understand eating patterns as they develop.

within hours after they had consumed a known menu. They found great error in the recall of food items and quantities; however, they did recognize that the complexity and unfamiliarity of the menu, as well as an interview technique which did not distinguish colors or portions of items, might have negatively influenced the students' responses.

By using the graduated food models, we avoided speaking in terms of household measures. In addition, a bright color wheel in the PIN enabled the children to identify specific colors of questionable food items and thereby helped to increase the accuracy of the recalls.

In large community studies, more than one interviewer is often needed. To limit the variability among interviewers, a protocol which standardizes the interview technique is essential. Nutritionists in this study did not feel bound word-for-word to the protocol; rather, they found it comforting to have a written guide. They were free to challenge and expand the probes. Voice tone and facial expression of interviewers cannot be controlled by a written protocol, and since these factors can influence a respondent, interviewers should periodically discuss their approaches.

Uniform use of the graduated food models further standardized the recalls obtained by different interviewers. An adequate description of each food on the recall form aided in selecting and checking identification numbers quickly and accurately.

The PIN, which became a very useful tool, was developed when we recognized that visual aids are needed to help the children recall snack foods. On the average, they remembered one to three more snack foods by using the PIN. To ensure that a child understood that he was to choose foods he actually ate and not those he liked, a careful probing with light conversation was planned.

At the onset of the school lunch analysis, the nutritionists learned that one cannot take for granted that all schools follow quantity recipes specified for Type A school lunch (USDA Food and Nutrition Service, 1974). Even within a city, school lunch managers alter the recipes to match available commodities, to allow for equipment shortages and production problems, and to suit the tastes of both children and staff. Therefore, nutritionists were on the scene to measure and weigh the food in each school lunch as it was prepared and served.

The school lunch measurement was an excellent way to check the child's memory. However, during the interview, we recorded only the foods he actually ate—not everything that the child remembered having on his tray. To test a child's ability to completely recall this meal, information about all items remembered should be coded on the dietary recall form.

COMMENT

Chemical analysis of food actually eaten would be the most accurate method for analyzing the diets of children, but this technqiue is not feasible for most nutrition staffs. An improved 24-hour dietary recall can be used by a small, well-trained staff to collect more reliable data on a large number of school children. Vigilant monitoring of school lunch operations, incorporation of known recipes in the ETNV, and organization of probing techniques are necessary to insure the reliability of the tool. The low coefficients of variation of duplicate recalls noted in the study indicate that the error of measurement between interviewers is small, if the tool is carefully tested before use in the field and if observers are carefully trained by a written protocol.

SUMMARY

Improved techniques, including special training of interviewers, the use of graduated food models, and detailed probing techniques, were incorporated into a 24-hour dietary recall method for interviewing children. Detailed school lunch data were collected on the day prior to the recall. A computerized food composition table was utilized for nutritional analysis of 58 dietary components.

The method was tested on a random sample of 76 students (21 white, 55 black). A test of reproducibility was performed on a subsample of duplicate recalls ($N = 10$). Low coefficients of variation of duplicate recalls indicated a small measurement error.

III. Anthropometry

8. Anthropometric and maturation observations on children, ages 2½ to 14 years

The association of anthropometric variables with coronary artery disease and hypertension has been well documented in epidemiologic studies (Kannel et al., 1967b, Klein et al., 1973; Dyer et al., 1975). Since these cardiovascular diseases may originate in childhood, it is important to elucidate the early onset of these associations. Of the many studies of growth characteristics, few have incorporated detailed observations of blood pressure and lipids in children. Such studies are needed in exploring the relationship of anthropometric variables and cardiovascular disease. Biologic changes occur more rapidly in infancy and childhood than in any other period of life, and the influence of those changes on known risk-factor variables that might correlate with subsequent disease requires further investigation.

Selected anthropometric measurements were obtained on 714 Bogalusa preschool children, ages 2½–5½ years, and 3,524 school children, ages 5–14 years in order to characterize the pediatric population and to form the core for subsequent epidemologic observations. Additionally, indices of external physical maturation were obtained on the 5- to 14-year-olds. Such measurements, collected in a standardized manner on all children, enable us to describe and compare the biologic and morphologic growth of children residing within a given geographic environment.

This chapter is intended to show the distribution of height, weight, triceps skinfold, upper-arm length and circumference, and external maturation indices in a total community of children. These observations will serve as a reference for corresponding measurements from comparable communities, provide current anthropometric and maturation data for assessing secular trends, contrast black and white children residing in the same community, and report the anthropometric and maturational variables that are being studied in relation to the early natural history of coronary artery disease and hypertension.

METHODS

Methods of measurement

All measurements were taken by trained observers carefully following a written protocol. For multiple readings, the examinee was newly positioned and studied each time, and the mean of a set of multiple readings represented the observation for a child. A random process determined the first sex to be examined each day and the order of examination for individuals within each sex. The children wore underpants, a short-sleeved examination gown, and socks. A summary of the protocols for each measurement follows:

Height (nearest 0.1 cm) was measured and recorded twice on each of two instruments: a manual height board built for our study by the Specialized Center of Research—Arteriosclerosis at the University of Iowa and an automatic height board modified from plans obtained from the Mayo Clinic. The automatic instrument was calibrated at three specified times during each screening day. For each child, measurements were taken first on the Iowa Height Board; we report here only the results for this instrument, since 98.1% of the automatic and manual height observations agreed within 1.5 cm.

At examination the child stood erect, firmly against the vertical backboard with his chin parallel to the floor and eyes forward. All children were requested to wear a flat hair style which would not distort the measurement. When necessary, the examiner stood on a pedestal to avoid parallax while reading the measurement.

Weight (nearest 0.1 kg) was measured and recorded twice on each of two instruments: a balance beam metric scale (physician's office scale, Detecto Scales Inc., Brooklyn, N.Y.) and an automatic electronic scale (National Controls, Inc., Santa Rosa, Calif.). The automatic scale was calibrated at three specified times during each day of screening; the manual scale was calibrated monthly or whenever the scale was moved. Each child was measured first on the balance beam scale. We report here only the results for the balance beam scale, since 99.9% of the weight observations agreed within 0.5 kg.

At examination the child stood still in the center of the scale platform. In these data no correction has been made for the clothing worn during examination, since it was standardized apparel with a weight range of 0.2–0.4 kg.

Right Upper-Arm Length (nearest cm) was measured from the acromion to the olecranon processes with the GPM Anthropometer (Siber Precision Inc., Carlstadt, N.J.), with the child's forearm raised to make a 90° angle. The midpoint between the acromion and olecranon was marked on the skin of the dorsal surface.

Right Upper-Arm Circumference (nearest cm) was measured with a cloth tape measure at the marked midpoint. While the child's arm hung loosely at his side, the examiner took the measurement without compressing the circumference.

Right Arm Triceps Skinfold Thickness (nearest mm) was measured with Lange Skinfold Calipers (Cambridge Scientific Industries, Cambridge, Md.). The instruments were calibrated monthly to a tolerance of 0.4 mm or better with precision-made steel standard blocks measuring 5, 11, and 20 mm.

For the measurement the child stood on an elevated platform, relaxed, and placed his partly closed right hand, palm up, into the loosely formed cup of his left hand. With the thumb and forefinger of his left hand, the examiner, standing behind the child, grasped the dorsal skinfold parallel to the long axis over the triceps muscle. Allowing the skinfold to slide free of muscle, the examiner gently compressed and measured the skinfold, then recorded the result. The measurement was repeated three times.

External Maturation (Tanner criteria (Tanner, 1962)) was visually assessed for the 5- to 14-year-old age group in a clinical setting. The examining physician, using Tanner photographs, noted the growth of pubic hair and development of female breasts and male genitalia; the observations were recorded by a nurse. The Tanner ratings range from 1 (no development) to 5 (complete development). For girls, the Tanner stage was recorded for each breast with the mean of the two scores being the observation for an individual.

Time of Onset of Menarche (month, year) was asked of the school-age girls.

Age (last birthday in years) was computed based on date of birth and date of examination.

Statistical analysis

The data were subjected to an analysis of variance (least squares analysis) for a two-factor experiment (Winer, 1971). For analysis of racial differences in maturation, Kärber's method was used (Irwin and Cheeseman, 1939; Cornfield and Mantel, 1950) as applied by Bryan and Greenberg (1952). Although only means and selected percentiles are reproduced in this chapter, additional data are tabulated in a publication of the National Heart, Lung, and Blood Institute (1978). The results for 15-year-olds, representing approximately two-thirds of the population for that age, are included in the graphs of this chapter for illustrative purposes only, since no special effort was made to examine school-age children outside the 5- to 14-year age range.

OBSERVATIONS OF PRESCHOOL-AGE CHILDREN

Height and weight

Figure 8–1 and Tables 8–1 and 8–2 show the cross-sectional growth pattern of the preschool-age children. The distribution of height is symmetrical within both races and sexes. An asymmetrical weight distribution is noted, however, for black children, with variability increasing with age. In boys, the median heights and weights between blacks and whites differed slightly, while black girls were generally taller and heavier than white girls (Fig. 8–1). Among all children, blacks averaged 2.0 cm taller ($p < 0.005$) and 0.6 kg heavier ($p < 0.01$) than their white age peers.

Skewness and variability in the weight distribution may simply reflect developmental differences in growth for children of the same chronological age. Therefore, we investigated the distribution of weight for children of the same height (Fig. 8–2). The children

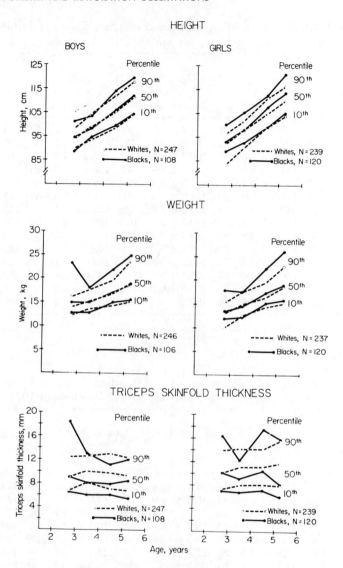

Figure 8–1. Height, weight, and triceps skinfold measurements of preschool children. Median, 10th, and 90th percentile values are shown according to age, race, and sex of the children.

showed an increase in the variability of weight, with increases of height as well as of age. Additionally, skewness is noticeable in this distribution for black girls, indicating a disproportionate amount of

Table 8–1. Number of children, mean, and standard deviation for height of children by sex, race, and age, September 1973–September 1974

Age at last birthday (yrs)	White boys n	$\bar{x} \pm S.D.$ (cm)	Black boys n	$\bar{x} \pm S.D.$ (cm)	White girls n	$\bar{x} \pm S.D.$ (cm)	Black girls n	$\bar{x} \pm S.D.$ (cm)
2.75[1]	37	93.9 ± 3.1	12	94.9 ± 3.9	33	90.9 ± 4.7	19	94.2 ± 4.0
3.50[1]	80	98.7 ± 4.7	32	98.9 ± 3.6	78	97.3 ± 4.4	38	98.4 ± 5.2
4.50[1]	89	105.2 ± 4.8	40	106.7 ± 5.4	86	105.1 ± 4.3	38	107.2 ± 4.7
5.25[1]	41	111.3 ± 4.8	24	111.8 ± 5.9	42	110.2 ± 4.5	25	113.6 ± 5.9
5	92	112.3 ± 5.3	45	112.0 ± 4.9	99	110.5 ± 5.1	38	113.4 ± 4.5
6	104	118.0 ± 5.0	54	118.0 ± 5.4	87	117.8 ± 5.3	58	118.7 ± 5.7
7	100	123.3 ± 5.8	56	125.2 ± 5.0	96	122.5 ± 5.1	61	124.4 ± 6.1
8	112	129.7 ± 5.8	65	130.3 ± 5.9	103	129.0 ± 5.8	56	131.7 ± 5.9
9	106	135.9 ± 5.8	82	134.7 ± 5.4	104	133.7 ± 6.3	59	134.9 ± 6.4
10	129	139.2 ± 6.1	75	140.4 ± 5.3	110	140.6 ± 7.3	62	142.5 ± 8.6
11	119	145.9 ± 7.4	75	146.1 ± 7.5	115	147.7 ± 8.1	70	149.4 ± 7.1
12	151	150.5 ± 8.3	87	151.1 ± 8.3	137	153.6 ± 7.6	81	156.5 ± 7.1
13	128	159.1 ± 9.9	75	159.0 ± 9.7	120	157.8 ± 6.9	74	158.9 ± 7.8
14	116	165.4 ± 8.6	68	165.3 ± 9.3	90	161.7 ± 6.4	63	161.6 ± 6.1

[1]Mean age at last birthday

Table 8–2. Number of children, mean, and standard deviation for weight of children by sex, race, and age, September 1973–September 1974

Age at last birthday (yrs)	White boys n	$\bar{x} \pm S.D.$ (kg)	Black boys n	$\bar{x} \pm S.D.$ (kg)	White girls n	$\bar{x} \pm S.D.$ (kg)	Black girls n	$\bar{x} \pm S.D.$ (kg)
2.75[1]	37	14.1 ± 1.5	11	15.4 ± 3.4	32	13.1 ± 1.9	19	14.0 ± 2.2
3.50[1]	80	15.5 ± 2.6	32	15.2 ± 2.0	77	15.0 ± 1.8	38	14.6 ± 1.9
4.50[1]	88	16.9 ± 2.1	40	17.7 ± 2.8	86	16.8 ± 2.0	38	18.3 ± 3.4
5.25[1]	41	19.1 ± 2.8	23	19.3 ± 2.8	42	19.2 ± 4.6	25	20.0 ± 4.8
5	90	19.9 ± 3.3	45	19.3 ± 2.9	99	18.9 ± 4.3	38	19.5 ± 2.4
6	102	21.9 ± 4.3	52	21.3 ± 3.4	87	21.7 ± 3.5	58	22.0 ± 4.0
7	100	24.3 ± 4.2	55	25.5 ± 4.5	96	24.0 ± 4.8	60	24.8 ± 4.7
8	112	28.0 ± 5.2	65	27.9 ± 6.0	103	28.3 ± 6.5	56	28.9 ± 6.7
9	107	31.7 ± 5.2	82	31.1 ± 6.4	104	30.1 ± 6.3	59	30.5 ± 7.0
10	129	34.7 ± 7.9	74	33.1 ± 5.6	110	35.2 ± 8.5	62	36.2 ± 11.2
11	118	38.5 ± 9.7	74	38.2 ± 9.2	115	40.7 ± 9.1	70	41.7 ± 8.8
12	151	43.3 ± 10.7	86	41.7 ± 10.0	136	46.0 ± 10.4	81	48.3 ± 12.1
13	128	49.8 ± 12.4	75	48.4 ± 13.1	119	49.0 ± 11.1	74	51.2 ± 12.4
14	116	55.3 ± 13.0	68	53.3 ± 12.2	90	53.5 ± 11.6	63	55.3 ± 14.1

[1]Mean age at last birthday

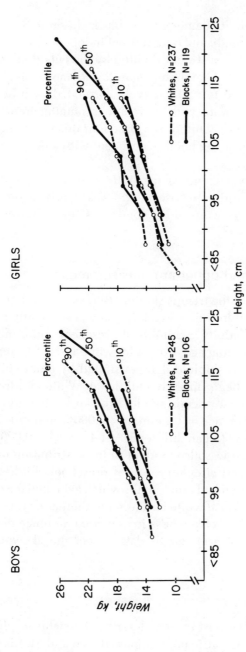

Figure 8–2. Weight per height interval for the preschool children at selected percentiles according to sex and race of the children.

weight for a given height among some black children. Since the relationship between weight and height is not independent, we employed the ponderosity index of weight divided by the cubed height (W/H^3), which is independent of height on theoretic and morphologic grounds. This index was found to be negatively correlated with height ($p < 0.001$) for this age group with correlations ranging from -0.47 for black girls to -0.63 for white boys. Based on this index, ponderosity decreased with increasing height consistent with a decrease in chubbiness from infancy.

Plots of selected percentiles for W/H^3 against height showed no separate group of children whose weight was clearly disproportionate to their height. Boys were more ponderous than girls of the same height.

Triceps skinfold and upper-arm measurements

In the distribution of the triceps skinfold thickness (see Fig. 8–1) only black preschool children displayed the skewness usually present for older children and adults. Skinfolds of preschool children tended to decrease with increasing age, except for white girls. The sex and race differences in triceps skinfold data, exhibited by older children and adults, are seen to begin in early childhood. White children of each sex had a greater mean triceps skinfold thickness than did the black children (mean difference = 1.2 mm, $p < 0.0005$), and girls had greater skinfolds than boys (mean difference = 1.4 mm, $p < 0.0005$).

A racial difference was also evident in the distribution of the right upper-arm length and circumference of preschool children (unpublished). Black children had arm lengths which averaged 0.8 cm greater ($p < 0.0005$) that those of white children but their arm circumferences were smaller by 0.2 cm. Skewness in arm circumference data and the relative symmetry of arm length data reflect the skewness in the triceps skinfold.

COMMENTS

Anthropometric data most clearly describe the status of physical development within pediatric populations (Roche and McKigney, 1976; Johnston and Beller, 1976) and serve as a background for studying other risk-factor variables noted in older children. Owen and Lubin (1973) reviewed current anthropometric data and concluded that while black infants were smaller with respect to lengths and weights at birth, by 24 months they surpassed white children in these measurements. Previous studies (National Center for Health Statistics, 1970; 1972; 1973c; 1974) have shown that through adolescence, black school-age children are generally taller, heavier, and have less subcutaneous fat than white children of the same age, even when matched on a socioeconomic status. However, only a few studies have supplied information about the preschool growth period. No subset of the preschool children could be clearly characterized as having a weight in excess of their height as judged by the ponderosity index (W/H^3). In contrast, among Bogalusa children 5–14 years of age (see below), measures of ponderosity indicated the existence of a group of children gaining weight disproportionately to their height (Foster et al., 1977). This emergence of a more ponderous subset among school children likely reflects the influence of environmental factors and altered patterns of eating.

Another measure of obesity, the triceps skinfold thickness, increased with age in the preschool group only for the white girls, while boys lost arm subcutaneous fat. A similar loss of fat by young boys was reported in the Ten-State Nutrition Survey (TSNS) (Garn and Clark, 1976) and was also observed in the Health and Nutrition Examination Survey (HANES) (Abraham et al., 1975). In general, the mean heights of Bogalusa children were greater than those of the TSNS but were similar to those observed in the Preschool Nutrition Survey (PNS) (Owen et al., 1974) and the HANES. Similar mean weights of girls were found in the three studies, but Bogalusa boys were lightest after age 3. The obvious racial difference in triceps skinfold thickness at this early age without corresponding racial difference in obesity clearly suggests a hereditary origin of differences in triceps skinfold thickness.

OBSERVATIONS OF SCHOOL-AGE CHILDREN

Height and weight

Figures 8–3 and 8–4 and Tables 8–1 and 8–2 show the age trends by race and sex for height and weight in the school-age group. With increasing age the distribution of height remains symmetrical and maintains a constant range of variability. In contrast, the distribution of

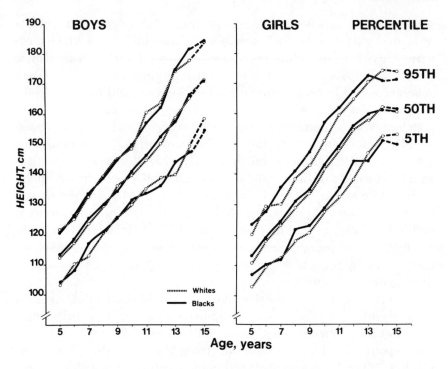

Figure 8–3. Height of children by age, sex, and race. Incomplete sample of
15-year-olds not included in totals. White boys, $N = 1,157$; black boys, $N =
682$; white girls, $N = 1,061$; black girls, $N = 622$.

weight is asymmetrical for both races and sexes and is accompanied
by an increase in variability with increasing age, resulting in a relative
excess of heavy children in the older age groups. On the average, boys
of both races differed only slightly in height and weight. Black girls
were 2 kg heavier than white girls ($p < 0.005$) and were also 2.8 cm
taller on the average. For girls, it appears that rates of growth, based
on annual cross-sectional means, begin to decrease around 12 years of
age, although complete leveling off of the growth rates was not observed since we did not follow this sample to adulthood. White girls
were generally shorter (except at ages 10–12) and lighter (except at
ages 8 and 10–12) than white boys, whereas the opposite relationship
was generally observed for black girls and boys.

Three questions arise from the observed increases in skewness and
in variability of the weight distribution as age progresses: a. Is there

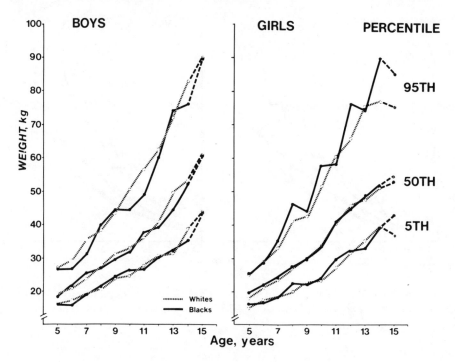

Table 8–4. Weight of children by age, sex, and race. White boys, N = 1,153; black boys, N = 676; white girls, N = 1,059; black girls, N = 621.

also an increase in the skewness and in the variability of weight as the *height* increases, resulting in a relative excess of heavy children among the tall? To answer this question, selected weight percentiles were plotted by height (Fig. 8–5), showing that the increase in the skewness and in the variability of weight for children of the same height is similar with increasing height and with increasing age; b. Is the median ponderosity, which is measured independently of height, increasing or decreasing with increasing height? c. Is the variability of the ponderosity increasing or decreasing with increasing height? To answer these questions, we used weight divided by the cube of height (W/H^3), an index of ponderosity which is independent of height on theoretic and morphologic grounds. For example, when a cube of a substance doubles its dimensions the weight increases eightfold, but W/H^3 remains constant. Plots of percentiles of this index by height showed a slight decrease in the median ponderosity index with in-

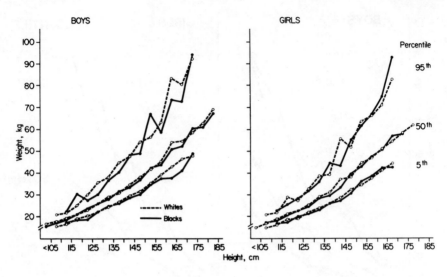

Figure 8–5. Weight per height interval of children by sex and race. White boys, $N = 1,152$; black boys, $N = 676$; white girls, $N = 1,059$; black girls, $N = 621$.

creasing height for all race-sex groups. However, at the 95th percentile, ponderosity increased with height. The variability and skewness of the ponderosity index increased with increasing height for all groups, indicating a "singling out" of those children who are gaining weight at a level inconsistent with their given height. In general, girls were less ponderous than boys of the corresponding height.

Triceps skinfold and upper-arm measurements

The results for triceps skinfold thickness are presented in Figure 8–6. Our data demonstrate that the skewness, known to exist in skinfold, increased with age for both races and sexes. The median value for boys of both races showed little change with age while the median for girls increased. Girls displayed a larger skinfold thickness than boys. White children consistently had triceps skinfold values 2.5 mm larger than black children. This distinct racial difference was also observed for adults by Newman (1956) and for children in the Health Examination Survey conducted by the National Center for Health Statistics (1972; 1974).

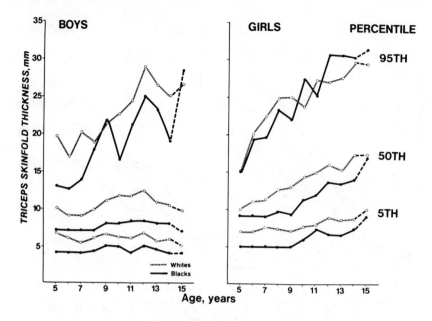

Figure 8–6. Skinfold thickness of right-arm triceps of children by age, sex, and race. White boys, $N = 1,157$; black boys, $N = 682$; white girls, $N = 1,061$; black girls, $N = 622$.

Percentiles for the right upper-arm length and circumference are shown in Figures 8–7 and 8–8. Black children, particularly girls, had longer upper-arm lengths by 0.7 cm than whites ($p < 0.0005$), while the arm circumference of whites exceeded that of blacks by 0.3 cm ($p < 0.025$). Skewness seen in arm circumference data is not unexpected since it reflects the dependence of arm circumference on body weight and triceps skinfold thickness.

Maturation and its relation to obesity

The pattern of external maturation as measured by the Tanner criteria for grading the growth of pubic hair and the development of male genitalia and female breasts is shown in Figure 8–9. The age of 50% transition between the respective maturation stages is summarized by race and sex in Table 8–3. Because of the limited age range of our population, not all children have progressed through the five Tanner stages. Therefore, we present the age of 50% transition from stage 1 to

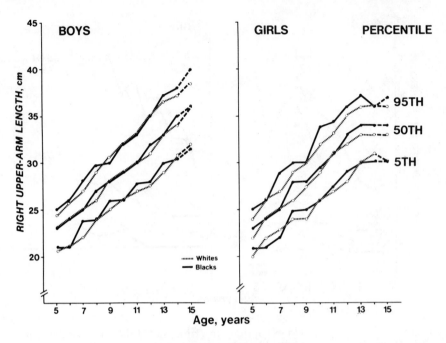

Figure 8–7. Right upper-arm length in children by age, sex, and race. White boys, $N = 1,157$; black boys, $N = 682$, white girls, $N = 1,061$, black girls, $N = 622$.

stage 2 for boys and for girls and from stage 2 to stage 3 for girls only. Note that calculation of the 50% transition points requires 0% and 100% response in the terminal age classes (Bryan and Greenberg, 1952). By age 14, over 93% but less than 100% of boys of both races had progressed to stage 2 of the Tanner criteria. Thus, the reported age underestimates the true age of 50% transition.

Maturation data in Figure 8–9 show that black children of each sex progressed through each Tanner stage at an earlier age than white children; similar results have been reported by Nankin et al. (1974). On the other hand, menarche as reported by the girls occurred later in the black than in the white girls. Among the 1,684 girls examined, 399 stated they had begun menstruation. Since not all girls remembered the month of occurrence of the menarche, for analysis we used only the year of age at onset. Figure 8–9 shows the age at menarche of girls, by race and percentage who reported menarche. Onset of menses

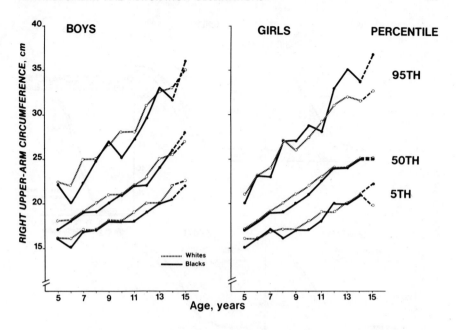

Figure 8–8. Right upper-arm circumference in children by age, sex, and race. White boys, $N = 1,157$; black boys; $N = 682$, white girls, $N = 1,061$; black girls, $N = 622$.

occurred earlier in white girls than in black girls. The age (±2 standard errors) of 50% transition for reported menarche occurred earlier for white girls than for black girls (Table 8–3). Again it must be noted that the age of 50% transition underestimates the true age, since by age 14 only 97% of white girls and 95% of black girls have reported menarche. Earlier menarche in white girls is also reflected in Table 8–4.

The means and the standard error of the ponderosity index at each maturation stage were calculated separately for each maturation characteristic, controlling for age and sex. In an analysis by 2-year age groups, girls showed a consistent positive association between maturation and ponderosity that was entirely absent in boys. These results were consistent for each race, and held true for pubic hair, male genitalia, female breast development, and menarche.

To determine if observations in this community are applicable to

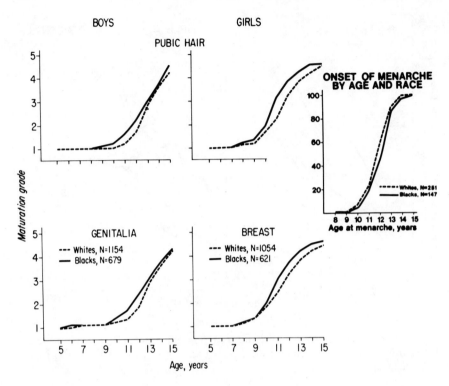

Figure 8–9. Mean maturation grade of children by age, sex, and race. For girls the arithmetic mean of the Tanner score for each breast was computed and used as the observation.

children in other American communities, we compared our data to that of the Health Examination Survey (National Center for Health Statistics, 1970; 1973a; 1973c), which was conducted (1963–70) on a probability sample of the noninstitutionalized children 6–17 years of age living in the United States. For each sex, differences in height and weight are very slight between the Bogalusa children and those of the national sample. Although the 95th percentile of weight describes Bogalusa girls as being increasingly heavier than the national sample after age 11, the one-tailed Kolmogorov-Smirnov two-sample test for large samples (Siegel, 1956) shows no significant difference between the two samples. Our results for the annual cross-sectional

Table 8–3. Age in years (±2 S.E.) of 50% transition[1] between the Tanner maturation stages by sex, race, maturation variable, and for menarche by race, September 1973–May 1974

Maturation		Boys		Girls	
Stage	Variable	White	Black	White	Black
1–2	Pubic hair	12.52 ± 0.17	11.72 ± 0.25	10.86 ± 0.19	10.13 ± 0.25
	Genitalia	11.82 ± 0.22	11.16 ± 0.27	—	—
	Breast	—	—	10.37 ± 0.21	10.22 ± 0.25
2–3	Pubic hair	—	—	11.66 ± 0.18	10.98 ± 0.24
	Genitalia	—	—	—	—
	Breast	—	—	11.60 ± 0.18	10.91 ± 0.24
—	Menarche	—	—	12.69 ± 0.17	12.83 ± 0.22

[1]Kärber's method (Irwin and Cheeseman, 1939; Cornfield and Mantel, 1950; Bryan and Greenberg, 1952).

observations of the triceps skinfold thickness are also similar to those of the Health Examination Survey.

Our data for onset of menarche, however, are at variance with data from the national sample. From Table 8–4 we see that at a given age, a larger percent of black than of white girls of the United States have reached menarche. Except at age 10, the opposite relation holds for Bogalusa girls. The racial difference in age at menarche as reported to us may be due to a racial difference in the perception or definition of menarche or may reflect hereditary and environmental factors, especially socioeconomic ones (Cagas and Riley, 1970). Poorer economic conditions are known to delay the onset of menarche. However, a recent study of Cuban girls (Laska-Mierzejewska, 1970) found no statistically significant difference in the reported age of menarche in girls from widely differing economic environments.

COMMENT

This survey has measured anthropometric and maturation variables in conjunction with factors known to increase the risk of cardiovascular disease in adults—obesity, hypertension, and hyperlipidemia. The relationship of obesity to hypertension and elevation of serum lipids in adults is now well known. Similar interrelationships have now been shown in children and are reported in detail (Chapters 18, 20, 22; Voors et al., 1976). Briefly, weight and height are closely related to

Table 8–4. Percent of Bogalusa girls reporting menarche, by race and age at last birthday, September 1973–May 1974, compared to the National Health Examination Survey (HES)[1]

Age at last birthday	Whites				Blacks			
	HES		Bogalusa Heart Study		HES		Bogalusa Heart Study	
	Sample total	Percent reporting	Sample total	Percent reporting	Sample total	Percent reporting	Sample total	Percent reporting
10	505	0.8	110	3.6	77	4.0	62	4.8
11	477	11.6	115	13.9	84	21.3	70	11.4
12	448	41.7	136	45.6	88	51.2	80	35.0
13	509	72.9	120	68.3	94	74.1	74	66.2
14	480	91.4	90	96.7	100	93.5	63	95.2

[1]National Center for Health Statistics, 1973a.

blood pressure levels in school-age children whose levels appear unrelated to age. Black children were observed to have higher blood pressure levels than white children. A relation between serum lipid levels and weight was also observed (Frerichs et al., 1978b). For example, white boys (and white girls to a lesser extent) showed a positive correlation between ponderosity and cholesterol and triglycerides, while black children exhibited this correlation only with triglycerides. The black children have higher serum cholesterol levels, which is related to their α-lipoprotein levels (Srinivasan et al., 1976a). These subtle differences, detectable from large population studies, may be influenced by diet-induced obesity. The ponderosity index presented in this material reflects deviations in weight that could influence hyperlipidemia or hypertension.

One measure of obesity, the triceps skinfold thickness, differed between races. As with adults, white children have a thicker triceps skinfold than black children. The thicker triceps skinfolds of whites may be the result of selective survival of genetic differences in the regulation of fat transport and deposition (Garn, 1971; Newman and Munro, 1955). Conversely, the longer extremities of blacks (see Fig. 8–7) may have facilitated heat conduction (Garn, 1971; Newman and Munro, 1955).

Girls and boys displayed different patterns of gaining subcutaneous fat at the triceps site, a finding well known from other studies. While skinfold values for boys reached a maximum at 12 years of age, the continuous increase in skinfold thickness of girls was interrupted from 12–13 years. The "preadolescent fat wave" noticeable in our white boys 11–13 years old was also observed by Tanner and Whitehouse (1975) and by Rauh and Schumsky (1968) in a sample of Cincinnati school children having a racial composition similar to our population. Tanner further noted a plateau from $10^{1}/_{2}$ to 12 years in the steady increase of triceps skinfold values of girls that was not observed in boys. The delayed skinfold plateau in Bogalusa girls may parallel a height spurt, as reported earlier (Tanner, 1962).

The other measure of obesity, the ponderosity index, has a skewed distribution when observed over fixed height intervals, which may indicate that some children gained weight disproportionately. If this excessive weight gain continues as the child grows taller, then a diagnosis at an early age of weight that is excessive for height could result in timely corrective measures.

Our observation of an earlier age of menarche in more ponderous girls has been reported by others (Reynolds, 1946; Wolff, 1955; Garn and Haskell, 1960; Tanner, 1962; Zacharias et al, 1970; Frisch, 1974). For Bogalusa boys the absence of a relation between ponderosity and maturation contrasts with the reports of others associating endomorphic boys with an earlier maturation than ectomorphic boys (Reynolds, 1946; Wolff, 1955; Hunt et al., 1958; Garn and Haskell, 1960; Tanner, 1962; Zacharias et al., 1970; Frisch, 1974). At least for girls, these results may indicate a link between environment and hormonal makeup, and could help clarify the possible relationships between obesity or stature and disease states (e.g., diabetes mellitus, hypertension, and mammary neoplasm (de Waard, 1975)). The interrelationships of these anthropometric and maturation characteristics with risk-factor variables, blood pressure, and serum lipids, may prove to be important indicators of susceptibility to cardiovascular diseases later in life. Longitudinal observations will be required to establish the relationship of these biologic variables to cardiovascular diseases which may originate in childhood.

SUMMARY

An epidemiologic survey of anthropometric and maturation variables was conducted on 714 Bogalusa preschool-age children and 3,524 school-age children, representing 80% and 93% of the respective biracial populations. For the school-age children, black boys differed slightly from white boys in height and weight; black girls were taller and heavier than white girls. The black children had longer upper-arm lengths and smaller upper-arm circumferences than the white children. The median ponderosity (weight divided by the cubed height) decreased with increasing height for the four race-sex groups, and the skewed distribution of ponderosity indicated an excess of heavy children among the tall. Based on the Tanner criteria for grading secondary sex characteristics, maturation occurred earlier in the more ponderous girls, although such was not the case for boys. While the Tanner secondary sex characteristics appeared earlier in black girls, white girls reported menarche earlier. The racial and sexual differences known to exist in triceps skinfold were observed for this population. No statistically significant difference was observed overall for height and weight between school-age children within this one community and those of the National Health Examination Survey. However, Bogalusa girls at the 95th percentile were heavier after age 11 than girls in the general survey. Also, there was a tendency for white girls in this community to report reaching menarche at an earlier age than black girls, which contrasts slightly with the national sample.

Among the preschool children, blacks were taller and heavier than whites, but white children exhibited greater skinfold thickness at the triceps site. Additionally, there was a marked negative correlation of a ponderosity index with height, which was not observed for the school-age children.

IV. Lipids

9. Serum lipids and lipoproteins in children—an overview

In the past two decades tremendous advances have been made in understanding serum lipids, especially in adults. This progress results from improved study techniques and their applications in numerous biochemical studies on individuals with aberrant forms of lipoproteins. A better understanding of the role of serum lipoproteins and their metabolism in health and disease indicates the need for similar information on children. Improved methods for analyses and standardization of serum lipids now make it possible to obtain studies on children in the general population. The following is an overview of serum lipid and lipoprotein study in children. For simplicity, the terms serum lipids and lipoproteins are used interchangeably.

GENERAL CLASSIFICATION AND PROPERTIES

The major lipids of plasma or serum are triglycerides, free cholesterol, cholesteryl esters, phospholipids, and free fatty acids (FFA). Except for FFA which are bound to albumin, the lipids circulate in the blood as lipid-protein macromolecular complexes, known as lipoproteins. In view of the functional interrelationship among these macromolecules, a definitive classification of lipoproteins is not possible at present. However, the varied physical and chemical properties of these lipoproteins permit an operational definition based on their size, floating densities in an ultracentrifugal field, or electrophoretic mobilities (Table 9–1) (Hatch and Lees, 1968; Lindgren et al., 1972; Eisenberg and Levy, 1975; Scanu et al., 1975).

The largest lipoproteins are called chylomicrons. The others have been classified as very low density (VLDL), intermediate density (IDL) or remnants, low density (LDL), and high density (HDL) lipoproteins. The surface properties of these macromolecules differ due to the nature of proteins and lipid–protein interactions. Therefore, on electrophoresis using an absorbing medium such as paper, or on agarose electrophoresis, chylomicrons remain at the origin, and LDL and HDL migrate as beta (β) and alpha (α) zones. While VLDL migrate between β and α zones (pre-β), IDL migrate to a so-called broad-β zone between the β and pre-β regions. Accordingly, the major lipoprotein classes are generally referred to as chylomicrons, β-, pre-β-, and α-lipoproteins. Because of our methodologic procedure, we will use the electrophoretic nomenclature in describing lipoprotein levels in children.

Recently, another system of classification was proposed based on the characteristics of the protein moieties (apoproteins) of lipoproteins (Alaupovic, 1971). According to this system, there are at least three major lipoprotein families in circulation (LPA, LPB, and LPC) having A, B, and C as their specific polypeptides. While apoproteins A (AI and AII) are the major apoproteins of HDL, apoprotein B is the major protein of LDL and is also present in chylomicrons and VLDL. Apoproteins C (CI, CII, and CIII) occur in VLDL and HDL. Serum lipoproteins are potent antigens whose reactivity is considered predominantly, if not exclusively, due to these apoproteins. Furthermore, apoproteins C and A are known to play a key role in the lipid-clearing activities of enzymes lipoprotein lipase and lecithin cholesterol acyltransferase (LCAT).

Although lipoproteins, as described above, differ in physicochemical properties, they represent a continuous spectrum of particles of changing composition rather than molecules of a discrete nature. This is especially so for lower density classes like chylomicrons, VLDL, and LDL. In general, chylomicrons predominantly contain triglycerides and are normally found in the serum only in the nonfasting state after a fatty meal. VLDL is also rich in triglycerides and in excess amounts, like chylomicrons, can render the serum turbid or milky in appearance due to its large particle size. While LDL predomi-

Table 9-1. General properties of human serum lipoproteins[1]

Parameter	Chylomicron	VLDL	IDL[2]	LDL	HDL₂[3]	HDL₃[3]
Hydrated density (gm/ml)	0.93	0.97	1.003	1.034	1.094	1.145
Solvent density of isolation (gm/ml)	<1.006	<1.006	1.006–1.019	1.019–1.063	1.063–1.125	1.125–1.21
Molecular weight	$(0.4$–$30) \times 10^9$	$(5$–$10) \times 10^6$	$(3.9$–$4.8) \times 10^6$	2.75×10^6	3.6×10^5	1.75×10^5
Diameter (nm)	>70.0	25.0–70.0	22.0–24.0	19.6–22.7	7.0–10.0	4.0–7.0
Electrophoretic mobility (paper, agarose)	origin	pre-β	β, pre-β	β	α	α
Composition (% by wt)						
cholesterol, unesterified	2	5–8		13		2
cholesterol, esterified	5	11–14		49		20
phospholipid	7	20–23		27		24
triglyceride	84	44–60		11		4
protein	2	4–11		23		50
Apoproteins						
A	+				+	+
B	+	+	+	+		
C	+	+	+		+	+

HDL₂₊₃

[1]The values have been compiled from many published results.
[2]Also known as LDL₁

[3]In addition to these subclasses, the HDL family has HDL₁ (hydrated density 1.05) and VHDL (hydrated density 1.25).

153

nantly carries cholesterol, on a mole basis HDL carries less (compared to LDL) but still a significant amount. Therefore, the level of HDL in serum should be taken into account in using serum cholesterol levels as an indicator of LDL. This is particularly so in children who have high HDL values, as discussed below. While LDL and VLDL are considered atherogenic, HDL is increasingly recognized as antiatherogenic, that is a negative risk factor (Miller and Miller, 1975). Gofman and co-workers as early as 1954, noted the importance of measuring different lipoprotein classes (Gofman et al., 1954). The lipoprotein phenotyping system subsequently developed by Fredrickson and colleagues advanced this concept and focused on the need to search for abnormal levels of lipoproteins (Fredrickson et al., 1967).

In addition to the above lipoprotein classes, another lipoprotein variant form known as LP(a) lipoprotein, or "sinking" pre-β-lipoprotein, occurs in serum, whose concentration among positive individuals varies from 2 to 76 mg/dl (Berg 1963). LP(a) has pre-β mobility by electrophoresis but is different from VLDL. This lipoprotein is cholesterol-rich (41.7%) and its protein moiety (27% contains apoprotein B, LP(a) apoprotein; and albumin. Its biologic significance in health or disease is not known except that it is heritable and certain families may follow autosomal dominant inheritance.

METABOLIC INTERRELATIONSHIPS IN FAT TRANSPORT

Although knowledge of physiologic function and fate of serum lipoproteins is far from complete, it is reasonably certain that lipoproteins do more than just render water-insoluble lipids soluble. Their functional interrelationship and biologic roles are intimately connected with triglyceride and cholesterol metabolism. Hence an understanding of this interrelationship is important in assessing the significance of lipid and lipoprotein profiles of an individual or of certain groups and in devising practical means to alter them if necessary. The lipoproteins undergo complex metabolic processes (Eisenberg and Levy, 1975; Greten, 1976). Unlike many other serum components that are mostly transferred from one point to the other as metabolites, the lipoproteins behave like organelles in which changes and exchanges continuously occur. The lipids of lipoproteins are derived from exogenous dietary fat and endogenous fats of hepatic origin. While the chylomicrons are synthesized in the intestine and carry dietary triglycerides, VLDL originates predominantly in the liver and transports endogenous triglycerides derived from dietary carbohydrates, FFA, and glycerol. The extrahepatic lipoprotein lipase at the capillary endothelial surface of adipose tissue and muscle hydrolyzes the triglycerides from these lipoproteins for storage or energy purposes; from this modification, remnants or IDL particles are formed. During this process, apoprotein C, phospholipids, and cholesterol (preferably unesterified) are removed and transferred to HDL. The remnant particles are further degraded, possibly by hepatic lipoprotein lipase, to form LDL.

Unlike triglycerides, cholesterol is not an energy-producing lipid and turns over far more slowly than triglycerides. Unfortunately, far less is known about its metabolism as related to lipoprotein metabolism. Recently, interest in understanding the factors that regulate the serum levels of LDL and HDL has grown, since these two lipoproteins, with relatively higher biologic half-lives than VLDL and chylomicrons, reflect the serum cholesterol levels. HDL is synthesized in both liver and intestine; its major role is as a reservoir of apoprotein C and acceptor of unesterified cholesterol from tissues and other lipoproteins. The enzyme LCAT bound to HDL converts the free cholesterol to cholesterol ester which in turn is transferred to LDL (Glomset and Norum, 1973). Eventually LDL and HDL are cleared from circulation by the tissues, and specific cell surface-binding sites have been implicated for LDL (Goldstein and Brown, 1974). It has been suggested that while the LDL may promote the flux of cholesterol into the cells, HDL may facilitate the transport of cholesterol from peripheral tissues to liver for subsequent catabolism and excretion as bile acids or free cholesterol (Bates and Rothblat, 1974; Miller and Miller, 1975). It is obvious, therefore, that any shift or defect in the highly integrated pathways of lipoprotein metabolism (due to heredity, environment, or disease) can influence the serum lipid and lipoprotein levels. Simpler methods of quantitating lipoproteins now allow studies to be performed on large numbers of persons, including children.

LEVELS IN INFANTS AND CHILDREN

Numerous reports have described the serum cholesterol and triglyceride levels in newborns, infants, and children (Hames and Greenberg, 1961; Starr, 1971; Fredrickson and Breslow, 1973; Dyerberg and

Hjorne, 1973; Fallat et al., 1974; Berenson et al., 1974b) but, unfortunately, these levels show marked variability which is in part due to methodologic differences in their determination. Until recently, most data have not been appropriately standardized on large numbers of children of different ages and different ethnic groups. The standardization programs for measuring lipids developed by Lipid Research Clinics (LRC) in collaboration with the U.S. Center for Disease Control in Atlanta is a step forward (Lipid Research Clinics Program, 1974). The data generated by the nationwide LRCs and by the Specialized Centers of Research-Arteriosclerosis epidemiologic surveys of well-defined pediatric populations in Bogalusa (La.), Muscatine (Iowa), and Rochester (Minn.) now provide valuable information on the distribution of serum lipid and lipoprotein levels in children (Lauer et al., 1975; Frerichs et al., 1976; Srinivasan et al., 1976a; Ellefson et al., 1978; National Heart, Lung and Blood Institute, 1978).

Selected percentiles for serum lipids and lipoproteins in children are given in Table 9–2. The abrupt increase in serum lipid and lipoprotein levels during infancy suggests both genetic and environmental influences. The importance of these two factors and their interaction need to be determined early in life, since the evolution of serum lipids in a child's first few years of life might have therapeutic implications.

The fractional distribution of serum cholesterol in different lipoprotein classes (Fig. 9–1) indicates that cholesterol at birth as well as during childhood is distributed predominantly in β- and α-lipoproteins, whereas the pre-β-lipoprotein remains low during childhood. In neonates or children it is not uncommon to find total serum cholesterol within acceptable "normal limits" (by any criteria) but elevated β-lipoprotein, or high total serum cholesterol but normal β-lipoprotein. This is due to the prevalence of high α-lipoprotein levels in children. Obviously, measuring individual lipoproteins rather than just measuring the serum cholesterol in children is imperative in terms of risk for atherosclerosis. Furthermore, the interrelationships among the different lipoprotein classes in children (Srinivasan et al., 1976a) as well as in adults (Miller and Miller, 1975) indicate that the α-lipoprotein level in serum is inversely proportional to both pre-β- and β-lipoprotein levels. This is attributed to the functional associations among the major classes of lipoproteins which, as mentioned earlier, apparently are related to the status of lipid metabolism

Table 9-2. Serum lipids and lipoprotein cholesterol levels (mg/dl) in children age 0–14 years[1]

	N	Total cholesterol	N	Triglycerides	Lipoprotein cholesterol		
					β-	pre-β-	α-
Neonates[2]	419	68 (42–103)	419	34 (14–84)	29 (17–50)	2 (1–12)	35 (13–60)
Infants							
6 mo	312	132 (89–185)	260[3]	80 (45–169)	73 (40–111)	9 (1–25)	51 (23–88)
1 yr	291	145 (99–193)	249[3]	73 (42–158)	81 (49–121)	7 (2–25)	51 (22–81)
Children							
2–14 yrs	4,140	162 (122–213)	3,838[3]	60 (34–124)	87 (57–130)	6 (1–21)	67 (32–102)

[1] The values represent median ("normal range," 5th–95th percentiles) levels observed in children of Bogalusa, La.
[2] Cord blood
[3] Fasting samples only

157

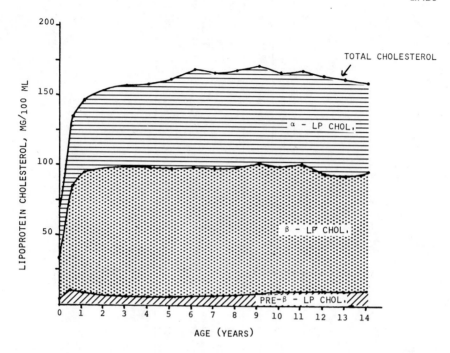

Figure 9–1. Fractional distribution of serum total cholesterol in children from birth to 14 years of age in different lipoprotein classes. Differentially shaded areas from top to bottom represent α-, β-, and pre-β-lipoprotein cholesterol, respectively. Note that serum total cholesterol during childhood is distributed mainly in β- and α-lipoprotein fractions

(Nichols, 1969; Eisenberg and Levy, 1975). Whether low levels of pre-β-lipoprotein (and triglycerides) and higher levels of α-lipoprotein reflect the status of lipid metabolism in children is not known.

FACTORS AFFECTING LIPID LEVELS

Since lipid transport by lipoproteins is a highly integrated, dynamic, and complex metabolic process, serum lipoprotein level could be affected in several ways. Both genetic and environmental factors help determine their concentration. The tremendous variability that exists, even among members of the same population, exposed to the same environmental factors, indicates that occurrence of hyper-or hypolipoproteinemia is subject to many different determinants. These discussions are mainly focused on well-defined studies in American populations. Some of the known factors that influence serum lipid and lipoprotein levels in children are briefly discussed below.

Genetics

Discrete genetic influences on serum lipid and lipoprotein levels have been demonstrated by several studies (Fredrickson and Levy, 1972; Jensen and Blankenhorn, 1972; Goldstein et al., 1973b; Fallat et al., 1974; Kwiterovich et al., 1974; Motulsky, 1976). Investigations of the heritability of lipid and lipoprotein levels have generally focused on aberrations in lipid metabolism which result in extremely high or low levels. Based on 95th percentile cut-off points in a normal reference population, estimates have been made that between 0.2 and 0.4% of the population carry the gene for familial hypercholesterolemia, 1% for familial hypertriglyceridemia, and 1–2% for familial combined hyperlipidemia (Goldstein et al., 1973b; Motulsky, 1976). With respect to coronary artery disease, three familial disorders are very important, as noted by Goldstein et al. who found them to be present in about 20% of all survivors of myocardial infarction (Goldstein et al., 1973a).

Familial hypercholesterolemia (hyper-β-lipoproteinemia) is the most well-recognized clinical entity in childhood which seems to result from a single abnormal autosomal gene (Fredrickson and Levy, 1972; Kwiterovich et al., 1974). On the other hand, for unknown reasons, familial hypertriglyceridemia is usually not completely expressed until the third decade in affected children (Fredrickson and Levy, 1972; Goldstein et al., 1973b; Fallat et al., 1974). Lipoprotein disorders related to lipoprotein lipase and LCAT enzyme deficiencies, Tangier's disease (α-lipoprotein deficiency), and abetalipoproteinemia are very rare genetic expressions (Fredrickson et al., 1967; Glomset and Norum, 1973; Eisenberg and Levy, 1975). In addition, there are reports of familial occurrence of hypo-β- and hyper-α-lipoproteinemia.

As is readily apparent, these extreme conditions do not help explain the role of genes in regulating the entire spectrum of lipids and lipoproteins. We have found that among full sibs ages 2–14, there is significant aggregation in values of each of the lipids and lipoproteins. Knowledge of one sib's lipoprotein level explained 1.4 to 12.3% of the variability in the lipoprotein levels of the remaining sibs. Whether this aggregation is due to common genes or to common environment is unknown. The lipid levels at birth and their evolution in subsequent years offer an interesting example of this dilemma. There is divergence of opinion on whether neonatal hyperlipidemia is genetically determined (Glueck et al., 1971; Darmady et al., 1972; Kwiterovich et al., 1973; Goldstein et al., 1974). The fact that the neonatal cholesterol levels do not reflect the values obtained in the same infants at 1 year of age (Darmady et al., 1972) indicates that the genetic determinants are also subject to profound and unrelenting environmental impact.

Age and sex

Over a lifetime, serum lipid and lipoprotein levels undergo continuous changes, more so in certain fractions than others. One can see (Fig. 9–1 and Table 9–2) a dramatic increase in lipids and lipoproteins during the first year of life. For example, the mean serum cholesterol levels increase from 70 mg/dl at birth to 155 mg/dl around the age of 3 years and remain relatively stable until 11 years of age (see Fig. 9–1). The dip in cholesterol between 11 and 16 years has been observed by many investigators (Lee, 1967; Starr, 1971; Dyerberg and Hjorne, 1973; Savage et al., 1976) and should be taken into account when monitoring the serum lipid profile of a child. Of the lipoprotein changes over time, β-lipoprotein levels consistently follow the serum cholesterol changes, including the downward trend during early adolescence.

Serum triglyceride levels exhibit a similar early pattern with a sharp increase from 40 mg/dl at birth to 83 mg/dl at 1 year of age. A peculiar overshoot appears to occur around 6 months to 1 year of age in triglyceride levels, which may possibly reflect the dramatic metabolic changes in early infancy, followed by a rapid growth spurt. The mean level then tends to decline to 61 mg/dl at 4 years of age, again gradually increasing to 77 mg/dl at age 14.

As expected, pre-β-lipoprotein reflects trends similar to those of the triglyceride changes. The absolute levels of α-lipoprotein almost double between birth and school age, at which time they remain relatively stable through age 11; then a decrease occurs through age 16, with an unusual decrease in white boys (Cresanta et al., 1979).

Compared to adults children have lower serum concentrations of total cholesterol, triglycerides, β-lipoprotein, and pre-β-lipoprotein and higher concentrations of α-lipoprotein (Frederickson et al., 1967; Barclay, 1972; Castelli et al., 1977a). The rate of increase in serum lipids differs considerably in children and adults; for example, Keys et al. (1950) estimated that the serum cholesterol level rises at the rate of 2.2 mg/dl/yr between the ages of 15 and 30. Ours and other studies of children and young adults suggest that between the ages of 17 and 20 a transition occurs (Berenson et al., 1972b; Dyerberg and Hjorne, 1973; Berenson et al., 1974b; Srinivasan et al., 1975a; Frerichs et al., 1976; Srinivasan et al., 1976a); unfortunately, little is known about the serum lipid changes during this period. Unlike changes in adults, the age-related increase is more pronounced in girls than in boys. The influence of gonadal hormones on lipid and lipoprotein metabolism may be the underlying reason for these differences (Furman et al., 1967; Barclay, 1972).

Race

Black children have greater total serum cholesterol and lower triglyceride levels than do white children (Frerichs et al., 1976). The cholesterol difference begins to appear during the preschool years and is clearly apparent during the school-age years. The increased level of α-lipoprotein in blacks accounts for the racial difference observed for total cholesterol.

From studies in Evans County, Ga., Tyroler and colleagues (1975) reported that in persons with identical levels of total cholesterol, black adults have proportionally more cholesterol as α-lipoprotein than do whites. Those authors speculated that this partly explains why blacks at a given level of cholesterol have a lower risk of coronary heart disease than do whites. If the lipoprotein implications are true, blacks may have a metabolic protective edge over whites, detectable as early as 4–5 years of age, and a dramatic difference around puberty.

Season

Seasonal variations are known to influence the serum lipid levels (Thomas et al., 1961; Bleiler et al., 1963; Doyle et al., 1965; Pincherle, 1971). An increase in serum cholesterol levels with decreasing temperature has been noted in several northern climates (Thomas et al., 1961; Pincherle, 1971). In men the serum cholesterol increases in winter and decreases in summer, whereas in women the reverse is noted (Bleiler et al., 1963). In the children of Bogalusa, La., we found little evidence of any relationship between air temperature and levels of serum lipids and lipoproteins. This could be due to the mild fluctuations in temperature common to the southern United States. Using a multiple linear regression analysis with the serum lipid or lipoprotein levels as the dependent variable and the daily temperature as the independent variable, we found that with a theoretic temperature reduction from 70 to 50°F, total cholesterol would increase by 2.5 mg/dl, triglycerides would remain unchanged, β-lipoprotein cholesterol would increase by 1.8 mg/dl, and α-lipoprotein cholesterol would increase by 0.3 mg/dl. While some of these changes are statistically significant and can be detected when a large number of observations (over 3,000) are made, the difference may be too small to indicate a biologic change in studies of a single person.

Diet

Currently, information suggests that diet could be a major determinant of serum lipid levels in infancy and childhood since other related factors are not expressed fully in early life. Unlike heredity, age, and sex, diet is subject to modification and has therefore received a great deal of attention (Wiese et al., 1966; Alfin-Slater, 1969; Kannel and Gordon, 1970; American Academy of Pediatrics, 1972; Ford et al., 1972; Keys, 1975; Nichols et al., 1976). In addition to the endogenous synthesis, serum lipid levels are governed by the dietary levels of fat, carbohydrate, protein, and cholesterol. Hormones like insulin, glucagon, epinephrine, adrenal and pituitary hormones, thyroid, hormone estrogens, androgens, and progesterone are vital in modulating the lipogenesis in the liver and mobilizing fatty acids from the peripheral tissues. Since serum lipids rise rapidly during infancy, opinions differ about whether diet modification or cholesterol challenge during infancy is required for better management of serum lipids in later years (Fomon, 1971; Friedman and Goldberg, 1972; Glueck and Tsang, 1972; Schubert, 1973). However, there is general agreement that the diet of American children is high in fat and cholesterol compared to the levels in other population groups that have less coronary artery disease later in life.

Numerous studies in adults have shown that within a single population, dietary components explain little of the variability observed in levels of the serum lipids (Kannel and Gordon, 1970; Keys, 1975; Nichols et al., 1976). Yet when individuals modify their diets, the concentrations of the serum variables are reduced (Galbraith et al., 1966; National Diet-Heart Study Research Group, 1968; Shorey et al., 1976). For example, cholesterol levels of adolescent boys were reduced by 15% after modification of the meals that were served by their boarding school (Ford et al., 1972). Special diets have also been recommended for children with familial hypercholesterolemia and familial hypertriglyceridemia (Fallat et al., 1974; Larsen et al., 1974). Interestingly, the relatively small dietary differences between the lower-income urban children and the rural children of Guatemala are reflected in serum cholesterol (Scrimshaw et al., 1957).

Although considerable dietary information has been collected on children, very few studies have focused on the relationship between nutritional components and serum lipids and lipoproteins within the context of a total community. Within Bogalusa, the mean caloric intake was 2,141 calories with 13% derived from protein, 49% from carbohydrates, and 38% from fats (Frank et al., 1978). Interestingly, 34% of the total consumed calories came from snacks, and sucrose constituted 18% of the total calories. Children with the lowest levels of serum cholesterol consumed significantly less fat (both total and per 1,000 calories) than those in the middle (25th to 75th percentile) or high (above 75th percentile) serum cholesterol groups. [No significant difference was observed in the intake of dietary cholesterol among the low, middle, and high serum cholesterol groups.] In addition, those children with longer eating spans consumed more calories and also had higher serum cholesterol levels.

Body habitus

Overweight and obesity in otherwise healthy adults are usually associated with excessive caloric intake and elevation in certain serum lipids and lipoprotein fractions (Galbraith et al., 1966; Barclay, 1972; Keys, 1975). Within a given individual, physical exercise and control of caloric intake are known to modulate both serum lipid levels and body weight (Mann et al., 1955; Galbraith et al., 1966). Little is known about the body habitus and serum lipid levels in normal, free·living children. From our studies, we know that obese children tend to have higher levels of triglycerides, pre-β-, and β-lipoproteins, and lower levels of α-lipoprotein than do lean children (Frerichs et al., 1978b.) Total cholesterol is not elevated in heavier black children except for the extremes, but does tend to be elevated in heavier white children, especially boys.

An example of the relationship between hypercholesterolemia, hypertriglyceridemia, and relative weight is shown in Figure 9–2. In general, the white children with high cholesterol and triglyceride levels tend to be heavier than average, most apparently among the white boys. Among the black children, those with high triglycerides are slightly heavier than the average, while those with high cholesterol levels cannot be distinguished from their peers. Interestingly, many of the hyperlipidemic children are among the leanest members of the population, indicating how difficult it is to categorize the indi-

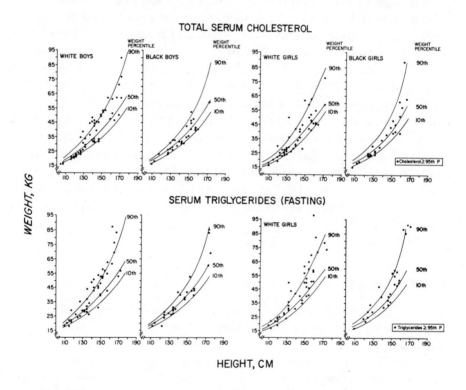

Figure 9–2. Relationship of hypercholesterolemia, hypertriglyceridemia, and relative weight. Serum total cholesterol and triglyceride levels at or above 95th percentile are related to height and weight measurements of children.

vidual based on average associations observed in the general population.

Disease states

Serum lipid levels are known to be altered in certain disease states, such as diabetes mellitus, hypo- and hyperthyroidism, nephrotic syndrome, biliary obstruction, pancreatitis, dysglobulinemia (including autoimmune hyperlipoproteinemia), and viral infections (Fredrickson et al., 1967; Barclay, 1972). In the presence of these states, alterations of lipoproteins must be evaluated as secondary disorders (Beaumont et al., 1970). Of these conditions, hyperlipidemia and diabetes mellitus in children need special attention since coronary artery disease is a major complication in diabetic adults. Alterations in fat transport which occur in diabetes relate to insulin levels in the metabolism of triglyceride-rich lipoproteins (Bierman and Porte, 1968; Olefsky et al., 1974). Abnormalities in insulin levels affect either production (obesity-related lipemia) or removal (diabetes-related lipemia) of triglycerides. Juvenile-onset diabetes, a condition which affects one school-age child per 1,000, is typified by a marked insulin deficiency and elevations of both serum cholesterol and triglyceride levels (Drash, 1975). Adult-onset diabetes exhibits a similar lipid profile. If 2% of the American population has diabetes mellitus, then that many children will eventually become diabetic. It is therefore important to know serum lipid levels in the asymptomatic children of diabetic adults.

Other factors

Factors like personality, stress, smoking, and use of contraceptive pills are also considered determinants of serum lipid levels in adults. In children, these factors warrant detailed investigation. Several drugs are known to affect lipoprotein levels (Steinberg, 1969) although their use is limited in children. Therapeutically, nicotinic acid and clofibrate, which block fat transport, tend to effectively reduce serum triglyceride and pre-β-lipoprotein levels; on the other hand, serum cholesterol and β-lipoprotein levels are affected by cholestyramine, plant sterols, and thyroxine, which predominantly enhance excretion processes (Bortz, 1974).

10. Serum lipids and lipoproteins at birth, 6 months, and one year

We have previously shown that lipid and lipoprotein levels of children by age 3 years already approach those of early adulthood (Berenson et al., 1972b; Srinivasan et al., 1975b; Srinivasan et al., 1976a; Frerichs et al., 1976; Berenson et al., 1978a). Furthermore, differences in lipid and lipoprotein levels between blacks and whites were noted in children (Frerichs et al., 1976; Srinivasan et al., 1976a) as well as adults (Tyroler et al., 1975), suggesting the possible influence of genetic factors. In newborns, however, there are diverging reports concerning sex or genetic differences in lipids and lipoproteins (Glueck et al., 1971; Darmady et al., 1972; Spellacy et al., 1974; Carlson and Hardell, 1977; Glueck et al., 1977).

Although the study of cord blood cholesterol has been suggested to be sufficient for the diagnosis of a genetic form of hypercholesterolemia (Glueck, 1971; Tsang et al., 1975), it is apparent that further studies of blood lipids and the lipoproteins are indicated, especially from a total population of black and white infants born in a geographically defined community (Frerichs et al., 1978a).

POPULATION SAMPLE

The study consisted of 440 infants (98.4%) from a total of 447 babies (38.5% black, 61.5% white) born between January 1, 1974, and June

30, 1975. All of the black infants and 97.5% of the white infants were included and the eligible population was subsequently verified using the county birth register.

At 6 months of age, 351 (88% of available population) were examined while at 1 year of age 316 (82.3% of available) were seen.

OBSERVATIONS

Weight, serum lipids, and lipoproteins

As observed in Figures 10–1 and 10–2, white children at birth, when compared to blacks, tended to weigh more and have higher serum levels of total cholesterol, triglycerides, β-lipoprotein, and α-lipoprotein. No racial difference was observed in levels of pre-β-lipoprotein. Ninety percent of all white infants weighed between 2,353 gm (5th percentile) and 4,186 gm (95th percentile) while for black newborns, the 5th and 95th percentiles were 1,962 gm and 3,989 gm, respectively.

The means and standard deviations for birthweight and weight at 6

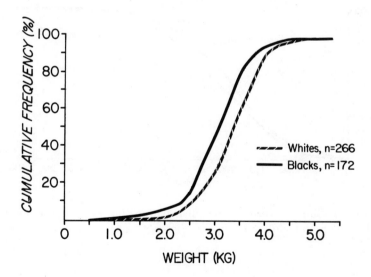

Figure 10–1. Cumulative frequency distribution for weight at birth of black and white Bogalusa newborns.

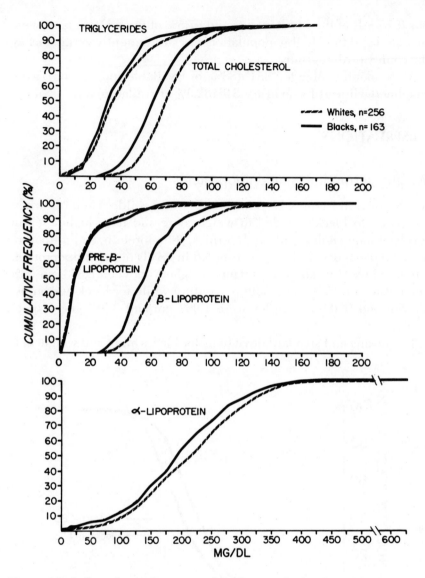

Figure 10–2. Cumulative frequency distributions for lipids and lipoproteins at birth of black and white Bogalusa newborns.

months and 1 year of age are shown in Table 10–1. The average birthweight for all infants was 3,228 gm, with whites weighing more than blacks. White boys were significantly heavier than the other three race-sex groups. At both 6 months and 1 year of age, boys were slightly heavier than girls for both races ($p < 0.0001$). Means, standard deviations, and 95th percentiles for the serum lipids and lipoproteins are given in Table 10–2. Mean levels of both total cholesterol and β-lipoprotein at birth were significantly greater in whites of both sexes than in blacks. White girls had the highest average levels among the four race-sex groups of total cholesterol, β-lipoprotein, and α-lipoprotein. With the exception of pre-β-lipoproteins, black boys consistently had the lowest observable levels of all the cord blood variables. For all children combined, 44% of the total cholesterol was found in β-lipoproteins (30.4 ± 10.3 mg/dl), 5% in pre-β-lipoproteins (3.6 ± 4.1 mg/dl), and 51% in α-lipoproteins (35.5 ± 14.8 mg/dl). Individual variability was marked. The average concentrations of the cord blood variables in Bogalusa newborns are in general agreement with those reported by other investigators (Glueck et al., 1971; Darmady et al., 1972; Glueck et al., 1973; Greten et al., 1973; Kwiterovich et al., 1973; Goldstein et al., 1974; Cress et al.,1977; Glueck et al., 1977).

Among 6-month-old infants, white children had significantly higher serum cholesterol, triglycerides, and pre-β-lipoprotein than black infants. At the 1-year stage the differences were significant only for triglycerides and pre-β-lipoproteins. No statistically significant sex-related differences were observed among the 6-month-old or 1-year-old children except that at 1 year, girls had higher β-lipoprotein than boys.

Our observation that the average level of total cholesterol at birth is higher in whites than in blacks is opposite to that reported in school-age children (Frerichs et al., 1976; Levy et al., 1976). White newborns have higher levels of total cholesterol and β-lipoprotein than black newborns. On the other hand, black Bogalusa children at school age have higher levels of total cholesterol than white children, due mainly to higher levels of α-lipoproteins. The mean levels of β-lipoproteins are essentially the same (Srinivasan et al., 1976a). Observed black-white difference in total cholesterol and β-lipoproteins at birth persisted even when comparing newborns of the same weight or socioeconomic status. The reason for difference is not apparent. Glueck et al. (1977) observed no such race-related difference in serum lipids in

Table 10–1. Mean, standard deviation and 95th percentiles for weights of infants, January 1974–June 1976

Weight (kg)	White boys		White girls		Black boys		Black girls		All children		
	N	$\bar{x} \pm$ S.D.	N	$\bar{x} \pm$ S.D.	N	$\bar{x} \pm$ S.D.	N	$\bar{x} \pm$ S.D.	N	$\bar{x} \pm$ S.D.	95th percentile
Birth[1]	133	3.4 ± 0.6	133	3.2 ± 0.6	84	3.1 ± 0.7	88	3.0 ± 0.6	438	3.2 ± 0.6	4.1
6 months	103	8.0 ± 0.9	105	7.3 ± 0.8	70	7.7 ± 1.1	72	7.4 ± 0.9	350	7.6 ± 1.0	9.1
1 year	90	10.2 ± 1.0	89	9.5 ± 0.9	66	10.0 ± 1.4	70	9.5 ± 1.1	315	9.8 ± 1.1	11.8

[1]Data not collected by SCOR-A.

Table 10-2. Mean, standard deviation, and 95th percentiles for serum lipids and lipoproteins of infants, January 1974–June 1976

Serum variable mg/dl	Age	White boys N	White boys x̄ ± S.D.	White girls N	White girls x̄ ± S.D.	Black boys N	Black boys x̄ ± S.D.	Black girls N	Black girls x̄ ± S.D.	All children N	All children x̄ ± S.D.	95th Percentile
Total cholesterol	Birth	129	70 ± 17	127	76 ± 17	79	62 ± 20	84	66 ± 17	419	70 ± 18[7]	103
	6 months	96	138 ± 25	94	137 ± 26	64	126 ± 37	58	135 ± 30	312	134 ± 29[3,5]	185
	1 year	85	144 ± 22	87	147 ± 28	59	143 ± 26	60	145 ± 30	291	145 ± 27	193
Triglycerides[1]	Birth	129	44 ± 26	127	39 ± 20	79	37 ± 19	84	38 ± 22	419	40 ± 22	84
	6 months	85	103 ± 55	78	94 ± 51	47	81 ± 32	50	82 ± 30	260	92 ± 47[6]	169
	1 year	78	85 ± 40	79	90 ± 39	45	71 ± 32	47	76 ± 37	249	82 ± 38[6]	158
β-Lipoprotein[1]	Birth	127	68 ± 22	125	70 ± 21	78	54 ± 18	82	62 ± 23	412	65 ± 22[7]	106 (50)[2]
	6 months	83	155 ± 38	76	159 ± 44	47	149 ± 52	50	165 ± 53	256	157 ± 46[3]	237 (111)
	1 year	72	170 ± 39	69	186 ± 51	41	172 ± 57	47	183 ± 49	229	178 ± 47[4]	259 (121)
Pre-β-lipoprotein[1]	Birth	127	18 ± 21	125	14 ± 16	78	16 ± 16	82	16 ± 19	412	16 ± 19	52 (12)
	6 months	83	57 ± 37	76	49 ± 35	47	34 ± 25	50	39 ± 27	256	47 ± 38[7]	113 (25)
	1 year	72	49 ± 39	69	46 ± 32	41	29 ± 21	47	38 ± 33	229	42 ± 34[6]	113 (25)
α-Lipoprotein[1]	Birth	129	200 ± 86	126	234 ± 83	79	196 ± 101	83	201 ± 77	417	210 ± 88	355 (60)
	6 months	85	310 ± 144	78	301 ± 108	47	303 ± 161	50	295 ± 101	260	303 ± 150	521 (88)
	1 year	77	319 ± 118	78	299 ± 105	45	331 ± 70	47	301 ± 115	247	311 ± 106	479 (81)

[1] Fasting children only

[2] Corresponding lipoprotein cholesterol values are given in parenthesis.

[3] Age differences between 6-mo- and 1-yr-old children significant at $p < 0.001$ (F-test)

[4] Sex differences among 6-mo- and 1-yr-old children significant at $p < 0.05$ (F-test)

[5,6,7] Race differences significant at $p < 0.05$, $p < 0.01$, $p < 0.0001$ (F-test), respectively.

171

neonates, although their study was hospital-based rather than community-based and therefore may not be comparable.

Interrelationship among serum lipids and lipoproteins

The interrelationships among the serum lipids and lipoproteins are shown by race in Table 10–3. Total cholesterol was highly correlated with both β- and α-lipoproteins, the two major carriers of cholesterol in the blood. Triglyceride, while significantly correlated with β-lipoproteins, was highly correlated with the major carriers of triglycerides in the sera, namely pre-β-lipoproteins. The association between triglycerides and pre-β-lipoproteins was significantly greater in whites than in blacks, with over 67% (r^2) of the variability in pre-β-lipoprotein levels explained by knowledge of the respective triglyceride levels. α-Lipoproteins were negatively correlated with both triglycerides and pre-β-lipoproteins. The proportion of total cholesterol carried in either α- or β-lipoproteins at birth is considerably different from the percentage in adulthood. In contrast to Framingham adults (age 50–59) in whom 21% of the total cholesterol is in α-lipoproteins and 66% in β-lipoproteins (Castelli et al., 1977a), the cholesterol at birth is almost equally distributed in α- and β-lipoproteins. The shifting of these proportions helps explain why at birth total cholesterol is highly correlated with both α- and β-lipoproteins, while during adulthood the correlation of total cholesterol is high with β-lipoproteins but not with α-lipoproteins (Castelli et al., 1977a). It is of interest to note that the positive correlations of cholesterol with β-lipoproteins and triglycerides with pre-β-lipoproteins and the negative correlation of triglycerides with α-lipoproteins are observed in adults (Castelli et al., 1977a), school-age children (Srinivasan et al., 1976a), preschool children (Berenson et al. 1978a), and newborns, suggesting that basic biochemical relationships between the lipids and lipoproteins are already established at birth.

That the positive relationships of total cholesterol with both β-lipoprotein and α-lipoprotein should be considered in evaluating hyperlipoproteinemia becomes clear when viewing those neonates with serum values at or above the 95th percentile. Of the 22 newborns with hypercholesterolemia, based on the 95th percentile level ($\geq$ 103 mg/dl), 7 (32%) also exhibited hyper-β-lipoproteinemia (β-lipoprotein cholesterol $\geq$ 49.7 mg/dl) while 10 (45%) were hyper-α-lipopro-

Table 10–3. Pearson product moment correlation coefficient between
serum lipids and lipoproteins by race in 252 white and 160 black
newborns, January 1974–June 1975

	Triglycerides	β-Lipoprotein	Pre-β-lipoprotein	α-Lipoprotein
Total cholesterol				
white	0.110	0.641[1]	0.068	0.729[1]
blacks	0.070	0.641[1]	0.017	0.804[1]
Triglycerides				
whites		0.435[1]	0.820[1,2]	−0.412[1]
blacks		0.391[1]	0.696[1]	−0.347[1]
β-Lipoprotein				
whites			0.270[1]	−0.012
blacks			0.139	0.103
Pre-β-lipoprotein				
whites				−0.399[1]
blacks				−0.329[1]

[1]Levels of significance: correlation coefficient different from zero, $p < 0.001$.
[2]Significant racial difference in correlation coefficients, $p < 0.01$

teinemic (α-lipoprotein cholesterol $\geq$ 60.2 mg/dl). On the other hand, of the 20 neonates with β-lipoprotein levels at or above the 95th percentile, 13 (65%) had serum cholesterol values which were below the 95th percentile.

Relationship between weight and serum lipids and lipoproteins

Within each race, all of the correlation coefficients between birth-weight and the respective serum variables were of a low order and none were statistically significant. The effect of birthweight on the serum variables was further analyzed by comparing within race the mean levels of serum lipids and lipoproteins in each of three birth-weight categories ($<$ 2.5 kg, 2.5–3.5 kg, and $>$3.5 kg). There were no statistically significant differences either black or white neonates in any of the lipid or lipoprotein categories. Within each weight category, whites persistently had higher levels of total cholesterol, β-lipoproteins, and α-lipoproteins than did blacks, indicating that the previously mentioned racial differences in the cord blood variables exist independent of birthweight.

When analyzing the mean levels within five birthweight categories ($<$ 1.8 kg, 1.8–2.5 kg, 2.5–3.5 kg, 3.5–4.0 kg, and $\geq$ 4.0 kg), we observed no significant differences in white neonates but some statistically significant differences were apparent in the black newborns, although of a low and inconsistent order. Interestingly, in blacks weighing less than 1.8 kg the mean triglyceride levels were significantly higher ($p < 0.05$) and mean α-lipoprotein levels significantly lower ($p < 0.05$) than in black infants with a birthweight between 1.8 and 2.5 kg, although neither of the serum variables in the lowest birthweight group differed significantly from the mean levels within the remaining three weight categories.

Effects of factors at time of delivery, socioeconomic status and season

After adjusting for the effects of race and sex, we compared the mean levels of the serum lipids and lipoproteins with respect to the type of delivery, stress at delivery, and the one-minute Apgar score. Whether the delivery was normal or abnormal (includes Caesarean) had no discernible effect on the lipid or lipoprotein values. In addition, no statistically significant differences were found in the mean levels of birthweight or the serum variables between those who had some stressful event at birth (fetal anoxia, prolapsed cord, premature separation of placenta, prolonged labor, or abnormal presentation) and those who did not. Only 342 of the 419 infants whose cord blood was sampled (82%) had an Apgar score. After dividing the population into three Apgar categories (1–7, 8, 9–10), we found no significant differences among the three groups in mean levels of any of the serum variables.

Other investigators have recently reported a higher prevalence of maternal-fetal problems in hypertriglyceridemic newborns than in a normal control group (Tsang et al., 1974b; Anderson and Friis-Hansen, 1976; Cress et al., 1977). When we compared the 42 Bogalusa newborns with triglyceride levels at or above the race-sex-specific 90th percentile with the remaining group ($n = 377$), we found no significant difference in the proportions of any factors associated with perinatal stress. Of the 42 hypertriglyceridemic newborns, only 34 (81%) were given an Apgar score and only one score was equal to or less than 6. This proportion is almost equal to that found in the remaining 377 newborns for whom 308 (82%) received an Apgar score of which 17 (6%) were equal to or less than 6.

The effect that socioeconomic factors have on cord blood variables was indirectly analyzed by comparing the mean values by race of children born in each of the two Bogalusa hospitals. One hospital is operated by the state of Louisiana and serves the indigent population, while the other is private and requires a fee for service. Of all cord bloods collected at the state hospital, 66% were from black newborns and 34% were from white newborns, while at the private hospital, the racial division was 19% black newborns and 81% white newborns.

At both hospitals, white neonates weighed significantly more than black neonates, while in both races those born at the private hospital weighed significantly more than those born at the public hospital. The average birthweight of blacks delivered at the private hospital was almost identical to the average birthweight of whites at the public hospital, suggesting that both socioeconomic and genetic factors influence the weight at birth.

In contrast, the previously observed racial differences in levels of the cord blood variables were not explained by socioeconomic differences between black and white neonates. There were no significant differences within each race between neonates born at the two hospitals in any of the mean levels of the serum variables, although racial differences in total cholesterol and β-lipoproteins were apparent within each of the two hospitals.

Since cord bloods were collected over an 18-month period, we were able to determine if the season of the year had any effect on lipid levels. Based on analysis of variance comparing mean values on four seasons of the year, we found no significant differences in any of the serum variables.

Relevance of neonatal hyperlipoproteinemia

Numerous studies have focused on the value of cord blood as a screening mechanism for identifying neonatal Type II hyperlipoproteinemia (Glueck et al., 1971; Darmady et al., 1972; Greten et al., 1973; Kwiterovich et al., 1973; Goldstein et al., 1974; Tsang et al., 1974a; Tsang et al., 1975; Ose, 1975). Familial hypercholesterolemia (monogenic inheritance, 0.4% of all births—Tsang et al., 1974a) can be identified at birth if one or more parents exhibits the trait (Kwiterovich et al., 1973; Tsang et al., 1975). However, the evidence is not clear for the remaining 99% of the general population as to the value of lipids and lipoproteins at birth for predicting levels within the same individual later in life.

Several investigators have reported that cord blood cholesterol levels appear to have little relation to levels at 1 year of age (Darmady et al., 1972; Greten et al., 1973; Ose, 1975), while others suggest that the evidence is far from conclusive (Kwiterovich et al., 1973; Tsang et al., 1974a; Tsang et al., 1975). Kwiterovich (1974) feels that cord blood β-lipoprotein cholesterol (or LDL cholesterol) has greater diagnostic power of subsequent hyperlipidemia than total cholesterol due to the prominent contribution made to cord blood cholesterol by α-lipoproteins. Ose (1975), however, did not find this to be the case when he compared at 1 year of age 42 infants with LDL cholesterol levels at birth equal to or above the 95th percentile with a control group of 39 infants with cord blood values below the 95th percentile; he found no differences between the two groups of 1-year-olds in either total cholesterol or triglycerides.

Persistence of levels over time for serum lipids and lipoproteins

Although we found little evidence that levels at birth for the serum lipids and lipoproteins were predictive of levels at 6 months or 1 year (Webber et al., 1978), we did note a significant tendency for the lipids and lipoproteins of an infant to remain consistent with respect to his peers from 6-months to 1-year of age. The distributions at 6 months and 1 year are shown in Figure 10–3 for those children measured at both times. Shaded areas are those children at 6 months of age who were above the 90th percentile. There is a tendency for them to remain high with 7 out of 23 (30%) still in the top decile and 14 out of 23 (61%) in the top three deciles at 1 year.

The most remarkable evidence of tracking was demonstrated for β-lipoprotein cholesterol (Fig. 10–4) in which 6 out of 15 (40%) who were in the top decile at 6 months remained there at 1 year. In addition, 12 out of 15, or 80%, were in the top three deciles. This tendency to track was also noted at the low end of the distributions.

Is it important to measure lipid levels at birth? We feel that the lipid and lipoprotein levels in cord blood provide baseline data for evaluating the evolution of lipoprotein profiles in children, at least for an epidemiologic study. Our subsequent studies show that values at birth lack correlation with levels at 6 months or 1 year, but those at 6 months significantly correlate with later levels (Webber et al., 1978; 1979c). By far, the most dramatic change in the lipids and lipoproteins over the

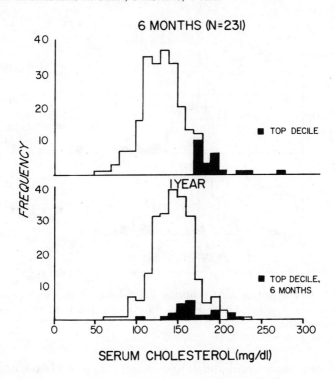

Figure 10–3. Frequency distributions for serum total cholesterol at 6-months and 1-year of age. Shaded areas show those children in the top decile at 6-months of age.

lifespan of an individual occurs during the first year of life and essentially approaches young adult levels by 2 to 3 years of age (Berenson et al., 1974b; Berenson et al., 1978a). If we can elucidate those factors which serve as determinants of lipid and lipoprotein levels during the first years of life, we may come closer to understanding the lipid regulatory mechanisms in the general population and thereby provide the necessary insight for programs aimed at primary prevention.

SUMMARY

The lipid profile—total cholesterol, triglycerides, and lipoproteins (β, pre-β, and α)—of cord blood is presented for 419 black and white infants (94% of the eligible population) born during an 18-month period in Bogalusa. At birth, white neonates of both sexes had higher average

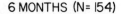

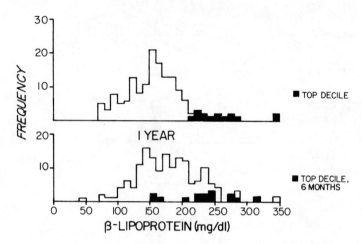

Figure 10–4. Frequency distributions for β-lipoprotein cholesterol at 6-months and 1-year of age. Shaded areas show those children in the top decile at 6-months of age.

levels of total cholesterol and β-lipoproteins than did black neonates. White girls among the four race–sex groups had the highest cord blood levels of total cholesterol, β-lipoproteins, and α-lipoproteins. Stress at delivery, birthweight, socioeconomic status, and season of the year had no observable effect on any of the lipid or lipoprotein levels. The magnitude and direction of the relationships between the respective lipids and lipoproteins in cord blood were similar to those we have observed in preschool and school-age children in the same community. Total cholesterol was highly correlated with both β- and α-lipoproteins; and triglycerides with pre-β-lipoproteins but inversely with α-lipoproteins. These observations suggest that basic biochemical relationships are already established at birth; however, observations at 6-months of age were more predictive of levels found at 1 year of age. Serum β-lipoproteins exhibited the greatest consistency with future lipoprotein levels.

11. Serum lipids and lipoproteins in preschool-age children

In an effort to study the early evidence of factors related to risk for coronary artery disease, many programs are focusing on school-age children. But it is as important to extend observations into the preschool years to broaden our information on the early natural history of arteriosclerosis. Numerous studies have characterized growth patterns from infancy onward, but there are few studies of child populations where serum lipid and lipoprotein data are collected. We studied the serum lipid and lipoprotein profile of Bogalusa's preschool population, ages 2 1/2–5 1/2 years. Of 898 eligible children, born 1969–71, 714 (80%) participated. Of those examined, 32% were black and 68% white.

GENERAL OBSERVATIONS

Serum lipid and lipoprotein levels in individual race-sex groups. The mean (± S.D.) levels by race and sex for serum lipids and lipoproteins are shown in Table 11–1. The values for serum total cholesterol included nonfasting children, since we observed little difference between fasting and nonfasting in school-age children (Frerichs et al., 1976). However, the values for triglycerides and lipoproteins are given only for children who were reported as fasting. Serum levels of

Table 11–1. Number of children, mean, and standard deviation for serum lipids and lipoproteins of children, ages 2½–5½ years, by race and sex, May–September, 1974

Serum variables (mg/dl)	White boys		White girls		Black boys		Black girls		All children	
	n	$\bar{x} \pm S.D.$	n	$\bar{x} \pm S.D.$	n	$\bar{x} \pm S.D.$	n	$\bar{x} \pm S.D.$	n	$\bar{x} \pm S.D.$
Total cholesterol	243	155 ± 24	231	158 ± 25	106	161 ± 26	114	158 ± 29	694	157 ± 25
Triglycerides[1]	229	63 ± 26[3]	216	69 ± 31[2,4]	101	57 ± 19	109	58 ± 22	655	63 ± 27
β-lipoprotein[1]	229	189 ± 44	216	197 ± 41	101	199 ± 52	109	199 ± 53	655	195 ± 46
Pre-β-lipoprotein[1]	229	28 ± 27	216	30 ± 27	101	25 ± 20	109	30 ± 25	655	29 ± 26
α-lipoprotein[1]	229	356 ± 107	216	353 ± 114	101	369 ± 116	109	346 ± 121	655	355 ± 113

[1] Fasting children only
[2] Sex differences significant at $p < 0.05$ (F-test)
[3,4] Race differences significant at $p < 0.05$, $p < 0.001$ (F-test)

total cholesterol, β-lipoproteins, and α-lipoproteins were slightly higher at all ages in black boys than in white boys. On the other hand, white boys showed slightly higher levels of triglycerides and pre-β-lipoproteins than black boys. Among girls, only triglycerides and β-lipoproteins showed such race-related trends, however, the observed differences due to race were statistically significant ($p < 0.001$) only with triglycerides. White girls had slightly higher levels of total cholesterol, triglycerides, β-lipoproteins, and pre-β-lipoproteins and lower levels of α-lipoproteins than white boys. Similar sex-related differences in lipid and lipoprotein levels were seen among black children only for triglycerides, pre-β-lipoproteins, and α-lipoproteins. None of the above variables showed a statistically significant sex-related difference except triglycerides ($p < 0.05$).

Changes in lipids and lipoproteins with age. Changes in serum lipid and lipoproteins levels (mg/dl, mean ± 2 S.E.) with age are shown in Figures 11-1 and 11-2. For the total preschool population, serum cholesterol tended to increase slightly with age, especially after age 3 (155 ± 3.4 at age 3 vs 159 ± 4.5 at age 5). Triglyceride levels were slightly higher at age 2 (67 ± 5.7) than at ages 3 through 5 (range of 61 ± 3.2 to 64 ± 5.5). Beta-lipoprotein decreased from a level of 203 ± 9.3 at age 2 to 194 ± 6.2 at age 3 and changed very little at age 5 (192 ± 8.4). The levels of pre-β-lipoproteins changed little between ages 2 and 4 (29 ± 5.0 vs 27 ± 3.2); however, there was a definite increase at age 5 (34 ± 5.6). Alpha-lipoprotein levels also increased, especially between ages 3 and 5 (348 ± 14.5 vs 363 ± 19.6). Regression analyses of serum lipids and lipoproteins with age indicated no significant increase in this three-year-age span except in α-lipoproteins. However, regression analyses may not accurately depict age-related trends if any of these variables tend to abruptly decrease or increase at certain age intervals, which appears to happen around ages 2 and 3.

Normal range (percentiles). The statistical normal limits for serum lipids and lipoproteins in these preschool-age children were estimated from their 5th, 50th (median), and 95th percentile values (Table 11-2). At the 95th (upper) percentile level, white children had 6% lower total cholesterol, 19% higher triglycerides, 13% lower β-lipoproteins, 8% higher pre-β-lipoproteins, and 6% lower α-lipoproteins than black children. Similar differences were seen at the 50th

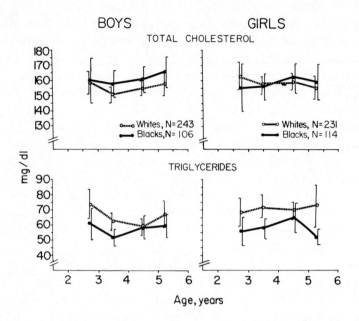

Figure 11–1. Serum cholesterol and triglyceride levels by age, race, and sex in the preschool-age children. As noted in older children (Frerichs et al., 1976), serum cholesterol levels tended to be higher in black children and triglycerides higher in white children.

(median) percentile levels with some exceptions (pre-β-lipoproteins and α-lipoproteins). The 5th (lower) percentile level did not reflect the differences of the 95th percentile level except in triglycerides. In general, the statistical upper normal limits (95th percentile) observed in this group of children are definitely lower than the currently recommended normal limits for serum lipids and lipoproteins (except α-lipoproteins) (Fredrickson et al., 1967). However, since normal limits are not well established, these data can serve as guidelines. The lipid values for school-age children in the Bogalusa Heart Study are comparable to those found by SCOR-A in Rochester, Minn. and by the Lipid Research Clinic, Cincinnati, Ohio (Ellefson et al., 1978; Morrison et al., 1978).

Interrelationship among serum lipids and lipoproteins. Table 11–3 shows that there was a weak correlation between total cholesterol and triglycerides in both races. A similar but somewhat stronger relation-

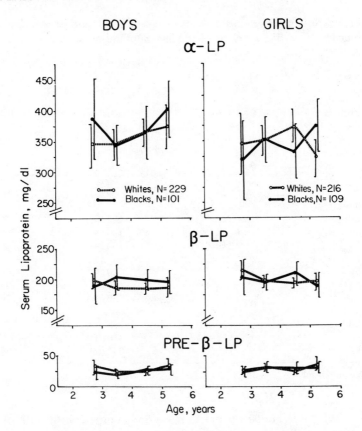

Figure 11–2. Serum α-, β-, and pre-β-lipoprotein levels in preschool-age children by age, race, and sex.

ship was observed between β- and pre-β-lipoproteins. In contrast, the α-lipoproteins were inversely related to β-lipoproteins and to a greater extent to both pre-β-lipoproteins and triglycerides. As expected, total cholesterol correlated highly with β-lipoproteins, and triglycerides with pre-β-lipoproteins. Interestingly, α-lipoproteins were highly correlated with serum total cholesterol, due to the fact that a considerable fraction of total cholesterol is derived from α-lipoproteins. When the lipoprotein concentrations were expressed in terms of their corresponding lipoprotein cholesterol values, it was found that in preschool-age children, α-, β-, and pre-β-lipoproteins contributed 40%, 58%, and 2% of cholesterol, respectively, to the serum total

184
LIPIDS

Table 11–2. Selected percentile levels for serum lipids and lipoproteins of children, ages 2½–5½ years, by race, May–September, 1974

Serum variables	5th	Percentiles (mg/dl) 50th	95th
Total cholesterol			
all children	116	157	198
whites	116	156	195
blacks	114	159	207
Triglycerides[1]			
all children	34	57	113
whites	35	59	117
blacks	29	54	98
β-lipoprotein[1]			
all children	124 (58)[2]	192 (90)	276 (129)
whites	126 (59)	190 (89)	265 (124)
blacks	119 (56)	195 (91)	306 (144)
Pre-β-lipoprotein[1]			
all children	4 (1)	20 (4)	79 (18)
whites	4 (1)	20 (4)	82 (18)
blacks	5 (1)	20 (4)	76 (17)
α-lipoprotein[1]			
all children	171 (29)	356 (60)	533 (90)
whites	172 (29)	359 (61)	527 (89)
blacks	163 (28)	347 (59)	562 (95)

[1]Fasting children only
[2]Corresponding lipoprotein cholesterol values are given in parentheses.

cholesterol pool. These observations were in agreement with our observations in school-age children (Frerichs et al., 1976; Srinivasan et al., 1976a).

Interrelationship of serum lipids with other variables. The interrelationship between the blood lipids and such factors as age, race, sex, and obesity was determined using multiple linear regression techniques (Table 11–4). In these studies an index of obesity, W/H^2, was calculated using the method of Benn, which calculates a value independent of height ($r = 0.04$) (Benn, 1971). This index is specific to our population and is highly correlated with an independent assessment of adiposity, namely the triceps skinfold ($r = 0.69$). Table 11–4 illustrates that of five independent variables, only a few are statistically significant when related to a specific serum lipid variable. None are significantly related to cholesterol.

For triglycerides there is a significant race effect (blacks lower than whites) and sex effect (males lower than females), as well as a relationship with weight relative to height (W/H^2). There is no independent relationship of triceps skinfold with triglycerides beyond the relationship with W/H^2. Both age and W/H^2 are weakly ($p < 0.05$) but positively associated with pre-β-lipoproteins. As stated earlier, there is no detectable relationship of lipids to blood pressure in this age group.

COMMENT

The serum lipid and lipoprotein levels in these preschool-age children showed a definite racial difference only in triglycerides. Although white children tended to have slightly higher pre-β-lipoprotein and lower α-lipoprotein levels than black children, the differences were not as striking as in the school-age children (5–14 years) from the same community. Whether the children tend to show a definitive race-related pattern only after a certain age due to genetic or environmental factors is not clear. For instance, any differences in dietary pattern and nutritional status among children of various age groups

Table 11–3. Pearson product moment correlation coefficients between serum lipids and lipoproteins by race in fasting children, 445 whites and 210 blacks, ages $2^{1}/_2$–$5^{1}/_2$ years, May–September, 1974

Variables	Triglycerides	β-lipoprotein	Pre-β-lipoprotein	α-lipoprotein
Total cholesterol				
whites	0.100[1]	0.735[3]	0.082	0.491[3]
blacks	0.188[2]	0.726[3]	0.162[1]	0.420[3]
Triglycerides				
whites		0.268[3]	0.799[3,4]	−0.408[3]
blacks		0.322[3]	0.593[3]	−0.288[3]
β-lipoprotein				
whites			0.269[3]	−0.193[3]
blacks			0.214[2]	−0.296[3]
Pre-β-lipoprotein				
whites				−0.497[3,4]
blacks				−0.293[3]

Levels of significance: correlation coefficient different from zero:
[1] $p < 0.05$
[2] $p < 0.01$
[3] $p < 0.001$
Significant racial differences in correlation coefficients:
[4] $p < 0.01$
[5] $p < 0.001$

Table 11–4. Stepwise multiple linear regression for serum lipids and selected variables in children, ages 2½–5½ years, May–September, 1974

Serum variable (mg/dl)	Number of children	Coefficient for multiple linear regression equation						
		Constant	Age (yrs)	Race[2] w,b,	Sex[2] m,f	Wt/Ht[2] wt=kg,ht=m	TSF[2] (mm)	Multiple R^2
Total cholesterol[1]	689	139.9	1.3	3.1	1.5	0.2	0.3	0.01
Triglycerides[1]	650	25.5	-0.1	-8.9[5]	4.9[3]	3.0[4]	-0.3	0.05
β-lipoprotein	650	184.5	-2.3	6.4	5.7	-0.0	0.3	0.01
Pre-β-lipoprotein[1]	650	-10.9	2.4[3]	-2.4	3.9	2.1[3]	-0.6	0.02
α-lipoprotein[1]	650	331.0	9.3	3.7	-12.8	-1.5	2.2	0.01

[1]Fasting children only
[2]w = white, b = black, m = male, f = female, wt = weight, ht = height, TSF = triceps skinfold thickness

Levels of significance (t-test):
[3]$p < 0.05$.
[4]$p < 0.01$.
[5]$p < 0.001$.

(preschool-age vs school-age) might affect the lipid and lipoprotein profiles.

Interestingly, the changes with age ($2^{1}/_{2}$–14 years) in the median levels of pre-β- and α-lipoproteins in children of this community indicated a progressive increase in differences (especially in pre-β-lipoproteins) related to race after age 7 or 8 (Srinivasan et al., 1976a). The sex-related changes in preschool-age children indicated a common tendency for girls (especially white girls) to have higher serum total cholesterol, triglycerides, and β- and pre-β-lipoprotein, but lower α-lipoprotein concentrations than boys.

Five major independent variables (age, race, sex, W/H^2, and triceps skinfold) help explain only 1–5% of the variance (as seen by the multiple R^2) in the serum lipid and lipoprotein levels, leaving 95% or more to be explained by other unnamed factors. To some extent these associations explain less variability than in children 5–14 years of age, and probably even less than in adults, suggesting that a transition occurs from childhood to adulthood with greater influence of environment over time. An inherent metabolic response to environmental factors controlled by genetic influences, mono- and/or polygenetic, seems to be paramount in accounting for this variability.

SUMMARY

Serum lipid and lipoprotein profiles in 716 children, ages $2^{1}/_{2}$ to $5^{1}/_{2}$ years, were studied. Serum levels of total cholesterol, β-lipoproteins, and α-lipoproteins were slightly higher in black boys than white boys. The reverse was true for triglycerides and pre-β-lipoproteins. For triglycerides, significant race and sex effects and a relationship with weight relative to height (W/H^2) were noted. Age and W/H^2 were positively associated with pre-β-lipoproteins.

12. Serum cholesterol and triglyceride levels in school-age children

Blood cholesterol has long been recognized as a major independent risk factor for coronary artery disease in adults (Tyroler et al., 1971; Kannel et al., 1971a; Stamler, 1973). More recently, the level of blood triglycerides has been incriminated as a coronary artery disease risk factor independent of cholesterol (Carlson and Bottiger, 1972; Rosenman et al., 1975) although the evidence for independence is not conclusive (Kannel et al., 1971a).

Earlier studies on limited numbers of children have shown that the mean serum cholesterol levels for children 3–4 years of age already approach levels found in young adults (Berenson et al., 1974b; Srinivasan et al., 1975a). The marked individual variability observed in these studies suggested a need for an epidemiologic survey of a larger defined population to detect subtle differences in serum cholesterol and triglycerides which might relate to race, sex, and early age. This chapter reports the serum cholesterol and triglycerides data from 3,446 children, ages 5–14 years. The details of the blind duplicate samples, the methodology for assessing measurement error, and the rationale for incorporating the laboratory controls in an epidemiologic survey are discussed in Chapter 4.

OBSERVATIONS

Effects of fasting on serum lipid levels

In order to determine the effect of a 12- to 14-hr fast on lipid levels, a comparison was made using Student's t-test of blood samples from 3,183 fasting children and 263 nonfasting children. The distributions of cholesterol and triglyceride levels were skewed. However, the large samples involved made it unnecessary to transform the data for analysis. (The data were analyzed in both the log transformed and nontransformed states. The results of hypothesis tests were equivalent.) Figure 12–1 illustrates that there is no statistically significant difference between mean serum cholesterol levels in fasting (165.3 mg/dl) and nonfasting (162.7 mg/dl) children, whereas the mean level of serum triglycerides is significantly lower in fasting children (68.7 mg/dl for fasting vs 87.7 mg/dl, $p < 0.0001$). Therefore, in all subsequent analyses, cholesterol values for fasting and nonfasting subjects are combined, but triglyceride values are presented for only fasting subjects.

Serum total cholesterol

The racial distributions of serum total cholesterol in the children are shown in Figure 12–2. Statistically significant differences were observed between levels in whites and blacks, the former tending to be lower (mean levels of 162 mg/dl vs 170 mg/dl, $p < 0.0001$; Student's t-test). For both races, serum cholesterol values appear to be normally distributed, although the median values are slightly lower than the means (median values of 160 mg/dl in whites and 168 mg/dl in blacks), indicating the distributions are shifted very slightly toward higher values. In addition, there is a slight increase in the number of black children with cholesterol values in the interval between 226 and 235 mg/dl. The lowest value for serum cholesterol was 77 mg/dl, while the maximum value was 346 mg/dl. As seen in Table 12–1, there was no significant difference between the races in serum cholesterol concentrations at every age interval, but the mean concentration over the ten-year span was higher for blacks than whites. No consistent differences were observed in cholesterol levels between boys and girls in either racial group.

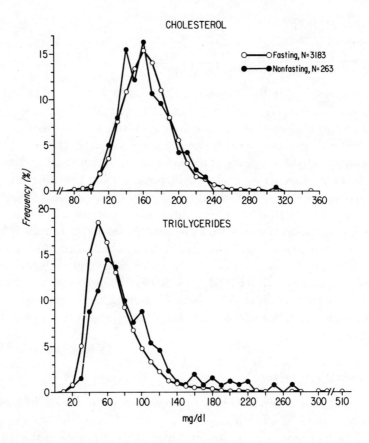

Figure 12-1. Distributions of total serum cholesterol and triglycerides in fasting and nonfasting children, ages 5-14 years.

The linear regression of cholesterol with age is shown in Table 12-2 for 5-10-year-olds and for 11-14-year-olds. The two age groups were selected to assess the age-related changes of cholesterol levels during both the preadolescent and the early adolescent years. No significant change with age is observed in the 5-10-year-old group. A negative slope is seen in children ages 11-14, but the correlation is significantly different from zero only in white boys; however, none of the correlation coefficients are large.

The median and selected percentile levels for serum cholesterol by age, race, and sex are shown in Figure 12-3. Cholesterol levels remain relatively constant in all children until ages 11 and 12, after

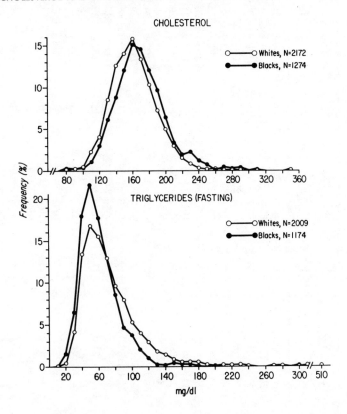

Figure 12–2. Distributions of total serum cholesterol and triglycerides (fasting) by race in children, ages 5–14 years.

which a slight reduction occurs, more pronounced in boys than in girls. At the median (50th percentile), blacks exceed whites at every age interval. This same difference in cholesterol levels between the races is even greater at the 95th percentile except for 12- and 13-year-old girls. Ninety-five percent of all black children have serum cholesterol levels below 225 mg/dl, whereas 95% of all white children are below 210 mg/dl. The 5th percentile levels for blacks and whites are 126 mg/dl and 121 mg/dl, respectively.

Serum triglycerides

The distributions of serum triglycerides (see Fig. 12–2) indicate that white children tend to have higher triglyceride levels than do black

Table 12-1. Mean, standard deviation, and range of total serum cholesterol levels in children by age, race, and sex

Age (years)	Black children				White children			
	Boys		Girls		Boys		Girls	
	N[1]	Mean ± S.D. (range) mg/dl	N[1]	Mean ± S.D. (range) mg/dl	N[1]	Mean ± S.D. (range) mg/dl	N[1]	Mean ± S.D. (range) mg/dl
5	42	169.5 ± 26.8 (115 – 237)	37	165.7 ± 22.1 (128 – 226)	89	160.8 ± 27.5 (107 – 253)	93	159.1 ± 25.5 (80 – 225)
6	53	169.8 ± 37.5 (112 – 286)	56	178.9 ± 31.8[3] (120 – 278)	103	167.5 ± 34.0 (84 – 293)	84	160.9 ± 31.2 (86 – 267)
7	54	170.3 ± 36.9 (104 – 276)	60	170.4 ± 32.4 (102 – 248)	99	160.6 ± 29.0 (90 – 257)	93	163.3 ± 28.3 (102 – 225)
8	64	164.7 ± 29.3 (82 – 231)	52	178.7 ± 33.2[2,3] (114 – 267)	111	161.7 ± 31.7 (107 – 346)	100	168.4 ± 26.9 (123 – 231)
9	82	177.2 ± 36.9 (108 – 293)	59	172.5 ± 29.7 (106 – 248)	106	166.2 ± 28.6 (112 – 291)	102	167.1 ± 26.5 (108 – 248)
10	74	169.0 ± 28.6 (105 – 259)	60	171.9 ± 32.1 (97 – 254)	127	162.5 ± 29.4 (94 – 282)	108	162.4 ± 24.7 (104 – 229)
11	74	171.0 ± 29.5 (77 – 254)	69	174.4 ± 32.9 (87 – 307)	119	163.8 ± 26.4 (95 – 215)	112	165.9 ± 26.6 (110 – 223)
12	85	173.3 ± 31.2[2,3] (77 – 254)	77	163.7 ± 24.0 (113 – 241)	147	162.4 ± 26.8 (104 – 241)	129	162.9 ± 28.1 (118 – 313)
13	74	160.3 ± 25.2 (116 – 251)	72	167.7 ± 25.2 (93 – 225)	125	157.4 ± 25.8 (109 – 227)	120	165.2 ± 25.9[2] (115 – 256)
14	67	164.9 ± 25.8[5] (120 – 236)	63	166.6 ± 28.5[3] (122 – 274)	116	150.6 ± 25.3 (104 – 226)	89	157.7 ± 26.8 (80 – 229)
Total	669	169.2 ± 31.2[5] (77 – 293)	605	170.9 ± 29.6[5] (87 – 307)	1,142	161.3 ± 28.7 (84 – 346)	1,030	163.5 ± 27.1 (80 – 313)

[1] Number of children in population
[2] Sex differences significant at $p < 0.05$ (F test)

[3,4,5] Race differences significant at $p < 0.05$, $p < 0.01$, and $p < 0.001$, respectively (F test).

Table 12–2. Linear regression with age of serum cholesterol and
triglycerides by race and sex in children, ages 5–14 years

	Correlation with age	Intercept[1] (mg/dl)	Slope[1] (mg/dl/yr)	Standard error of the slope (mg/dl)
Cholesterol (ages 5–10 yrs)				
boys, black, n = 369	0.018	167.5	0.36	1.03
white, n = 635	0.024	159.8	0.42	0.69
girls, black, n = 324	−0.001	173.5	−0.02	1.02
white, n = 580	0.062	155.8	0.97	0.65
Cholesterol (ages 11–14 yrs)				
boys, black, n = 300	−0.129	210.2	−3.29	1.46
white, n = 507	−0.182	213.5	−4.23[4]	1.02
girls, black, n = 281	−0.082	193.4	−1.96	1.42
white, n = 450	−0.093	192.1	−2.24	1.13
Triglycerides (ages 5–14 yrs)[2]				
boys, black, n = 609	0.099	49.3	0.95	0.38
white, n = 1,033	0.111	54.9	1.37[3]	0.38
girls, black, n = 565	0.032	60.7	0.28	0.37
white, n = 976	0.179	52.7	2.42[4]	0.43

[1]Equation for the indicated line (serum lipid levels = intercept + slope × age).
[2]Blood samples only from fasting children
[3]$p < 0.001$
[4]$p < 0.0001$

children (means of 73 mg/dl vs 61 mg/dl, $p < 0.0001$; Student's t-test)
in direct contrast to the observations of cholesterol noted above. The
triglyceride levels, however, are definitely skewed toward high
values in the distributions of both blacks and whites. As a reflection of
the skewness, the median value is less than the mean by 8 mg/dl in
white children, and by 6 mg/dl in black children. The range for triglyceride values in all fasting children was between 8 mg/dl and
506 mg/dl.

Because the distributions are skewed, statistical analyses were performed on untransformed and $\log_{10}$ transformed data in line with other
investigators (Goldstein et al., 1973a). The results from the two sets of
analyses were essentially identical. The central limit theorem states
that for a random sample from a distribution with finite variance, the
distribution of a sample mean approaches normality as the sample size
increases. Hence, only the analyses of untransformed data are presented.

Serum triglyceride levels in children tend to increase with age in all

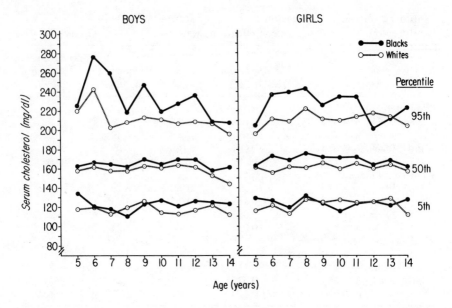

Figure 12–3. Percentiles for serum cholesterol by race and sex in children, ages 5–14 years.

race-sex groups (Table 12–2), although this increase is very slight in blacks. All children ages 5–14 years were combined since the onset of adolescence appeared to have a minimal effect on triglyceride levels. Although the slopes for white children are significantly different from zero, the proportion of variance of serum triglycerides explained by linear regression on age is only between 1.2 and 3.2% (r^2). In a comparison of four race-sex groups, white children have significantly higher levels of serum triglycerides than do black children (Table 12–3), and girls have higher levels than boys in both racial groups, although these differences are not maintained throughout each age interval.

Three sets of percentile levels for serum triglycerides are shown in Figure 12–4. The lack of uniformity at the 95th percentile is due to the high variability at the extremes. The levels for all groups at the 95th percentile vary from a low of 91 mg/dl in 7-year-old black boys to a high of 181 mg/dl in 11-year-old white girls. Discounting any sex differences or increases of age, the triglyceride values of 90% of the white children are between 36 mg/dl (5th percentile) and 136 mg/dl

Table 12–3. Mean, standard deviation and range of serum triglyceride levels in fasting children by age, race, and sex

Age (years)	Black children				White children			
	Boys		Girls		Boys		Girls	
	N[1]	Mean ± S.D. (range) mg/dl	N[1]	Mean ± S.D. (range) mg/dl	N[1]	Mean ± S.D. (range) mg/dl	N[1]	Mean ± S.D. (range) mg/dl
5	30	55.6 ± 20.2 (34 – 118)	31	67.1 ± 29.4 (29 – 176)	71	69.4 ± 27.1 (30 – 150)	88	64.8 ± 23.7 (31 – 138)
6	44	57.0 ± 21.3 (21 – 109)	50	61.1 ± 21.7 (30 – 145)	91	64.1 ± 32.0 (28 – 243)	77	66.5 ± 30.4 (26 – 175)
7	49	52.8 ± 19.1 (19 – 108)	52	59.1 ± 21.9 (25 – 117)	96	62.5 ± 25.1[5] (8 – 135)	91	74.2 ± 33.5[3,6] (28 – 193)
8	61	56.9 ± 26.4 (22 – 165)	50	63.4 ± 20.3 (32 – 112)	102	62.8 ± 31.1 (28 – 228)	96	69.2 ± 31.1 (19 – 183)
9	80	61.5 ± 31.2 (24 – 172)	55	62.2 ± 24.8 (23 – 160)	99	66.1 ± 31.3 (26 – 236)	98	73.4 ± 29.9[5] (32 – 178)
10	71	53.3 ± 20.1 (24 – 119)	60	66.5 ± 37.9[2] (22 – 305)	123	69.2 ± 34.2[6] (14 – 210)	105	80.8 ± 41.9[5] (22 – 234)
11	70	64.3 ± 24.3 (22 – 148)	64	67.2 ± 24.5 (24 – 146)	114	75.3 ± 46.9 (24 – 315)	111	87.1 ± 60.8[6] (27 – 506)
12	81	60.3 ± 22.3 (24 – 162)	74	62.4 ± 17.1 (28 – 114)	134	68.2 ± 33.9 (20 – 200)	122	84.8 ± 34.7[4,7] (28 – 220)
13	68	60.5 ± 28.1 (27 – 196)	69	65.2 ± 23.4 (33 – 154)	110	72.7 ± 29.3[6] (28 – 160)	106	82.3 ± 32.4[2,7] (28 – 230)
14	55	65.5 ± 25.6 (33 – 154)	60	63.2 ± 19.5 (29 – 120)	93	78.2 ± 32.4[6] (34 – 222)	82	83.3 ± 30.6[7] (25 – 192)
Total	609	59.2 ± 24.8 (19 – 196)	565	63.7 ± 24.3[2] (22 – 305)	1033	68.9 ± 33.5[7] (8 – 315)	976	77.3 ± 37.6[4,7] (19 – 506)

[1]Number of children in population

[2,3,4]Sex differences significant at $p < 0.05$, $p < 0.01$, and $p < 0.001$, respectively (F test).

[5,6,7]Race differences significant at $p < 0.05$, $p < 0.01$, and $p < 0.001$, respectively (F test).

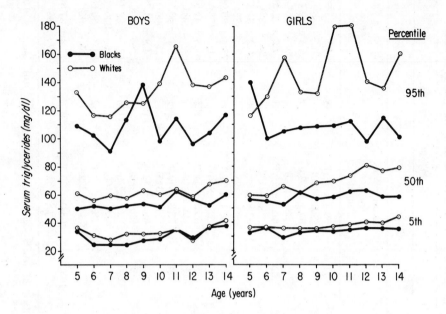

Figure 12–4. Percentiles for serum triglycerides (fasting) by race and sex in children, ages 5–14 years.

(95th percentile), whereas the values for the same percentage of black children are between 32 mg/dl (5th percentile) and 105 mg/dl (95th percentile).

COMMENT

The levels of both serum cholesterol and serum triglycerides are highly variable within a population and require large numbers of people before subtle differences become statistically significant. Obviously, care must be taken in the interpretation of these results since in a large sample size, group differences which are statistically significant may or may not be important from a biologic standpoint. Our mean levels of cholesterol agree relatively well (within 10 mg/dl) with values found by numerous investigators in the United States (Hames and Greenberg, 1961; Hodges and Krehl, 1965; Johnson et al., 1965; Baker et al., 1967; Clarke et al., 1970; Friedman and Goldberg,

1973) although the values reported from the Muscatine study (Lauer et al., 1975) are a notable exception with a mean serum cholesterol level reported (uncorrected to the Abell-Kendall method) in white children 20 mg/dl higher than in our comparable population. Our values are lower by more than 30 mg/dl than levels reported in Swedish or Australian children (Godfrey et al., 1972; Dyerberg and Hjorne, 1973; Hickie et al., 1974), but many of these studies are not directly comparable because of different analytical methods. (Schwartz and Hill, 1972).

Analytical variation is also a major consideration when comparing triglyceride levels in different study populations (Fletcher, 1972). Although studies of blood triglycerides in children are scarce, our mean levels in Bogalusa are in close agreement (within 10 mg/dl) with those of other investigators analyzing blood from fasting children (Godfrey et al., 1972; Dyerberg and Hjorne, 1973; Hickie et al., 1974). A major exception was reported by Hodges and Krehl (1965) for nonfasting Iowa girls between 14 and 17 years who had a mean value of 45 mg/dl, almost half the level of the oldest group of fasting white girls in Bogalusa.

Because of technical limitations, it is important to appreciate potential errors which can occur in the field as well as in the laboratory. Detailed analyses of our data for sources of measurement error (see Chapter 4) show that the 95% confidence interval for a single analysis of serum cholesterol and triglycerides is approximately ± 18 mg/dl. Given this range of potential error, it is important to note how difficult it is to derive an accurate lipid profile for a given individual from a single blood sample, even in a rigidly controlled research laboratory.

The age-related changes in blood lipid levels are important, although they cannot be clearly explained at this time. The progressive increase in triglycerides, most obvious in white girls, suggests a relative increase in body fat, possibly resulting from overeating or underexercise (Johnson et al., 1956). In contrast, however, there is a tendency for a decrease in cholesterol around puberty, more obvious in boys, which likely reflects marked hormonal influences. A similar decline in serum cholesterol at this stage of sexual maturation in boys has been observed in other cross-sectional studies (Johnson et al., 1965; Starr, 1971; McGandy, 1971). From our knowledge of serum cholesterol and triglyceride levels in adults, we can assume that the trend of triglyceride concentrations to increase with age should continue, whereas the slight negative trend in serum cholesterol levels in children 11–14 years old should be reversed and start to increase during late adolescence and continue upward through adulthood.

The differences between the races in blood cholesterol or triglycerides were not noted in New York (Baker et al., 1967) or in Evans County, Ga. (Hames and Greenberg, 1961), however, neither study's sample size was as large as the Bogalusa sample.

The differences between the races in Bogalusa are likely due to genetic influences, although environmental factors such as diet and socioeconomic status may contribute. Education and occupation data were collected on the children's household head by a mailed questionnaire. Based upon our initial analyses, there was little association between the household head's social status and the lipid levels of the children. Further, although slight differences were noted in dietary intake based on race and sex, these do not seem to account for racial and sexual differences in lipid levels.

SUMMARY

Serum lipid profiles of 3,446 (91% of population) children, ages 5–14 years, were determined. Black children had significantly higher mean levels of serum cholesterol than did white children (170 mg/dl vs 162 mg/dl, $p < 0.0001$). On the other hand, significantly lower levels of triglycerides were found in black children (61 mg/dl vs 73 mg/dl, $p < 0.0001$). Girls had higher levels of triglycerides than boys in both races (blacks, 64 mg/dl vs 59 mg/dl, $p < 0.001$; whites 77 mg/dl vs 69 mg/dl, $p < 0.001$). The racial differences in serum cholesterol and triglyceride levels were even more apparent at the 95th percentile. The serum cholesterol level remained relatively constant in all children until ages 11 and 12 years, after which a slight reduction occurred. This reduction was more pronounced in boys than in girls. In contrast, a significant increase in the level of triglycerides with age was observed in all children except black girls, the increasing slope being most pronounced in white girls.

13. Serum lipoprotein profiles in school-age children

There has been a surge of interest in identifying problems associated with hyperlipoproteinemia in children and in comparing lipoprotein levels of parents and their children (Rafstedt, 1955; Tamir et al., 1972; Levy and Rifkind, 1973; Glueck et al., 1974; Kwiterovich et al., 1974). Serum lipids in free-living children have been studied mostly in terms of cholesterol and triglycerides. Recently serum lipoprotein profiles have been reported in only a limited number of free-living children (Dyerberg and Hjorne, 1973; Berenson et al., 1974b; Srinivasan et al., 1975a). It was apparent from these studies that the extreme individual variability in lipoprotein levels makes larger samples necessary to detect subtle differences possibly related to race, sex, and early age. Serum lipoprotein profiles of 3,182 children, ages 5 to 14 years, are described here.

OBSERVATIONS

Distribution of serum lipoproteins

The distribution by race of serum β-, pre-β-, and α-lipoproteins in children 5–14 years old is presented in Figure 13–1. Whereas the distribution of β-lipoproteins showed no racial difference (mean level of

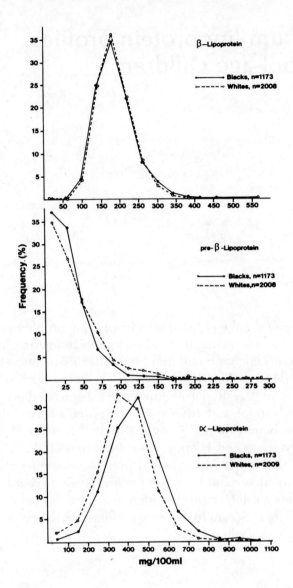

Figure 13–1. Distributions of β-, pre-β-, and α-lipoproteins by race in children, ages 5–14 years.

190 mg/dl in black children compared to 189 mg/dl in white children), both pre-β and α-lipoprotein distributions indicated a consistent racial difference. White children tended to have higher pre-β-lipoprotein levels than black children (mean level of 40 mg/dl in white children vs 33 mg/dl in black children, $p < 0.001$). On the other hand, black children tended to have higher α-lipoprotein levels than white children (mean levels of 436 mg/dl and 384 mg/dl, $p < 0.0001$). In both racial groups the mean values for β-lipoprotein (184 mg/dl for both races) and α-lipoprotein (431 mg/dl in white children and 389 mg/dl in black children) were only slightly different from the corresponding mean values. The median values for pre-β-lipoprotein, however, were 21.7 and 23.8% less than the mean values in black and white children, respectively. The distributions of α-, pre-β-, and β-lipoproteins were unimodal, but a chi-square goodness-of-fit test indicated that none were normally distributed.

Serum lipoprotein levels in individual race-sex groups

Serum β-, pre-β-, and α-lipoprotein levels were compared among the four race-sex groups at every age. The results are shown in Tables 13–1, 13–2, and 13–3. All statistical analyses were performed on the logarithmically transformed data, although the arithmetic mean and standard deviation values obtained from the untransformed data are presented in the tables. The β-lipoprotein levels given in Table 13–1 showed no significant race difference among children ages 5–14 except among 5-year-old girls. Although girls from both races tended to have a slightly higher level of β-lipoproteins than boys (black children $p < 0.05$; white children $p < 0.01$), these differences were not statistically significant for each age interval. Furthermore, a decrease in β-lipoprotein concentration was noticeable after age 11 in all children irrespective of sex or race. White children of both sexes showed a higher pre-β-lipoprotein level than black children (Table 13–2); however, a statistically significant racial difference was observed only in girls ($p < 0.01$), especially in the 12- to 14-year age group. Interestingly, like β-lipoprotein, the pre-β-lipoprotein levels were generally higher in girls than in boys in both racial groups (black children $p < 0.01$; white children $p < 0.001$), although the differences were not significant for each group. α-Lipoprotein levels (Table 13–3) in children differed markedly between races in both boys ($p < 0.001$)

Table 13–1. Serum β-lipoprotein levels (mg/dl, mean ± S.D.) in children by age, race, and sex

Age (yr)	Black children				White children			
	N	Boys	N	Girls	N	Boys	N	Girls
5	30	206 ± 54	31	201 ± 41[3]	71	193 ± 48[1]	88	179 ± 39
6	44	192 ± 58	50	209 ± 46	91	191 ± 51	77	198 ± 44
7	48	192 ± 48	52	192 ± 45	96	187 ± 49	91	197 ± 47
8	61	188 ± 43	50	205 ± 60	102	188 ± 54	96	196 ± 48
9	80	197 ± 60	55	194 ± 51	99	200 ± 52	98	203 ± 51
10	71	179 ± 38	60	196 ± 56	123	185 ± 51	105	198 ± 50[1]
11	70	190 ± 55	64	204 ± 49	114	190 ± 50	111	198 ± 52
12	81	185 ± 48	74	179 ± 39	134	181 ± 47	122	183 ± 40
13	68	169 ± 46	69	176 ± 40	110	175 ± 46	105	184 ± 42
14	55	184 ± 41	60	190 ± 50	93	177 ± 45	82	182 ± 45
5–14	608	187 ± 50	565	193 ± 49[1]	1033	186 ± 50	975	192 ± 47[2]

Sex differences:
[1]$p < 0.05$ (F test after conversion to $\log_{10}$ β-lipoprotein).
[2]$p < 0.01$ " " " " " " "
Race differences:
[3]$p < 0.05$ " " " " " " "

Table 13–2. Serum pre-β-lipoprotein levels (mg/dl, mean ± S.D.) in children by age, race, and sex

Age (yr)	Black children				White children			
	N	Boys	N	Girls	N	Boys	N	Girls
5	30	26 ± 20	31	29 ± 29	71	32 ± 28	88	28 ± 25
6	44	20 ± 13	50	30 ± 22	91	28 ± 27	77	27 ± 25
7	48	23 ± 14	52	27 ± 22	96	28 ± 25	91	38 ± 35
8	61	30 ± 27	50	36 ± 26	102	28 ± 33	96	33 ± 26[1]
9	80	33 ± 27	55	31 ± 21	99	37 ± 32	98	39 ± 33
10	71	29 ± 27	60	34 ± 29	123	38 ± 33[4]	105	49 ± 48
11	70	35 ± 25	64	43 ± 31	114	40 ± 36	111	49 ± 38[1]
12	81	34 ± 27	74	32 ± 22	134	38 ± 33	122	53 ± 38[3,5]
13	68	35 ± 32	69	36 ± 23	110	42 ± 33	105	51 ± 31[1,5]
14	55	37 ± 31	60	40 ± 27	93	48 ± 30[4]	82	56 ± 33[5]
5–14	608	31 ± 26	565	34 ± 26[2]	1033	36 ± 32	975	43 ± 36[3,5]

Sex differences:
[1]$p < 0.05$ (F test after conversion to $\log_{10}$ pre-β-lipoprotein).
[2]$p < 0.01$ " " " " " " "
[3]$p < 0.001$ " " " " " " "
Race differences:
[4]$p < 0.05$ " " " " " " "
[5]$p < 0.01$ " " " " " " "

Table 13–3. Serum α-lipoprotein levels (mg/dl, mean ± S.D.) in children by age, race, and sex

Age (yr)	Black children				White children			
	N	Boys	N	Girls	N	Boys	N	Girls
5	30	401 ± 113	31	395 ± 110	71	369 ± 120	88	399 ± 135
6	44	458 ± 150	50	429 ± 159	91	424 ± 163	77	372 ± 135
7	48	447 ± 163	52	445 ± 128[3]	96	394 ± 119	91	366 ± 125
8	61	414 ± 140	50	435 ± 121	102	393 ± 127	96	413 ± 115
9	80	459 ± 124[3]	55	439 ± 124[3]	99	388 ± 128	98	378 ± 126
10	71	463 ± 153[2]	60	427 ± 171[3]	123	399 ± 123[1]	105	342 ± 123
11	70	436 ± 127	64	406 ± 137	114	387 ± 134	111	364 ± 132
12	81	467 ± 146	74	430 ± 108[2]	134	410 ± 120	122	376 ± 120
13	68	438 ± 131	69	452 ± 104[2]	110	385 ± 105	106	398 ± 103
14	55	425 ± 105[4]	60	406 ± 100[2]	93	341 ± 118	82	358 ± 112
5–14	608	444 ± 137[4]	565	428 ± 128[4]	1033	390 ± 127[1]	976	376 ± 124

[1]Sex differences at $P < 0.05$ (F test after conversion to $\log_{10}$ α-lipoproteins).
Race differences:
[2]$p < 0.05$ (F test after conversion to $\log_{10}$ α-lipoprotein).
[3]$p < 0.01$ " " "   "   " "   "
[4]$p < 0.001$ " " "   "   " "   "

and girls ($p < 0.001$), with black children tending to be higher than white children. This trend was consistent throughout the ten-year age span (except in 5-year-old girls). Though the overall (ages 5–14) mean levels of α-lipoproteins were slightly higher in boys than in girls, the differences were significant only among white children ($p < 0.05$).

When the lipoprotein concentrations were expressed in terms of their corresponding lipoprotein cholesterol values, the α-lipoprotein cholesterol (with mean levels of 74 mg/dl in black children and 65 mg/dl in white children) constituted as much as 44 and 40% of the total lipoprotein cholesterol (serum total cholesterol) in black and white children, respectively.

Statistical normal limits (percentiles)

To estimate the normal limits for serum lipoproteins in this pediatric population, the 5th, 50th (median), and 95th percentile values by race and sex were calculated and are given in Table 13–4. Since serum lipoprotein concentrations are generally being measured and reported

Table 13–4. Selected percentile levels by race and sex for serum lipoproteins in children 5–14 years old

| Serum lipoproteins | Percentiles | | |
	5th	50th	95th
β-lipoprotein			
boys, black	119 (56)[1]	181 (85)	286 (134)
white	119 (56)	181 (85)	272 (127)
girls, black	128 (60)	188 (88)	284 (133)
white	126 (59)	188 (88)	278 (131)
Pre-β-lipoprotein			
boys, black	4 (1)	24 (5)	79 (18)
white	4 (1)	27 (6)	106 (24)
girls, black	6 (1)	27 (6)	83 (18)
white	5 (1)	35 (8)	113 (25)
α-lipoprotein			
boys, black	231 (39)	440 (75)	673 (114)
white	182 (31)	392 (67)	596 (101)
girls, black	230 (39)	425 (72)	637 (108)
white	171 (29)	382 (65)	575 (98)

[1]The corresponding lipoprotein cholesterol values are given in parentheses.

in terms of corresponding lipoprotein cholesterol, the percentile values for the individual lipoprotein cholesterol were also included in the table. The 5th and 95th percentile levels for this group of children showed very little difference between boys and girls within each race. Although the percentile levels for β-lipoproteins were very similar in both races, the upper 95th percentile level for pre-β-lipoprotein in black children was about 26% lower than in white children. For α-lipoprotein, the upper 95th percentile levels in white children were about 10% lower than in black children.

The three sets of percentile values by sex and race are also presented for every age in Figures 13–2, 13–3, and 13–4. The median and selected percentile levels of β-lipoproteins (Fig. 13–2) indicated no consistent racial differences at each age interval in either boys or girls. Although no definite age-related trend could be ascertained from these percentile levels, the median and upper 95th percentile levels indicated a decrease in β-lipoprotein between ages 11 and 14. For pre-β-lipoproteins (Fig. 13–3), the median level for white children exceeded that for black children at every age interval between the ages of 9 and 14; this difference was more pronounced in girls than in

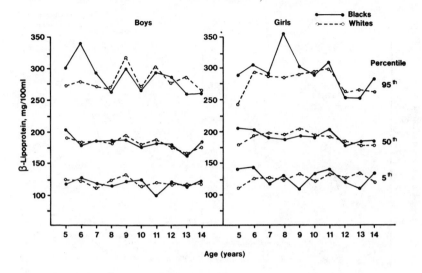

Figure 13–2. Selected percentile values (5th, 50th, and 95th) for serum β-lipoprotein by age, race, and sex in children.

boys due to a strong age-related increase in pre-β-lipoprotein levels in white girls. The difference between the races in pre-β-lipoprotein levels was even greater at the 95th percentile level except for 13- and 14-year-old boys and 6- and 8-year-old girls. Interestingly, black children exceeded white children at every age interval in their median α-lipoproteins level (Fig. 13–4).

Effect of age

To assess the effect of age on serum lipoprotein levels in these children, regression analyses were made by race and sex. The summary of the results is given in Table 13–5. In view of the skewed distribution of the serum lipoproteins, regression analyses were made after logarithmic transformation of the data as in the mode of previous reports (Goldstein et al., 1973a; Kwiterovich et al., 1974). Since β-lipoprotein levels showed a definite tendency to decrease after age 11 (Table 13–1), the regression analyses were made separately on children of age groups 5–10 and 11–14. Although β-lipoprotein levels decreased slightly with age in all children (except white girls between ages 5 and 10), the decreasing trend, as shown by the negative correla-

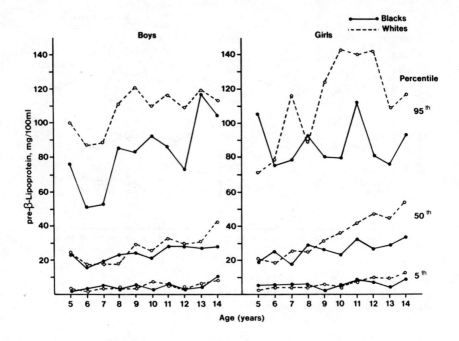

Figure 13–3. Selected percentile values (5th, 50th, and 95th) for serum pre-β-lipoprotein by age, race, and sex in children.

tion, was stastistically significant ($p < 0.05$) only between ages 11 and 14 (except in black boys). Interestingly, the β-lipoprotein levels in white girls between ages 5 and 10 increased slightly with age ($p < 0.05$). A highly significant ($p < 0.0001$) increase in pre-β-lipoprotein levels with age was observed in all children, and the rate of increase with age (coefficient of linear regression) was higher in white children than in black children. There was little correlation with age in the case of α-lipoprotein levels on all four race-sex groups studied.

Interrelationship among serum lipoproteins and lipids

The interrelationship among serum lipoproteins and lipids in black versus white children is presented in Table 13–6. In both the races, β- and pre-β-lipoproteins were positively correlated. A similar relationship was observed for serum total cholesterol and triglycerides, both of which were measured independently. In contrast, the α-lipoprotein

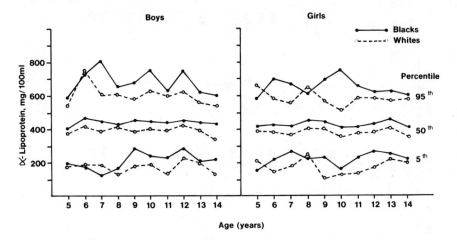

Figure 13–4. Selected percentile values (5th, 50th, and 95th) for serum α-lipoprotein by age, race, and sex in children. The decrease in α-lipoprotein levels becomes rather marked in white boys (noted in our subsequent studies) through age 17.

was negatively correlated with β-lipoprotein and to a greater extent with pre-β-lipoprotein, suggesting an inverse relationship between these lipoprotein classes. It should be noted that the α-lipoprotein was negatively correlated with serum triglycerides as well. The serum total cholesterol correlated with β-lipoproteins and triglycerides with pre-β-lipoproteins. The absolute values of the above correlations were generally greater in white children than in black children. On the other hand, the correlation coefficient between total cholesterol and α-lipoprotein was higher in black children than in white children.

Frequency of hyperlipoproteinemia

Since the three forms of hyperlipoproteinemia common in our population consist of elevated β- and/or pre-β-lipoproteins, their frequency in this pediatric population was calculated based on the currently recommended upper normal limits (Fredrickson et al., 1967). Table 13–7 shows that only 0.5% of black and white children exceeded the upper β-lipoprotein cholesterol level of 170 mg/dl and could be considered hyper-β-lipoproteinemic (Type IIa). On the other hand, 1.7% of black children and 4.7% of white children showed hyper-pre-β-

Table 13–5. Summary of regression analyses with age of serum lipoproteins in children by race and sex

Serum lipoproteins[1]	Correlation with age (r)	Coefficient of linear regression	Intercept (y)	Standard error of the slope
β-lipoproteins, *ages 5–10*				
boys, black, N = 334	−0.08	−0.0060	2.32	0.004
white, N = 582	−0.01	−0.0008	2.27	0.003
girls, black, N = 298	−0.08	−0.0051	2.33	0.004
white, N = 555	0.09[2]	0.0058	2.23	0.003
ages 11–14				
boys, black, N = 274	−0.06	−0.0057	2.32	0.006
white, N = 451	−0.12[2]	−0.0117	2.39	0.005
girls, black, N = 267	−0.13[2]	−0.0114	2.41	0.005
white, N = 420	−0.12[2]	−0.0112	2.40	0.004
Pre-β-lipoprotein, *ages 5–14*				
boys, black, N = 608	0.17[3]	0.0254	1.08	0.006
white, N = 1033	0.21[3]	0.0331	1.05	0.005
girls, black, N = 565	0.17[3]	0.0213	1.19	0.005
white, N = 975	0.32[3]	0.0476	0.99	0.004
α-lipoprotein, *ages 5–14*				
boys, black, N = 608	0.01	0.0007	2.61	0.003
white, N = 1033	−0.02	−0.0018	2.57	0.003
girls, black, N = 565	0.01	0.0005	2.60	0.003
white, N = 976	−0.02	−0.0017	2.55	0.003

[1]The regression analyses were done after conversion to $\log_{10}$ lipoproteins.
[2]$p < 0.05$.
[3]$p < 0.0001$.

Table 13–6. Correlation coefficients (r) for serum lipoprotein and lipid variables by race in children, ages 5–14 years

	β-lipoprotein	Pre-β-lipoprotein	α-lipoprotein	Total cholesterol
Pre-β-lipoprotein				
Black, N = 1173	0.231[2]			
White, N = 2008	0.393[2,5]			
α-lipoprotein				
Black, N = 1173	−0.093[1]	−0.359[2]		
White, N = 2009	−0.231[2,4]	−0.505[2,5]		
Total cholesterol				
Black, N = 1174	0.727[2]	0.097[1]	0.595[2,5]	
White, N = 2009	0.745[2]	0.206[2,3]	0.441[2]	
Triglyceride				
Black, N = 1174	0.282[2]	0.667[2]	−0.286[2]	0.127[2]
White, N = 2009	0.442[2,5]	0.798[2,5]	−0.422[2,5]	0.253[2,4]

Level of significance for (r):
[1] $p < 0.01$.
[2] $p < 0.0001$.

Race differences:
[3] $p < 0.01$.
[4] $p < 0.001$.
[5] $p < 0.0001$.

209

Table 13–7. Frequency in hyperlipoproteinemia in children ages 5–14 years, as defined by the recommended upper normal limits[1]

Lipoprotein elevation	Frequency[2]	
	Blacks	Whites
Hyper-β-lipoproteinemia alone β-lipoprotein cholesterol > 170 mg/dl	0.5 (6)	0.5 (9)
Hyper-pre-β-lipoproteinemia alone pre-β-lipoprotein cholesterol > 25 mg/dl	1.7 (20)	4.7 (94)
Both β-lipoprotein cholesterol > 170 mg/dl pre-β-lipoprotein cholesterol > 25 mg/dl	0.1 (1)	0.1 (3)

[1]Fredrickson et al., 1967.
[2]Percent (number).

lipoproteinemia (pre-β-lipoprotein cholesterol level >25 mg/dl) without associated hyper-β-lipoproteinemia (Type IV). Combined hyperlipoproteinemia, with both β- and pre-β-lipoprotein cholesterol levels exceeding the cut-off points above, was seen in only 0.1% of black and 0.1% of white children. Although α-lipoprotein levels are not considered when classifying hyperlipoproteinemias, it should be mentioned that 62% of black children and 46% of white children exceeded the suggested upper limits for α-lipoprotein cholesterol (male: 65 mg/dl; female: 70 mg/dl) (Fredrickson et al., 1967).

COMMENT

A striking racial difference was observed in the lipoprotein makeup of these children with the black children having relatively higher α-lipoprotein levels and lower pre-β-lipoprotein levels than the white children. White children in the same group had lower serum cholesterol and higher triglyceride levels than did black children (Frerichs et al., 1976). The differences in pre-β-lipoprotein levels in these two groups seem to be in agreement with their triglyceride levels, since in the fasting state serum triglyceride exists predominantly as a component of pre-β-lipoprotein (Fredrickson et al., 1967; Nichols, 1967). The higher concentration of cholesterol observed in the black children could be attributed to the differences in their α-lipoprotein levels, because the β-lipoprotein levels were very similar in both groups. Although serum cholesterol is generally considered to reflect the β-lipoprotein concentrations (Fredrickson et al., 1967; Nichols, 1967), the present study as well as earlier studies clearly show the need for quantitating individual lipoprotein classes rather than extrapolating them from serum cholesterol and triglyceride values (Berenson et al., 1972b; Kwiterovich, 1974; Srinivasan et al., 1975a). Recently, Tyroler et al. (1975) reported that black adults had more α-lipoprotein cholesterol than did a comparable group of white adults. These observations suggest that the racial differences in lipoprotein makeup are likely to persist from childhood through adulthood.

The sex- and age-related changes in this group of children indicated a common tendency for girls to have higher β- and pre-β-lipoprotein and lower α-lipoprotein concentration than boys. The pre-β-lipoprotein showed a progressive increase with age, β-lipoprotein showed a slight tendency to decrease with age, especially between ages 11 and 14, and α-lipoprotein remained relatively unchanged. Dyerberg and Hjorne (1973) reported that though girls tended to have higher lipid and lipoprotein levels than did boys, the sex and age differences were generally indistinct. Kwiterovich et al. (1974) observed no age-related change in any of the lipoprotein fractions within sex, although β-lipoprotein cholesterol decreased slightly with age when the sexes were combined. The tendency for decrease in β-lipoprotein concentrations and pronounced increase in pre-β-lipoprotein concentrations around puberty could be due to the influence of gonadal hormones on lipid and lipoprotein metabolism (Furman et al., 1967; Salhanick et al., 1969; Barclay, 1972; Tyroler et al., 1975). It should be mentioned that a clear-cut pattern of age- and sex-dependent changes in the serum lipoprotein concentrations around puberty may be less apparent from a cross-sectional study because of the differences in sexual maturity among individuals of a given age group. The studies of Lee (1967) indicate that a distinct pattern of change can be observed when the lipid levels of individual children are examined longitudinally. (Our most recent studies, extended through age 17, show decreases of β- and α-lipoproteins to about the same extent, except in white males. The white boys show a relatively greater decrease of α-lipoproteins and beginning increase of β-lipoproteins, thus establishing the adult pattern).

It is apparent from this study that the age- and sex-related differences in individual lipoprotein classes differ markedly from the adult pattern. In general, adult males (above 20 years of age) show higher levels of pre-β- and β-lipoproteins and lower levels of α-lipoproteins than do females; the increase in pre-β-lipoprotein with age is more pronounced in males than in females (Fredrickson et al., 1967; Nichols, 1969; Barclay, 1972). The transition from the infantile to the adult pattern for lipoproteins has been reported to occur between the ages of 16 and 20 in males and after the age of 20 in females (Dyerberg and Hjorne, 1973), however, these observations were based on a limited number of persons from an undefined population. Further studies are needed to ascertain at what age the characteristic adult patterns of lipoprotein develop.

The level of α-lipoprotein (cholesterol) observed in children was consistently higher than that found in young adults 23–25 years of age (using the same methodology) (Berenson et al., 1974b; Kwiterovich, 1974). Interestingly, Kornerup (1950) found significantly higher phospholipid levels in children ages 1–15 than in adults above the age of 20, even though there were no significant differences in serum cholesterol levels between these two groups. Since α-lipoproteins are rich in phospholipids, the high levels found in children could reflect this class of lipoproteins. However, these observations are at variance with other studies using a heparin-Mn^{2+} precipitation method for quantitating α-lipoprotein cholesterol (Fredrickson et al., 1967; Kwiterovich et al., 1974). The use of Ca^{2+} or Mg^{2+} in the precipitation methods is more specific and quantitative than Mn^{2+}, which is known to coprecipitate other serum proteins, including α-lipoproteins (Burstein et al., 1970; Srinivasan et al., 1970b). More recent studies on serum lipoprotein–heparin interactions indicated that, among the subclasses of high-density lipoproteins (HDL), 40% of HDL_2 and 10% of HDL_3 could be precipitated in the presence of Mn^{2+} (Srinivasan et al., 1975b). Therefore, the degree of difference between methods using Ca^{2+} and those using Mn^{2+} is likely to be determined by the proportion of each of the HDL subclasses (HDL_1, HDL_2, and HDL_3) present in the sera.

The interrelationship among different classes of lipoproteins indicates that the α-lipoprotein level in serum is inversely proportional to both pre-β- and β-lipoprotein levels. This is in agreement with the findings in an adult population by Nichols (1969) and Miller and Miller (1975). The observed interrelationship among different classes of lipoproteins and lipids was attributed to the functional associations among the major classes of lipoproteins which apparently are related to the status of triglyceride metabolism (Nichols, 1969). Interestingly, the body (tissue) cholesterol pool increased with decreasing serum α-lipoprotein levels, and low levels of α-lipoprotein have been associated with the incidence of coronary artery disease (Miller and Miller, 1975).

SUMMARY

Serum lipoprotein profiles in 3,182 children, ages 5–14, were studied. White and black children showed similar mean levels of β-lipoproteins. Pre-β-lipoprotein levels, however, were significantly higher in white children, while significantly higher levels of α-lipoprotein were found in black children. Girls had generally higher levels of β- and pre-β-lipoprotein and lower levels of α-lipoprotein than boys, although the differences were not significant at each age group. A significant increase in pre-β-lipoprotein levels and a slight but significant decrease in α- and β-lipoprotein levels occurs between 11 and 14 years. (Subsequent studies extending to 17 years of age show an unusual decrease of α-lipoproteins in white males.) The correlation of α-lipoprotein was negative with β-lipoprotein, and even more so with pre-β-lipoprotein. The above inverse relationships were significantly greater in white children than in black children, suggesting differences in lipoprotein profiles in the two groups. Lipoprotein values from a total community study are now available for comparison with the currently recommended (World Health Organization) upper normal limits for lipoproteins.

V. Blood Pressure

14. Blood pressure in children—an overview

It is well known that general mortality rates increase exponentially with age, so that for each additional ten years the mortality rate approximately doubles (Grove and Hetzel, 1968). As age progresses, the distribution of causes of mortality shifts more and more toward the cardiovascular disease, including diabetes mellitus. Nearly two-thirds of all deaths in the United States are due to cardiovascular disorders. Hypertension plays a dominant role among the identified precursors of death. It is therefore important to describe the natural history of blood pressure levels to aid our understanding of the onset of essential hypertension at a stage when hypertension may still be reversible.

Among hypertensive pediatric patients from clinic populations, secondary hypertension is traditionally believed to be predominant. (Loggie, 1975; Dustan, 1976). However, recently, primary hypertension has been found to underlie elevated blood pressure in a large majority of children screened from a general population (Londe et al., 1971). Hence, secondary hypertension in the general population may be rare relative to primary hypertension even at a young age.

Hypertension in its early stages is poorly understood. Perhaps this is due partly to our limited understanding of the disease and its subclinical manifestations and to the scanty information concerning the time-course changes of blood pressure. Furthermore, since there is a lack of satisfactory criteria for diagnosis, the true prevalence of hyper-

217

tension in children remains to be established. For example, in contrast to the clinical and anatomic manifestations in adults, similar effects and early damage to tissue are undetectable in children. Simply stated, the *early natural history of primary hypertension*, the evolution from youth, needs to be investigated.

Determinants of blood pressure

High blood pressure is an important cause of decreased life expectancy and health (Society of Actuaries, 1959; Kannel, 1974), and in adulthood it seems to be associated in part with the preceding blood pressure levels of adolescence (Miall and Lovell, 1967; Mathewson et al., 1972; Harlan et al., 1973; Miall and Chinn, 1973). Therefore, an assessment of the association of hypertension with potential determinants during adolescence may suggest preventive measures. What induces long-term changes in blood pressure as the body grows? What causes the blood pressure to rise during growth and development? Answers to these questions may not only delineate the criteria needed to assess the existence of subsequent hypertension, but may identify health determinants as well.

In analyzing the long-term correlates of human blood pressure control, it is necessary to distinguish conceptually between those blood pressure determinants for which other factors compensate within minutes or hours after their impact, resulting in negative feedback control, and those upon which the blood pressure equilibrium finally depends (Guyton et al., 1974). The latter, which determine the basal or fundamental blood pressure level, are of interest here, since in youth the basal blood pressure seems to predict future hypertension better than casual blood pressures (Harlan et al., 1973).

To search for possible determinants of blood pressure in the growing child, we attempted to measure basal blood pressures in children by systematic avoidance of anxiety states. We attempted to reduce the influence of the emotional state of the child on blood pressure by a. elaborate preliminary information and demonstration, b. a network of local volunteers as guides, c. sedentary waiting periods between the multiple measurements, d. observers trained for comparability of reading and intent upon creating a continuously friendly and relaxed atmosphere, e. encouraging the children to void prior to the blood pressure measurements, and f. observance of the blood pressure at the end of a sequence of other examinations. Replicability and validity of measurment were emphasized. Similar general principles apply in an office setting to obtain resting and relaxed blood pressure measurements.

Methods of Measurement

The evolution of blood pressure in a child below the age of six years is largely unknown, since blood pressure for the preschool population has rarely been assessed. In this age group the methodology of indirect blood pressure measurement is crucial: Korotkoff sounds are barely audible by stethoscope, cuff bladder size has a larger impact on the blood pressure reading than in older subjects, and the child's mood—a strong determinant of measured blood pressure—is less easily controlled. Clearly, some degree of automation in the blood pressure measurement of this age group would be beneficial.

At school age, the methodology becomes simpler: the Korotkoff sounds are loud enough for the stethoscope in conjunction with the mercury sphygmomanometer, and the child is able to sit still at this age so that recordings with automatic equipment become feasible.

"Tracking" of blood pressure

Clearly, not only the long-term but also the shorter-term variations of blood pressure levels in children need to be elucidated. The nature of such changes is not known; they may relate to the development of essential hypertension. Although hospital-based clinicians have repeatedly stated that essential hypertension is rare in children, evidence is evolving that essential hypertension begins in childhood (Londe et al., 1971). Our own observations suggest that primary hypertension begins early in life. Conversely, it may be assumed that prevention of essential hypertension would be more successful if the disease process were aborted in an early stage. If "tracking" of blood pressure occurs (i.e., if the child's relative rank of blood pressure among his peers remains constant) an early stage of hypertension becomes diagnosable, provided due attention is given to the details of measurement methodology. Obviously then, documentation of tracking of blood pressure in children has direct clinical application. Our studies (Webber et al, 1979b) along with others show that tracking does begin early in life. Our observations also indicate that with several blood pressure observations, a very high prediction of future levels is possible.

Determinants of essential hypertension

What are the determinants of essential hypertension? According to Miall et al. (1968), a distinction in determinants of hypertension can be made between (a) conditioning factors acting in childhood and adolescence and (b) perpetuating factors acting later in life. The distinct shift in the trend of blood pressure levels at the age of incipient adult stature (Fig. 14–1) (Stocks, 1924; Robinson and Brucer, 1939;

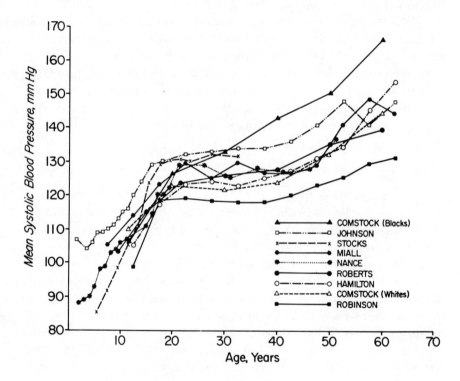

Figure 14–1. Blood pressure surveys of populations containing both children and adults. In all surveys, systolic blood pressure distinctly levels out at the age of incipient adult stature (ages 18–20). Later in life the blood pressure rise follows an almost exponential pattern. This example shows data for males. Females show similar changes.

Hamilton et al., 1954; Comstock, 1957; Nance et al., 1965; Miall and Lovell, 1967; Johnson et al., 1973; Roberts and Maurer, 1976) supports the concept of early conditioning factors and later perpetuation of hypertension.

Interest in basal blood volume as a long-term determinant of blood pressure dates back to Aygen and Braunwald (1962) and Borst and Borst (1963), who studied Starling's Law of the Heart in this context. Guyton et al. (1973) supported this concept more recently. The above-described shift in the trend of blood pressure level during the age when bone growth ceases fits the postulate of a major influence of basal blood volume on blood pressure levels at a young age. Obviously many factors are involved and these have been detailed by Guyton (1977).

Applications of studies of children

Although the concepts listed above should be subject to testing by epidemiologic studies, the lack of uniformity in the methodology of blood pressure measurement remains a stumbling block. A variety of large studies of American children have shown vast discrepancies (Fig. 14–2; Table 14–1) (Faber and James, 1921; Graham et al., 1945; Moss and Adams, 1962; Johnson et al., 1965; Londe, 1968). "Standard" grids of blood pressure by age were recently introduced as a guide for the practicing physician (Blumenthal et al., 1977). The objective of encouraging pediatricians to take blood pressures in children is important, but the observations are only as good as the methodology used to collect the data (Berenson et al., 1978b). Suggested methods of measurement are listed in the Appendix at the end of the chapter (Nuessle, 1957; Ertel et al., 1966; King, 1967; Pickering, 1968; Golden et al., 1974; Voors, 1975; Corns, 1976), and representative levels from our studies are given in the Appendix at the end of the book.

Studies of blood pressure in a total population of children are critical to understanding the early natural history of hypertension. Since hypertension is so common in the adult population and can be defined by accepted criteria, it becomes necessary to look at free-living children, especially over time, in an effort to observe the early onset of hypertension and to be able to define essential hypertension as a disease in early life.

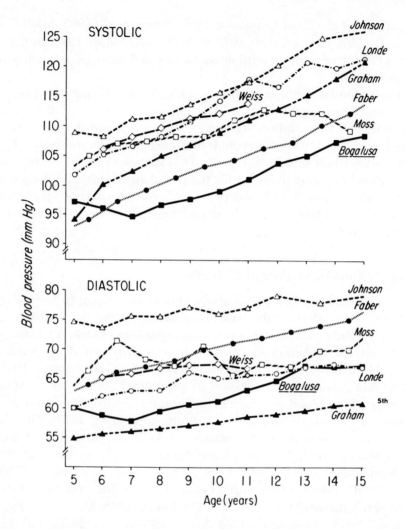

Figure 14–2. Comparison of indirect blood pressure measurements of white school children, by age, among selected studies in the literature. Graham used the fifth Korotkoff phase for determining diastolic blood pressure. The other studies used either fourth or a combination of fourth and fifth Korotkoff phases. The low values obtained on the Bogalusa children suggest a relaxed state. Such observations are quite reproducible and aid in following levels over time.

Table 14–1. Characteristics of selected population studies of blood pressure in children

	Faber and James (1921)	Graham et al. (1945)	Johnson et al. (1965)	Moss and Adams (1962)	Weiss et al. (1973)	Londe (1968)
Population	School children	Chisholm, Minn. school children	Tecumseh, Mich. community		Representative sample of U.S.	Office, clinic
Place of examination	Office?	School	Office?	Office?	Mobile Office	Office
Age	3–17	5–16	<1–80	2–18	6–11	3–15
N	1,101	3,580 (annually repeated)	8,380	1,022	7,119	1,593
Position of examinee	Seated	Seated	Seated?	Seated?	Supine	Supine
First Korotkoff phase	X	X	X	X[2]	X	X
Fourth Korotkoff phase	X		X	X	—[3]	—[3]
Fifth Korotkoff phase		X	X	X	X	X

[1] Health Examination Survey, National Center for Health Statistics.
[2] Adjusted according to height and arm circumference of child.
[3] Recorded only if fifth Korotkoff phase was not obtainable.

Our observations of a biracial population are also beginning to detect subtle differences between the black and white children and between children with high and low levels that reflect on the multiple mechanisms—renal, hormonal, and neurogenic—involved in controlling blood pressure (Berenson et al., 1979a; Voors et al, 1979b). The recognition of these differences may aid in identifying children susceptible to hypertension and in understanding mechanisms related to the high incidence of the disease in blacks (Berenson et al., 1979d).

RECOMMENDATIONS FOR OBSERVING BLOOD PRESSURES IN CHILDREN

The need to record basal blood pressure

The factors controlling blood pressure in the healthy person can be divided into at least two groups: a. factors that influence the pressure over short time intervals (reactions to immediate external influences, over the long term counterbalanced by negative feedback mechanisms—Guyton et al., 1974) and b. factors that influence the pressure on a sustained basis. The latter group determines the pressure taken under resting, basal conditions.

Since the basal pressure in adolescents and young adults seems a better predictor of essential hypertension in adulthood than "casual" blood pressure (Smirk, 1957; Harlan et al., 1973), we prefer to measure blood pressure under simulated basal conditions rather than depend upon casual observations. The latter are often influenced by undefined stresses experienced by a child under conditions in a physician's office. Such conditions, however, can be modified. Our own measurements of children resulted in mean values approaching known clinical basal values for children of comparable ages (Voors et al., 1976), and indicate that similar measurements can be obtained in actual practice in school or office setting.

Considerable tracking of blood pressure has been noted, especially with the observations of relaxed or basal-like measurements. Consequently, the occurrence early in life of essential hypertension as a disease is likely. It then becomes important to record blood pressures of children whenever practical. The initial entry into elementary school seems a useful time, and observations should be obtained whenever a child is subsequently examined. The importance of serial observations over time must be emphasized. Although in this text the data presented are of relaxed-resting values, which are most useful because of reproducibility and better predictive values, pressure variability from moment to moment under daily living conditions would also be useful.

Attention to examination, environment, and selection of examiners

Certain conditions attendant to recording blood pressures in children are needed to obtain consistent, basal blood pressure readings. A relaxed and unhurried atmosphere is important. One key aspect is to familiarize the child in advance, reducing the anxiety associated with the measurement procedure and the anticipation of other examination procedures. Completeing other examination procedures before blood pressure is recorded and seeing other children examined similarly may help relax a child. A female nurse is preferable as the blood pressure examiner.

Prior to his blood pressure measurements, the child should be allowed to void. The observations should be interspaced by pauses and occasional elevation of the arm to diminish venous engorgement. Obtaining repeated measurements is important. If the first one or two measurements is more than 2–3 mm Hg higher than subsequent readings, further measurements should be recorded. It is not unusual for a specific observer to affect the patient so that blood pressure readings are higher because of that interaction. A "white coat" anxiety often occurs when blood pressures are recorded by a hurried physician. Consequently, recordings in a relaxed atmosphere by a female observer may yield results that approach a resting state. Of utmost importance is the training of examiners in the art of recording indirect blood pressure readings.

Validity and precision of blood pressure measurement

Choice of instrument. For children approximately 7 years of age and older, routine use of the mercury sphygmomanometer in conjunction with a bell stethoscope is acceptable for obtaining valid measurements. However, in younger and smaller children, although reproducible blood pressures can be obtained, the stethoscope and sphyg-momanometer method has several disadvantages: a. the audible Korotkoff phases are difficult to distinguish because of the reduced intensity of the sounds; b. the low-frequency "sounds" from the artery under the cuff are relatively more important at low pressures and are not audible by the stethoscope (especially when a diaphragm stethoscope is used); and c. the relative narrowness of the rubber cuff bladder—due to the necessity to leave space for the stethoscope at the elbow crease—results in over-reading of the pressure, especially when pressures are low. In our observations of preschool-age children with an instrument using the Doppler effect, the blood pressure levels were also suggested to be spuriously high (Chapter 15). For these reasons we recommend using the Infrasonde (Marion Scientific Corp., Costa Mesa, Calif.) for ages 6 years and younger. Although not ideal, reasonable indirect systolic blood pressures can be obtained with the aid of a low-frequency transducer. Unfortunately, excessively low diastolic levels were obtained using this instrument in the preschool-age group. We feel reliable indirect blood pressures can be obtained in children beginning around 7 years of age with the standard equipment.

Choice of cuff size. Standard Baumanometer cuffs (W. A. Baum Co., Inc., Copiague, N.J.) are now available with calibrations to warn the physician when the arm circumference is too large for the cuff size. We recommend using the "adult-size" cuff *below* the "acceptable range" as printed on the cuff, and switching to "large adult-size" as soon as the calibration is *within* the "acceptable range" (although we are in favor of this method of calibration, longer and wider cuff bladders are needed than those defined in the "acceptable range"). The Infrasonde provides an "adult-size" cuff with a built-in bladder which we found satisfactory for children, three to five years old, provided that sponge rubber is adapted around the transducer to equalize the pressure exerted by the cuff on the skin.

Choice of diastolic Korotkoff phase. In children, we were unable to obtain consistently reproducible results with the fifth Korotkoff phase. The fifth-phase values were approximately 19 mm Hg less than fourth-phase values. Fifth-phase values included some 6% of children for whom no discrete fifth phase was recorded due to sounds persisting to 0 mm Hg. Although simultaneous indirect and direct measurements in children have been inadequately compared, some studies have suggested that the fourth-phase measurements may more closely approximate intra-arterial values. Our nurses recorded both fourth- and fifth-phase values when possible and obtained reasonably reproducible results for both, but fourth-phase values were consistent. We therefore recommend use of the fourth phase. For self-evaluation, it is helpful to record both phases routinely. A more detailed discussion on the choice of diastolic Korotkoff sounds is given in Chapter 6.

Decreasing the measurement error. Various steps are recommended to decrease measurement error in recording indirect blood pressures. These are listed in an Appendix at the end of this chapter. Taken together, these steps should decrease the likelihood of misclassifying a child, especially for purposes of managing elevated blood pressure levels. In the Bogalusa Heart Study we observed that the measurement error was about 4 mm mercury for both systolic and diastolic pressures. An approximate 95% confidence interval around the level of 100/65 (average of three readings) should be from 105/70 to 95/60 mm Hg.

Need for replicate measurements

Repeated measurements taken during a single examination are needed not only to insure a relaxed state during the measurements, but also to avoid recording fluctuations of pressures. In our study, we recorded three measurements by each of three nurses, two using mercury sphygmomanometers and the third using an automatic instrument. For practical purposes it would seem that three blood pressure readings by one nurse, or preferably replicate readings by two nurses, would obtain a good approximation of the child's blood pressure at one point in time.

APPENDIX TO CHAPTER 14
SUGGESTED METHODS TO DECREASE MEASUREMENT ERROR

INSTRUMENT
Maintenance. Check the functioning of blood pressure instruments at regular intervals, and perform required maintenance (Corns, 1976).

Adjust mercury. In case the amount of mercury in the sphygmomanometer reservoir needs adjustment, use a plastic syringe or a medicine dropper and add mercury (Corns, 1976).

Recalibrate aneroid manometer. Recalibrate the aneroid manometer frequently with a mercury column. A reserve manometer is useful (Corns, 1976).

Correct cuff bladder size. A choice of rubber cuff bladder sizes is needed. Use the widest size that fits the particular arm. Each bladder should have sufficient length for its width. These precautions will help avoid excessively high pressure readings (King, 1967; Voors, 1975).

Application of cuff to arm. When using the instrument, apply the deflated rubber bladder and cuff evenly and snugly around the arm, in order to avoid excessively high pressure readings (Nuessle, 1956).

Stethoscope acoustics. Use either a bell stethoscope without diaphragm or an electronic transducer with amplification of the 10–80 Hz band in order to increase the audibility of the crucial low-frequency components of the Korotkoff sounds. These are weak in young children (Ertel et al., 1966; Golden et al., 1974).

EXAMINER

Audiometric testing. Perform audiometry tests on examiners of blood pressures. Avoid selection of examiners with impaired hearing in the frequency range of the Korotkoff sounds.

Self-instruction. Acquire instructional audio tape of normal Korotkoff sounds (Ravin, distributed by Merck, Sharp and Dohme) to avoid misinterpretation of sounds.

Auscultatory pause. Avoid misdiagnosis of an auscultatory pause through proper inflation techniques; include pulse palpation.

Venous engorgement. Avoid softness of the Korotkoff sounds due to venous engorgement of the lower arm, by elevating the arm, exercising the forearm muscles, repositioning the arm, and rapidly reinflating the cuff bladder.

Avoid parallax. Maintain eye level at the mercury meniscus or with the aneroid needle, in order to avoid misreading due to parallax.

Hydrostatic pressure error. Keep the patient's brachial artery at the heart level in order to avoid bias in pressure measurement due to the weight of the blood.

Child diastolic pressure. The fourth Korotkoff phase in measuring the diastolic pressure of children is recommended.

EXAMINEE

Urinary bladder pressor effect. Urge child to void before blood pressure is measured. An elevation of blood pressure can be caused by distension of the urinary bladder (Pickering, 1968).

Child apprehension. Efforts should be made to reduce apprehension. Keep the examination nonthreatening by removing objects associated with pain and discomfort. Demonstrate the measurement procedure ahead of time. Take multiple measurements interspaced by 1- or 2-min pauses. Use a female examiner in a relaxed environment, and allow the child to see examinations on other children, if possible.

Intrasubject variability. Take several measurements and base level on measurements taken at serial examinations. This will avoid misdiagnosis due to the variability of the child's pressure.

15. Blood pressure in preschool-age children

A description of blood pressure in the growing child could provide clues to the early development of essential hypertension. After the age of 6, the increase in pressure with time appears constant until adult stature is reached; then the pressure curve levels off, to rise again in later life (Stocks, 1924; Robinson and Brucer, 1939; Hamilton et al., 1954; Comstock, 1957; Johnson et al., 1965; Nance et al., 1965; Miall and Lovell, 1967; Weiss et al., 1973; Roberts and Maurer, 1976). Clearly, there must be differences in blood pressure determinants between childhood and adulthood (Miall et al., 1968).

The evolution of blood pressure in a child below the age of 6 is largely unknown, since blood pressure for the preschool populations has rarely been assessed. Robinow et al. (1939), interpreting data on indirect measurements, believe that blood pressure between ages 1 and 12 years remains relatively constant. Allen-Williams (1945) found that children age 4 and 5 had higher systolic pressures by 3 mm mercury and equal diastolic pressures compared to children age 1 and 2.

This chapter presents the distribution characteristics of blood pressure in preschool-age children as assessed by various indirect methods, examines the relationship of blood pressure to other body characteristics, and evaluates the observations in relationship to the early natural history of essential hypertension.

LIMITATIONS OF RECORDING INDIRECT BLOOD PRESSURE IN PRESCHOOLERS

The inflatable bladder in the arm cuff should be sufficiently wide (Hansen and Stickler, 1966) and long (Voors, 1975) as indicated by studies of school children. Yet, it is likely that the lower the blood pressure level, the stronger the exaggerating effect of a small cuff bladder on blood pressure readings, especially since the upper arm tends to be short and chubby at this age (Breit and O'Rourke, 1974; Voors, 1975; Voors et al., 1976). The irritability of the child does not encourage an even, snug, and tight application of the deflated cuff bladder around the arm, and this may further exaggerate the pressure readings (Nuessle, 1956). The strong influence of emotions at this age almost precludes obtaining near-basal blood pressure levels.

The crucial changes in vascular sound components, occurring when the periarterial pressure is in the range of systolic and diastolic pressures, have frequencies mainly in the 10–80 Hz band (Golden et al., 1974). These sounds are virtually filtered out by the stiff diaphragm of the stethoscope (Johnston and Kline, 1940; Ertel et al., 1966) and are insufficiently audible through the bell stethoscope. The problem is even more acute at lower levels of blood pressure, as occur in shock and at the preschool age (Whitcher, 1969; Maurer and Noordergraaf, 1976). These considerations make selective electronic amplification of the 10–80 Hz Korotkoff sound components desirable for instrumentation in obtaining blood pressures at this age.

METHODS

Variation of children. The examinations in Bogalusa were similar to those described in Chapters 2 and 6 for school-age children. Emphasis was placed on a quiet atmosphere designed to keep the child relaxed and free from anxiety. The examination included approximately 25–30 children per day; the children received a physical examination, and blood samples were taken for analysis of lipids and hemoglobin. Blood pressure measurement was the final examination procedure, at which time the mood of the child was rated from 0 to 8, respectively, for asleep, lethargic, hypoactive, calm, alert, hyperactive, irritable, excessively frightened, and crying. This was done separately for each in-

strument. The various measurements and methods of observation are
described in detail elsewhere (Berenson et al., 1978a).

Flow of blood pressure examinations and instruments. Blood pressure was measured in a designated random order at each of three separate stations. Each station used a different instrument—the mercury
sphygomanometer, the Infrasonde 3000 (Marion Scientific Corp.,
Costa Mesa, Calif.), and the Arteriosonde 1010 (Roche Medical Electronics, Inc., Cranbury, N.J.). As discussed above, the Korotkoff
phases are difficult to discern in this age group; hence we included
two electronic instruments with transducers and amplification of the
vascular sounds and the Korotkoff signals. The Infrasonde 3000 amplifies the 10–80 Hz component of the sound spectrum with a low-frequency transducer, and the Arteriosonde 1010 amplifies the entire
audible range of the sound spectrum through the Doppler effect. Both
instruments produce audible signals by loudspeaker or earphone and
indicate cuff pressure by an aneroid manometer. To decrease the time
of examination, two teams were used, each team having three stations.
Both observers and children were randomly allocated to the teams and
to the three stations within each team. Three readings were made with
each instrument, totaling nine measurements per child. For each reading, first, fourth, and fifth Korotkoff phases were recorded.

Cuff bladder problems. For each instrument, the size of the rubber
cuff bladder was selected as large as feasible to avoid a small-cuff artifact (Table 15–1). For the sphygmomanometer, the width of the cuff
bladder is restricted by the need for free space for the stethoscope at
the elbow skin crease. Since the transducers used by both electronic
instruments for Korotkoff signal pickup have flat surfaces, they can be
slipped between the skin and the cuff, and hence permit the width of
the bladder to cover the elbow. The transducers of the electronic instruments, about 6 mm thick, were not flush with the inner surface of
the cuff bladder, and this thickness could produce a local compression
and influence the pressure readings. Therefore, sponge rubber was
adapted to encircle the transducers. This rubber was at the center of
equal thickness as the transducer (6 mm), and tapered off to zero mm
toward the periphery of the bladder.

Analysis. To observe relationships of these blood pressure levels to

Table 15–1. Cuff Bladder Selection for Children, Ages 2½–5½ years

Instrument	Upper-arm length[1](cm)	Bladder dimensions (cm)
Hg sphygmomanometer	16.9	5.8 × 17.8
	17.0–21.9	7.0 × 21.6[2]
	22.0+	9.5 × 21.6
Infrasonde	All	13.0 × 23.5
Arteriosonde	All	9.5 × 21.6[2]

[1]Acromion-olecranon distance measured by anthropometric caliper.
[2]Nonstandard cuff bladder sizes.

the other characteristics measured, the latter were entered as independent variables into a multiple regression analysis with blood pressure as the dependent variable. This was done separately for systolic and diastolic (fourth phase) pressures on each instrument.

In order to study the validity of the measurements by the three instruments, the difference between mean instrument readings for each child was assessed for pairs of instruments (Arteriosonde-Infrasonde, Sphygmomanometer-Arteriorsonde, Sphygmomanometer-Infrasonde) and entered as the dependent variable in a multiple regression analysis, using as independent variables those measured characteristics which conceptually relate to blood pressure (Voors, 1975).

The results were compared to those from the same geographic population of school-age children (Voors et al., 1976) to see whether the results in both age groups were biologically consistent.

GENERAL OBSERVATIONS

Levels of blood pressure

The use of three different instruments in this survey allowed observations on the attributes of each. *A priori* advantages and disadvantages of each instrument type have been noted.

Pressures by age. Mean blood pressures are plotted against age for the three instruments (Fig. 15–1). For both systolic and diastolic (fourth phase), Infrasonde pressures were the lowest and the sphygmomano-

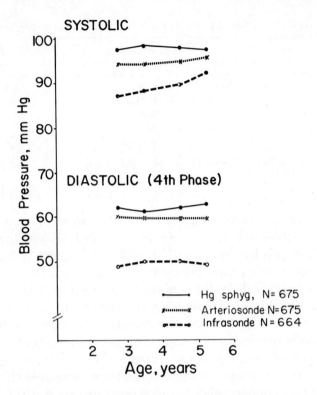

Figure 15–1. Comparison of mean blood pressure in children, ages 2½–5½ years, as measured on three instruments. This graph does not take into account the mood of the children, which was more excitable at the younger age. Controlling for mood, therefore, tends to increase the slopes.

meter pressures were the highest. The difference in mean readings of blood pressure levels between each pair of instruments is statistically significant ($p < 0.001$, F-test), both for systolic and for diastolic pressures. An unequivocal age gradient is shown only for the systolic pressures on the Infrasonde.

A comparison of blood pressure percentiles between children age 2½–5½ years and 5–14 years is given in Figure 15–2 for two categories of instruments: a. the sphygmomanometer and b. the electronic instruments with the infrasonic transducers: the Physiometrics automatic blood pressure recorder (Sphygmetrics, Inc., Woodland Hills, Calif.) for the school-age child and the Infrasonde for the preschool-age. (The Infrasonde, a nonrecording instrument, was used since au-

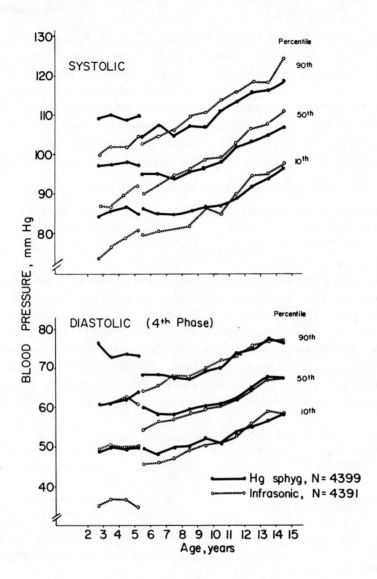

Figure 15–2. Comparison of blood pressures obtained with a low-frequency transducer with those recorded with a mercury sphygmomanometer in children ages 2½–14 years.

tomatic recording is difficult at this young age.) Beginning at age two, the infrasonic readings, systolic and diastolic, show consistent increases with increasing age. The sphygmomanometer readings, on the other hand, show U-shaped curves, rising only after the age of eight years. On both instruments the diastolic blood pressure variability is higher at the young age. Slight discontinuities in means between the two groups of children may be attributed to the fact that they were not examined simultaneously, and also that different instruments were used.

Correlates of blood pressure. The results of regression analysis of the blood pressure data with the various other characteristics (listed in Table 15–2) are presented in Table 15–3, which shows in order of decreasing magnitude all effects significant at the 0.01 level. The mood score had a universal effect with a magnitude of 2 mm mercury systolic pressure per scoring unit and 1 mm mercury diastolic (fourth phase) pressure per scoring unit. Some measure of body mass was the second most consistent correlate of blood pressure. There was no association with age, nor with serum lipids. For the diastolic sphygmomanometer pressure readings, individuality of observer had a notable effect. The large effect on systolic Arteriosonde pressures by Observer 3 was likely caused by technical misuse of the instrument. Together,

Table 15–2. Independent variables for multiple regression analysis

Demographic	Age
	Race[1]
	Sex[1]
Anthropometric	Height
	Ponderosity[2] = weight/height^3
	Upper-arm circumference[2]
	Triceps skinfold thickness[2]
Mood	Score ranging from *asleep* to *crying*
Laboratory	Total cholesterol[2]
	Triglycerides[2]
	Pre-β-lipoprotein[2]
	β-lipoprotein[2]
	Pre-β-lipoprotein + β-lipoprotein[2]
	Pre-β-lipoprotein/(pre-β + β-lipoprotein)[2]
	Hemoglobin
Blood pressure observers[1]	

[1]Entered as dummy variables.
[2]Logarithmic transformation.

Table 15–3. Stepwise multiple regression[1] of blood pressure on three instruments, in children ages 2½–5½ years

Instrument	Systolic	Diastolic (fourth phase)
Hg	Mood	Observer 8
sphygmo.	Arm circumference	Observer 7
	Observer 3	Mood
	Observer 7	Arm circumference
	Total cholesterol	Observer 3
		−Observer 1[2]
	$R^2 = 0.18$	$R^2 = 0.25$
Infrasonde	Mood	−Observer 2[2]
	Height	−Observer 8[2]
	−Observer 4	Mood
	Observer 6	Arm circumference
	Sex	
	$R^2 = 0.25$	$R^2 = 0.13$
Arteriosonde	Mood	Mood
	Observer 3	−Observer8[2]
	Arm circumference	Arm circumference
	−Observer 8[2]	Observer 3
	Height	Hemoglobin
		Black race
		−Observer 2[2]
	$R^2 = 0.29$	$R^2 = 0.21$

[1]Independent variable listed in order of acceptance by model.
[2]Negative regression slope.

these characteristics could explain 12 to 25 % of the pressure variability, considerably less than observed for the school-age children.

Correlates of instrument differences. In order to compare the measurements by the three instruments, the difference between mean instrument reading for each child was assessed for each pair of instruments. This difference was entered as the dependent variable in a new multiple regression analysis. We used certain characteristics of conceptual relevance, as independent variables: systolic pressure average for the combined instruments, diastolic average, triceps skinfold thickness, percent of arm circumference not covered by the shortest cuff bladder, percent of the upper-arm length not covered by the narrowest bladder (the "narrowness of this bladder"), and race.

We found that narrowness of the Baumanometer cuff bladders correlated positively with a relative excess in pressure readings. In one

instance, triceps skinfold thickness also correlated with this difference. These correlations, although statistically significant, explained
only 4–7% of the variability in pressure.

COMMENT

The different levels of blood pressure recorded with different instruments show the difficulty in obtaining valid measurements at this age.
The crucial changes of the arterial sounds under the deflating cuff
bladder occur in the 10–80 Hz component of the sound spectrum and
are of low intensity (Ertel et al., 1966; Ur and Gordon, 1970). Because
the Infrasonde amplifies this part of the sound spectrum, and because it permits use of the largest bladder size, which improves measurement validity, readings from the Infrasonde seem *a priori* to be
the most valid of the three instruments used, at least for systolic pressures.

We found that besides mood score, some measure of body size is a
correlate of blood pressure in this preschool-age population. The relationship to height and weight conforms to our observations on the
school-age children (Voors et al., 1977b). A gradual rise in the basal
blood pressure from birth to the attainment of a mature adult stature,
as found by readings of the Infrasonde, is *a priori* more likely than a
sudden rise after birth to levels equal to those of adolescents, as produced by the mercury sphygmomanometer (Robinow et al., 1939).

For the purpose of strict comparability of examination flow between
the school-age children (Voors et al., 1976) and the present preschool-
age population, venipuncture was performed early in the examination
and blood pressure assessment later. In a separate study (unpublished) in which blood pressure was measured both before and after
the venipuncture, we have assessed the impact of the venipuncture
both on the child's mood and on the blood pressure while controlling
for mood. We found that the mood was affected: the mood was more
excitable after the venipuncture, and, controlling for mood, the average increment in systolic blood pressure was 4.5 mm Hg; for diastolic
pressure this increment was 1.5 mm Hg.

The study of blood pressure in preschool-age children can yield
clues to the etiology of essential hypertension. Basal blood pressures
are difficult to measure at this age, apparently partly because the
child's mood varies during the examination. Both mercury sphygmo-

manometric and automatic blood pressure measurements are more difficult to obtain in preschool than in older children; nevertheless we found a relationship between weight or body size and blood pressure. In the future we hope to assess whether relatively high blood pressure in these children predicts future hypertension, since we did find considerable tracking in school children, even in those as young as five years of age (Voors et al., 1979a); whereas others have found that higher blood pressure levels in young adults determine future hypertension (Paffenbarger et al., 1968; Harlan et al., 1973; Sneiderman et al., 1976).

It is possible to obtain reproducible observations, at the preschool age, but further studies are needed to determine valid levels. It is important to obtain measurements in these children since this age seems to denote a strategic stage in this disease process.

SUMMARY

Eighty percent of all identified children 2$^1/_2$–5$^1/_2$ years old in a total geographic community were examined for cardiovascular disease risk factor variables, including blood pressure, anthropometric measurements, and blood lipids. Blood pressure was measured by three instrument types, each with three readings, according to a rigid, randomized design. Results from the three instruments were compared, and potential biases for each instrument are listed. The Infrasonde, which amplifies lower sound frequency components, has the theoretical advantage of best Korotkoff phase discrimination. Both automatic instruments permit use of over-sized cuff bladders.

All observations on the children were analyzed by multiple regression with blood pressure as the dependent variable. After controlling for the mood of the child, we found that some index of body size was positively related to blood pressure, whereas age, race, and serum lipids were not consistently related.

The basal or fundamental reference blood pressure is likely to rise gradually from birth to the age of incipient adult stature, and to be linearly related to height and to log weight. More information is needed on young children—particularly changes observed over time—to relate blood pressure levels in childhood to the early natural history of essential hypertension.

16. Blood pressure levels in school-age children

The measurement of blood pressure in a young age segment of a total geographic American community, especially of the school age, offers the opportunity of delineating normative values specific for age, race, and sex, and serves as a background for observing early hypertension in a free-living population. At the same time, a community-wide study of blood pressure offers the opportunity for concomitantly describing other characteristics that act as determinants of blood pressure. This chapter describes detailed blood pressure measurements on a biracial population of children, ages 5 through 14 years. The age group is a convenient one from the standpoint of a survey and reproducible and probably valid indirect blood pressure measurements can be obtained at this time. Further, the age seems to be one optimum for consideration of methods of primary intervention of hypertension in a general population.

Instruments

During the school year 1973–74, indirect blood pressures were obtained on 3,524 children ages 5–14 by the mercury sphygmomanometer (Baumanometer) and by the Physiometrics automatic blood pressure recorder. The automatic instrument is an electronic infrasonic device that records on a paper disk rotated by an aneroid manometer in open communication with an oversized rubber cuff bladder entirely encircling the upper arm. Selection of the bladder sizes for the Baumanometer cuff was based on arm measurement criteria recommended by Karvonen et al. (1964), Simpson et al. (1965), and King (1967), but with the restrictions that are commonly available bladders were used and that shorter arms require a narrower cuff in order to leave room for the stethoscope at the elbow skin crease (see appendix at end of chapter).

Blood pressure measurement

The children were encouraged to void before the blood pressures were measured, and volunteer workers guided them through a designated random sequence for examination. The blood pressure was determined for each child by three trained observers in the randomized sequence, each observer independently measuring three consecutive blood pressures per child. Although all of the blood pressure observers were white, black and white staff and volunteer escorts participated in the examinations. Two of these observers each used a well-illuminated mercury sphygmomanometer placed at eye level and the third a Physiometrics recorder; each instrument was assigned randomly on a daily basis, as were the observers to the instruments. The Physiometrics instrument was calibrated daily before use with the mercury column of the sphygmomanometer. Under quiet conditions, in a screened-off corner, observers recorded the first and fourth Korotkoff phases to determine the right-arm blood pressure while each child was resting and seated. The fifth phase was also recorded with sphygmomanometer readings, but these readings were less consistent and are not part of this report (but are discussed in Chapter 6). Care was taken to cover the brachial artery with the center of the rubber bladder. Physiometrics disks were read blindly by the same observer throughout the entire study period.

Analysis

In order to describe the detailed observations of blood pressure for the large population of children, certain questions were asked: a. What are the blood pressure levels related to age, race, and sex? b. Among all variables measured, which have a statistically significant effect on blood pressure? c. What variables relate to the differences in observations between the sphygmomanometer and the automatic Physiometrics recorder?

Measures of central tendency and dispersion of blood pressure levels by age, race, and sex subgroups were compared. An apparent difference in racial prevalence within the highest 5% of blood pressure ranks was tested by chi-square technique.

A multiple regression analysis was conducted with individual mean levels of blood pressure as the dependent variable and all other measured variables of relevance as independent variables. Logarithmic transformation was applied to independent variables except for age, height, hemoglobin, maturation, and the nominal variables. A ponderosity index (weight/height^3) was chosen as a measure of obesity because of its high correlation with body fatness (Allen et al., 1956). The logarithm of the ponderosity index was used in place of the logarithm of weight as an independent variable, in order to avoid artifacts resulting from the highly positive correlation between height and weight. For the same reason, the logarithm of triceps skinfold thickness, which is highly correlated with the ponderosity index and with weight, was not entered in the final analysis.

The difference between readings by sphygmomanometer and Physiometrics techniques was analyzed by selecting this difference as a dependent variable in a multiple regression analysis.

OBSERVATIONS

Levels of blood pressure and variation by age, sex, and race

The mean and standard error of mercury sphygmomanometer blood pressures for the children by age and sex are given in Figure 16–1. The relatively higher levels in 5- and 6-year-old children may be attributed to a small-cuff artifact (see Comment below). Since the difference in blood pressure between the sexes was not impressive (except for systolic pressures in the older children), the values for both sexes are combined in the remaining figures. Tables 16–1 and 16–2 give summary statistics for mercury sphygmomanometer systolic and diastolic pressures by age for all children studied (race and sex combined), including mean, standard deviation, percentiles, and range.

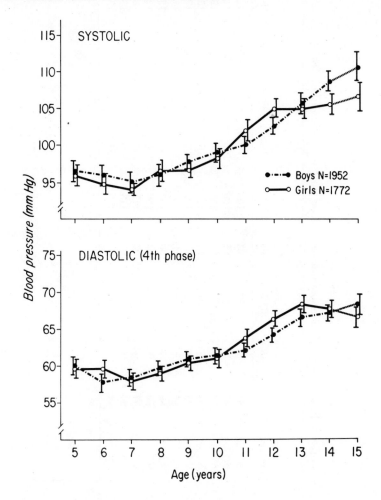

Figure 16–1. Mean mercury sphygmomanometric blood pressures ±2 S.E. in school children, by age, for boys and girls.

Blood pressure obtained by automatic instrument

Blood pressures by age and race obtained on the Physiometrics instrument are indicated in Figure 16–2. A difference clearly exists between the races for all ages by this instrument.

The difference in measurement between the two instruments (Fig. 16–3) is larger for black than for white children. Racial differences in

Table 16–1. Distribution characteristics of systolic mercury sphygmomanometric blood pressures of children by age

Age (at last birthday)	Number of children[1]	Mean	Standard deviation	Percentiles							Min	Max
				5th	10th	25th	50th	75th	90th	95th		
5	274	96.2	8.2	84	87	90	95	102	105	112	76	126
6	302	95.4	8.6	83	85	89	95	100	108	112	75	128
7	311	94.6	8.4	82	85	88	94	100	105	109	75	125
8	336	96.3	8.7	83	85	91	96	101	107	114	76	128
9	351	97.2	8.2	85	87	92	97	102	107	111	74	129
10	375	98.6	9.4	85	87	93	98	104	111	116	75	135
11	378	101.0	9.2	86	89	94	100	107	114	117	75	132
12	453	103.8	9.3	89	92	98	104	109	116	119	75	138
13	397	105.4	9.8	91	94	99	105	111	116	122	79	150
14	335	107.4	8.5	94	97	101	107	113	119	123	83	134
15	212[2]	108.8	9.9	94	96	102	108	115	121	125	88	150

[1] 13 observations deleted due to missing values
[2] Incomplete population sample

Table 16–2. Distribution characteristics of diastolic mercury sphygmomanometric blood pressures of children by age

Age (at last birthday)	Number of children[1]	Mean	Standard deviation	Percentiles							Min	Max
				5th	10th	25th	50th	75th	90th	95th		
5	274	59.8	6.8	49	50	56	60	64	69	72	41	80
6	302	58.6	7.9	47	48	53	58	64	68	72	36	80
7	311	58.2	7.1	46	50	54	58	63	67	69	33	75
8	336	59.4	6.6	48	51	55	60	64	67	70	41	79
9	351	60.7	6.5	50	52	56	61	65	69	72	44	80
10	375	61.3	7.9	49	51	56	61	66	71	75	35	88
11	378	63.0	7.6	50	54	58	63	68	74	76	42	83
12	453	65.3	7.6	53	55	60	65	70	75	78	46	89
13	397	67.5	7.9	55	57	62	68	73	77	80	46	92
14	335	67.4	7.0	55	58	62	68	72	77	79	44	89
15	212[2]	67.6	7.2	56	58	62	67	72	77	81	51	90

[1]13 observations deleted due to missing values
[2]Incomplete population sample

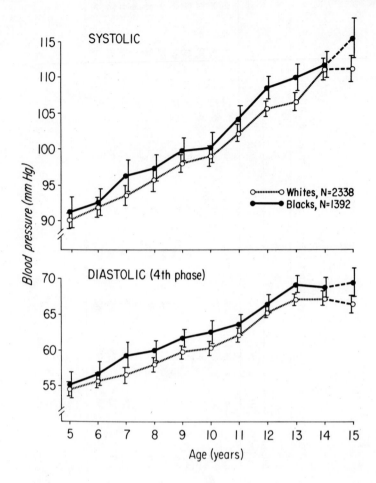

Figure 16–2. Mean (±2 S.E.) Physiometrics instrument blood pressures in school children, by age and race.

the means were more apparent on the Physiometrics recorder, where greater consistency was achieved for each age than on the sphygmo-manometer. The age trend of pressures for the 5- and 6-year-old children obtained by Physiometrics recordings differed from that obtained by sphygmomanometer; because of this difference slightly larger cuffs are used in subsequent studies (see appendix at end of chapter).

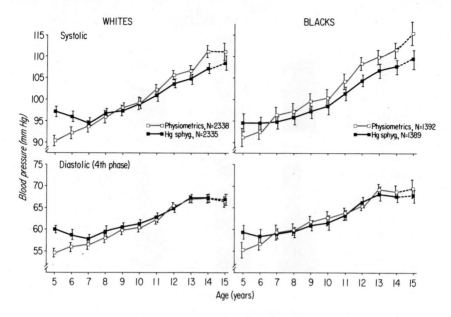

Figure 16–3. Comparison of mean Physiometrics (±2 S.E.) versus mercury sphygmomanometric blood pressures in school children, by age for each race.

Is the racial difference in blood pressure limited to the upper percentiles?

As indicated above, a significant racial difference in blood pressure (Fig. 16–2) may be limited to the upper 5%. In order to investigate this question, the mean of systolic and diastolic pressures on each individual was determined; the blood pressure values were ranked accordingly, separately for each year of age, for the sphygmomanometer and for the Physiometrics readings. The ranks were categorized into groups of 5%, and for each group ages 5–9 and 10–14 were combined. Within the resulting groups (4 sets of 20) the observed racial distribution was compared by chi-square tests, separately for each of the two age groups and each of the two instruments. We found that only in the upper 5% did the observed racial distribution differ from the expected. This departure from expected distribution was statistically significant for both age groups on the Physiometrics instrument, but on the sphygmomanometer only for ages 10–14, as shown in Figure 16–4.

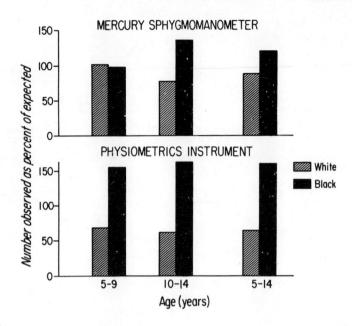

Figure 16–4. Racial distribution in the upper 5% of mean blood pressure for school children, by age group and by instrument. Mean blood pressure = ½ (systolic + fourth-phase pressure). On the mercury sphygmomanometer the racial difference at ages 5–9 was nonsignificant, and the significance for age groups 10–14 and 5–14 was at the 1% and 5% level, respectively. On the Physiometrics instrument the levels of significance were all beyond the 0.05% level (chi-square test).

Determinants of blood pressure level

Stepwise multiple regression analyses with blood pressure level as the dependent variable and other characteristics (Table 16–3) as independent variables were made separately for systolic sphygmomanometer, diastolic sphygmomanometer, systolic Physiometrics, and diastolic Physiometrics blood pressure readings. Because of the potential relationship between blood pressure and lipid levels, 263 children were excluded from these analyses because they had not fasted prior to the examination; an additional 164 were omitted due to missing data for sphygmomanometer analysis and 167 for Physiometrics analysis.

Table 16–3. Measured variables entered into the multiple regression equations

Description	Units of measurement
Dependent Variables	
Systolic pressure: mean of 6 sphygmomanometer readings	mm mercury
Diastolic pressure: mean of 6 sphygmomanometer readings	mm mercury
Systolic pressure: mean of 3 Physiometrics measurements	mm mercury
Diastolic pressure: mean of 3 Physiometrics measurements	mm mercury
Independent Variables	
Demographic	
age (exact calendar age[1])	years
race[2]	white = 1, black = 2
sex[2]	male = 1, female = 2
Anthropometric	
body height	cm
ponderosity index[3] = (body weight) / (body height)^3	kg/cm^3
upper-arm circumference[3]	cm
triceps skinfold thickness[3]	mm
external maturation index (pubic hair score plus breast development or male genitalia score)	Score range 2–10
Laboratory	
serum total cholesterol[3]	mg/dl
serum triglycerides[3]	mg/dl
serum pre-β-lipoprotein[3]	mg/dl
serum β-lipoprotein[3]	mg/dl
(serum pre-β-lipoprotein) + (serum β-lipoprotein)[3]	mg/dl
(serum pre-β-lipoprotein) / (serum pre-β + β-lipoprotein)[3]	—
blood hemoglobin	gm/dl
Blood pressure observers No. 1–8[2]	Yes = 1, No = 2

[1]Age of last birthday when entered as a constant
[2]Entered as dummy variables
[3]Logarithmic transformation

Tables 16–4 and 16–5 present the resulting regression coefficients with their levels of significance and standardized partial regression coefficients for all variables contributing to the blood pressure variation at the 1% level of significance, listed in the order of acceptance by the model. For the blood pressures obtained with the mercury sphygmomanometer shown in Table 16–4 and for those recorded by the Physiometrics instrument shown in Table 16–5, approximately 35% of the variation of blood pressure was explained by all of the independent variables entered into the regression analysis. We found

Table 16–4. Stepwise multiple regression for sphygmomanometer blood pressure[1]

Systolic		
Source	Regression coefficient	Standardized partial regression coefficient
Mean	285.73	
Height	0.28[a]	0.49
Pond. Index[2]	46.36[a]	0.29
Maturation	0.69[a]	0.18
Observer 4	1.41[a]	0.07
Observer 3	2.08[b]	0.06
Male sex	1.17[b]	0.06
Age	−0.51[b]	−0.14
Hemoglobin	0.51[b]	0.06
Observer 8	−0.94[c]	−0.04

Multiple correlation coefficient squared is 0.35

Diastolic		
Source	Regression coefficient	Standardized partial regression coefficient
Mean	3.13	
Upp Arm Cir.[2]	33.21[a]	0.30
Maturation	0.65[a]	0.21
Observer 7	2.64[a]	0.16
Observer 4	2.63[a]	0.15
Observer 3	3.34[a]	0.11
Hemoglobin	0.72[a]	0.10
Black race	0.86[a]	0.05
Observer 1	0.96[c]	0.05

Multiple correlation coefficient squared is 0.31

[1] 427 out of 3,524 children not analyzed due to nonfasting or missing data
[2] Log_{10}
a = $p < 0.0001$
b = $p < 0.001$
c = $p < 0.01$

Table 16–5. Stepwise multiple regression for Physiometrics blood pressure[1]

Systolic			Diastolic		
Source	Regression coefficient	Standardized partial regression coefficient	Source	Regression coefficient	Standardized partial regression coefficient
Mean	190.80		Mean	73.04	
Height	0.36[a]	0.53	Height	0.26[a]	0.52
Pond. index[2]	31.49[a]	0.17	Pond. index[2]	12.39[a]	0.09
Observer 4	3.51[a]	0.10	Observer 4	2.35[a]	0.08
Male sex	2.11[a]	0.09	Black race	1.95[a]	0.11
Black race	2.03[a]	0.08	Hemoglobin	0.82[a]	0.10
Hemoglobin	0.59[b]	0.06			
Observer 1	−1.76[b]	−0.04			
Maturation	0.34[c]	0.07			
Triglyceride[2]	2.62[c]	0.04			

Multiple correlation coefficient squared is 0.40   Multiple correlation coefficient squared is 0.32

[1]430 out of 3,524 children not analyzed due to nonfasting or missing data
[2]Log$_{10}$
[a] = $p < 0.0001$
[b] = $p < 0.001$
[c] = $p < 0.01$

251

that the variables which most consistently provided contributions to the associated variation were ponderosity index, body height, blood hemoglobin, external maturation, sex, and race (the latter on the Physiometrics instrument mainly).

It is apparent in Tables 16–4 and 16–5 that the influences of *body height and ponderosity index* were both very strong and in most instances overrode the apparent influence of age. This finding may be illustrated by the bivariate Pearson coefficients of correlation between body weight and blood pressure which were, respectively, for sphygmomanometer and Physiometrics, 0.54/0.48 and 0.61/0.53 (systolic/diastolic). The combined significance of the effects of the ponderosity index and body height may well support the premise of Alexander (1963) that systolic blood pressure increase is related to increase in blood and plasma volume.

Although the influence of hemoglobin on blood pressure is small, it is statistically highly significant and consistently present. This influence may be explained by a relative increase in blood viscosity, as in polycythemia (Fogarty et al., 1967). A similar relationship between hematocrit and blood pressure has been found by McDonough et al. (1965) in an adult population of Evans County, Ga.

The influence of *maturation* on blood pressure was seen in each instance except for the diastolic sphygmomanometer readings. Tanner (1962) has previously described this.

The positive effect of male *sex* on blood pressure was of low order and was significant in the systolic readings only.

The positive effect of black *race* was highly significant for the Physiometrics instrument but less so for the sphygmomanometer values. The influence of instrument on blood pressure readings is analyzed below.

For all practical purposes, each of eight *observers* examined an approximately equal number of children, twice as often by sphygmomanometer as by Physiometrics instrument. It was found that the largest effect due to *observer* had a magnitude of 3.5 mm Hg. The observer effect noted by the Physiometrics levels is consistent with interpersonal influence on the child, since measurement bias was excluded through blind reading of the disks.

There was no association of blood pressure with age nor with serum lipid levels, after controlling for the other variables.

Determinants of the difference between Baumanometer and Physiometrics blood pressure instruments

Stepwise multiple regression analysis for difference in reading by the two instruments as the dependent variable was made separately for the systolic and diastolic pressures. Independent variables were selected for conceptual relevance (Voors, 1975). The strongest determinant of the reading difference was the deficient coverage of the arm circumference under the bladder, followed in magnitude by level of blood pressure, and by triceps skinfold thickness. Race contributed slightly to the variation of this difference.

In total, 21% of the difference in systolic pressure readings and 9% of the difference in diastolic readings were explained by the independent variables.

COMMENT

An objective of these studies was to obtain reliable and reproducible resting blood pressure measurements in children. Attempts to reduce the variation of blood pressure readings included selection of observers shown to have normal hearing acuity by audiometric testing, careful training and monitoring of the observers as a group, strict adherance to a blind randomized design, multiple blood pressure measurements, utilization of automatic recordings with an oversized cuff bladder to avoid exaggerated readings, and blindness of reading the automatic blood pressure records.

The data presented in Table 16–6 suggest that the racial contribution to the difference between sphygmomanometer and Physiometrics readings as observed in Figure 16–3 is likely to be explained by the existing racial difference in upper-arm circumference (a mean difference between white and black children of 4–5 mm was observed, the whites having larger dimensions) and in triceps skinfold thickness (white children have a mean difference that is 2 mm larger than that of black children). A similar racial difference in skinfolds has been found in the National Health Examination Survey (Johnston et al., 1974). This explanation is consistent with the studies by Irvine, who artificially increased the skinfold thickness by the application of rubber straps (Irvine, 1967), and with work by Karvonen et al. (1964), Simpson et al. (1965), and King (1967). Therefore, the simplest explanation of the absence of racial difference in mercury sphygmomanometric readings is that the sphygmomanometer readings in white children are elevated relative to sphygmomanometer readings in black children with equal "true" blood pressure. An actual racial difference in blood pressure may be obscured; however, this difference seems to be preserved by the Physiometrics instrument.

The reason for the statistical correlation between pressure level and reading difference between sphygmomanometer and Physiometrics readings on a child is not clear. In the higher range of pressures, true blood pressures may be higher than mercury sphygmomanometer pressures. In 9 studies surveyed, the direction of the mercury sphygmomanometer deviation was similar to ours (considering Physiometrics pressure as true pressure) for the systolic readings, and in 7 out of 9 instances the same was true for the diastolic (fourth Korotkoff phase) readings (Ragan and Bordley, 1941; Steele, 1942; Van Bergen, et al., 1954; Roberts et al., 1958; Holland and Humerfelt, 1964; Moss and Adams, 1965; King, 1967; Raftery and Ward, 1968; Nielson and Janniche, 1974). Apparently, the human ear is unable to detect the first infrasonic signals (Whitcher, 1969; Golden et al., 1974) of the arterial wall vibration (Ur and Gordon, 1970) as the cuff pressure approaches the systolic pressure from above.

In the lower range of pressures, true blood pressures may be equal to or lower than mercury sphygmomanometer pressures. Since it is known that for the mercury sphygmomanometer an excess pressure reading is caused by the compliant motion of the periarterial tissues (Steinfeld et al., 1974), we conjecture that, under low cuff pressure corresponding to low intra-arterial pressure, these tissues will move relatively easily, but that this compliance will be impeded under high cuff pressure (corresponding to high intra-arterial pressure) (Voors, 1975). Embedding of the Infrasonde transducer in the cuff bladder permitted the Physiometrics instrument to have cuff bladders of ample size, thereby avoiding this excess pressure reading.

With these considerations, the discrepancy in instrument readings of Figure 16–3 may be partly explained. For 5- and 6-year-old children our protocol often called for an infant-size cuff bladder, which did not completely surround the arm (see appendix at end of chapter). For these ages, the sphygmomanometer-minus-Physiometrics reading difference is largest, and hence is likely to be caused by both cuff-bladder-length deficiency and low pressure level (Voors, 1975). For ages 11–14 years, the Physiometrics readings are higher than the sphygmomanometer readings, probably due to the differential sensitivity of the two instruments for the pressure wave frequency spectrum.

We attempted to reduce the influence of the emotional state of the child on blood pressure by a. elaborate preliminary information and demonstration; b. a network of local volunteers as guides; c. sedentary waiting periods between the multiple measurements; d. observers trained for comparability of readings and intent upon creating a continuously friendly and relaxed atmosphere; e. encouraging the children to void prior to the blood pressure measurments; and f. observance of the blood pressure at the end of a sequence of other examinations. There are no data to establish the potential effect of white observers on black children in this study.

We were unable to find studies on repetitive blood pressure measurement in recent literature on school-age children. Such studies obtained for adults (Diehl and Lees, 1929; Glock et al., 1956; Clark et al., 1956; Armitage and Rose, 1966) have shown that many repeated measurements (12 or more on small numbers of subjects) are on the average lower than the "casual" measurements in population studies (Bøe et al., 1957; Kagan et al., 1959; Gordon, 1964; McDonough, et al. 1964; Miall, and Lovell 1967). Taking age into account, the repetitive measurements were on the average 25 mm Hg lower than the casual population measurements for the systolic pressures and 15 mm Hg for the diastolic pressures (see Chapter 14, Fig. 14–2). Results from the National Health Survey are intermediate; three measurements per individual were taken instead of the usual one measurement (Gordon, 1964). Initial pressures in repetitive studies were on the average 2–14 mm Hg higher than the last measurements. In Bogalusa the first measurements differed from the later ones by an average of 2 mm Hg. One explanation for the low levels of blood pressure seems to be that subjects of repetitive measurements are generally less excited because of their familiarity with the procedure (Ayman and Goldshine, 1940).

The mean age-specific levels of blood pressure as observed in the present study are very similar to the basal blood pressures reported by Shock (1944). Harlan et al. (1964), in their 18-year follow-up of 350 naval flight students, found that basal blood pressures predicted subsequent pressures in the same individual better than did casual pressures. In their 30-year follow-up report (Harlan et al., 1973), they concluded that ". . . minimizing extraneous influences probably increases the validity and predictive capacity of blood pressures recorded early in life." The Bogalusa Heart Study, which included some annual follow-up examinations to observe trends over time, was designed to obtain observations on relaxed children which might serve as baseline measurements.

It has been frequently stated that essential hypertension is rarely found in childhood, and that most cases of hypertension in children are of a secondary nature (Singh and Page, 1967; Loggie, 1971). Recent observations by Londe et al. (1971), after extensive efforts to exclude secondary causes, fail to support this viewpoint. Although elaborate studies have recorded blood pressure in free-living children, interpretation of these observations in terms of disease is difficult. From our studies it becomes obvious that standard methods to obtain reproducible and baseline levels are needed, and that the level of the higher percentiles for a given population may be used at this time only as an approximate guide for making a diagnosis of hypertension. The natural history of primary hypertension will not be understood until the evolution of blood pressure levels is known, early changes in the cardiovascular system are recognized, and the determinants are identified, including the influence of familial and environmental factors. At such time it may become possible to predict whether a child will develop disease, and to begin meaningful prevention.

SUMMARY

Nine blood pressures were taken on each of 3,524 children by trained observers with mercury sphygmomanometers (Baumanometer) and Physiometrics automatic recorders in a rigid randomized design in a relaxed atmosphere with other children present. The pressures observed were low compared to data published previously. Black children had significantly higher blood pressures than white children. This difference, starting before age 10, was largest in the children in the top 5% of the pressure ranks. Stepwise multiple regression analysis revealed that this racial difference was significant when measured by an automatic recorder. Body size, expressed by height and by weight/height^3 index, was found to be a strong determinant of blood pressure level. Other positive determinants were blood hemoglobin and external maturation.

APPENDIX TO CHAPTER 16

Cuff Selection Protocol
1. Measure as "right upper-arm length" the acromion-olecranon distance. Use the "anthropometer" caliper.
2. Measure the right upper-arm circumference midway between the acromion and olecranon. Use centimeter tape measure.
3. Refer to the tables for cuff selection determined by upper-arm length and circumference.

Table 16–A. Cuff size to be selected, present study

Upper-arm circumference (cm)	Acromion-olecranon arm length (in cm)			
	0–23	24–27	28–31	32+
0–26	S(infant)	M(child)	M(child)	M(child)
27–29	S(infant)	M(child)	A(adult)	A(adult)
30+	S(infant)	M(child)	A(adult)	L(obese)

Table 16–B. Cuff size to be selected, recommendation

Upper arm circumference (cm)	Acromion-olecranon arm length (cm)			
	0–21	22–27	28–31	32+
0–26	T(toddler)	M(child)	M(child)	M(child)
27–29	T(toddler)	M(child)	A(adult)	A(adult)
30+	M(child)	A(adult)	A(adult)	L(obese)

Table 16–C. Rubber bladder dimensions for standard blood pressure cuffs (in cm)[1]

Cuff size	Bladder length	Bladder width
Infant (S)	12	7
Toddler (T)	21½	7
Child (M)	21½	10
Adult (A)	24	12½
Obese (L)	33 or 42	15

[1]As specified by a certain supplier; in reality measures deviated 0–2 cm.

17. Blood pressure in children measured over successive time periods

The variations of blood pressure levels in children over time need to be elucidated since these changes are probably related to the development of essential hypertension. Although it has been stated (Loggie, 1975; Dustan, 1976) that essential hypertension is rare in children, evolving evidence suggests that it begins in childhood (Londe et al., 1971; Voors et al., 1977a). It may also be assumed that hypertension could be more successfully prevented if the disease process were aborted early. Hence, for early diagnosis we need to know the time course of blood pressure levels and whether "tracking" occurs, i.e., to what extent a child with relatively high blood pressure levels will persist with relatively high levels, especially since the level of blood pressure during adolescence and young adulthood has been found to be predictive of later hypertension (Smirk, 1957; Miall and Lovell, 1967; Paffenbarger et al., 1968; Harlan et al., 1973; Sneiderman et al., 1976). Conventional impressions emphasize the lability of blood pressures at the early phases of hypertension (Goldring and Chasis, 1944; Fishberg, 1954; Pickering, 1968; Frohlich et al., 1970; Genest, 1974). However, these early phases of hypertension are often defined by casual blood pressure measurements, which are less predictive of future hypertension than basal pressures (Smirk, 1957; Harlan et al., 1973). Lability here may merely mean that the measured pressures of individuals exceed defined abnormal cutpoint levels more often by virtue of being close to this cutpoint or by virtue of a state of excitability. In the first case they are not truly labile, and in the second they are not truly hypertensive.

To help clarify these points data are needed from an entire geographic population of free-living children rather than from hospital-based patients and nonrepresentative selected individuals; data obtained by standardized methodolgy are also required. The community-wide examination of school-age children in the Bogalusa Heart Study has yielded pertinent information about the change of blood pressure over successive time periods.

Little is known about the persistence or determinants of high blood pressure levels in children. If a child's level of blood pressure ranks high, how likely will this ranking persist after an hour, a month, a year? What causes basal blood pressures to persist or to change over the short term? Answers to these questions are basic to understanding the early onset of essential hypertension.

GENERAL METHODS

Study populations

The major study population of 3,524 children comprised 93% of all children in the community. In one of the participating schools, 69 children in the fifth grade were reexamined for blood pressure once a month for eight consecutive months. Thirty-five of these children attended all eight sessions.

Children 5, 8, 11, and 14 years of age during the first examination in the study were reexamined after one year. A total of 1,101 children (83% of the 1,326 eligible) were examined twice.

Analysis

Relation between variability and level of blood pressure. When the blood pressure of a child is measured several times, any gross deviation in measurement from the true level will influence both the mean and the variation of the child's measured blood pressure: if the variant measurement overstates the true pressure, the mean will rise and the variation will rise, while a variant measurement which understates the true pressure will lower the mean while the variation still rises. This confounding, if it occurs, will therefore tend to create a spuriously high variability at both ends of the observed (not of the true) blood pressure range in the population (Oldham, 1968). In our analysis, we therefore used only the sphygmomanometer measurements to compute the variability. The mean of three Physiometrics measurements, taken independently for each child, were used to assess his mean *level* of blood pressure. The latter instrument may have produced blood pressure levels more valid than the sphygmomanometer, since larger cuff bladders were used (Voors, 1975), infrasonic amplification was applied (Golden et al., 1974), and permanent records were produced that could be read without observer bias (Webber et al., 1977).

Determinants of blood pressure variability. Individual variability of blood pressure (expressed as the standard deviation about the six sphygmomanometer readings) was entered as the dependent variable into a multiple regression analysis, and all other measured characteristics, including individual mean blood pressure levels, were entered as independent variables. Logarithmic transformation was applied to the independent variables—except age, height, maturation, hemoglobin, and the nominal characteristics—in order to approach Gaussian distributions. A ponderosity index (weight/height^3) was chosen as a measure of obesity for theoretic and morphologic reasons (see Chapter 8 and Foster et al., 1977). This ponderosity index was used instead of the body weight as an independent variable in order to avoid artifacts resulting from the highly positive correlation between height and weight.

Regression of initially high blood pressure toward the mean. In order to compute the amount of regression toward the population mean blood pressure as experienced by a child above the 90th percentile for his age, we used the statistical model of Gardner and Heady (1973), which requires knowledge of the interchild and intrachild variability. The interchild variability was obtained from the same population for which we developed percentile charts (National Heart, Lung, and Blood Institute, 1978). The intrachild variability (Dixon and Massey, 1969) was computed by pooling the intrachild variances for the 35 fifth-graders examined monthly.

Tracking of blood pressure in children originally in the extreme deciles. In the study population with two complete examinations one year apart, children in the upper and lower decile of blood pressure (mean of six sphygmomanometer measurements) for the initial exam-

ination were identified and their blood pressures (mean of six sphygmomanometer readings) were observed after one year. After reducing
the regression toward the mean to zero in a statistical adjustment, the
average reexamination pressures were compared to the original upper
and lower decile pressures in order to obtain quantitative insight into
the amount of tracking of the blood pressure.

Determinants of blood pressure level. The determinants of systolic
and diastolic blood pressure level upon reexamination were ascertained by stepwise multiple regression analysis in which blood pressure was the dependent variable. Independent variables were all currently measured characteristics plus the blood pressure level obtained
one year earlier.

OBSERVATIONS

Bivariate correlations

Bivariate Pearson coefficients of correlation between mean sphygmomanometer pressures for various time intervals are shown in Figure
17–1. Correlation coefficients approximated 0.80 for systolic and 0.50
for diastolic pressures.

The annual reexamination data are specified by age, race, and sex
in Table 17–1. Correlation coefficients approximated 0.70 for systolic
and 0.50 for diastolic pressures. No consistent differences in the correlation coefficients by race and sex were observed.

Relation between variability and level of blood pressure at initial examination

For each child the intrachild standard deviation of the six systolic and
diastolic sphygmomanometer pressures was computed. Mean (± 2
S.E.) intrachild standard deviations of systolic sphygmomanometer
pressures are presented by intervals of five mm Hg Physiometrics
pressure level in Figure 17–2. There was no statistically significant
relationship between these two variables (test for linear regression of
standard deviation on level by analysis of variance procedure) at the
0.05 level. Mean (± 2 S.E.) intrachild standard deviations of diastolic
sphygmomanometer pressures are also presented in Figure 17–2.
Here, the association is negative (test for linear regression of standard
deviation on level by analysis of variance procedure, $p < 0.0001$).

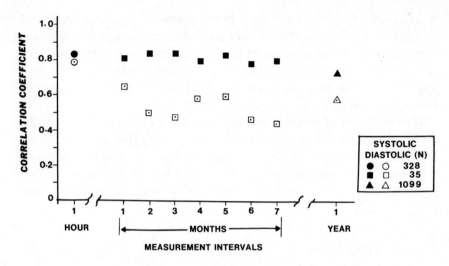

Figure 17–1. Intrachild correlation coefficients of blood pressure (mercury sphygmomanometer) for different time periods. Blood pressure measurement on rescreenees after an approximate 1-hr interval, over monthly time intervals, and over two successive years are shown.

Determinants of blood pressure variability at initial examination

Time-order in which measurements were taken. Means for the first three of the nine measurements taken from each child are presented in Table 17–2 for each instrument. For systolic readings, the difference between first and second measurement was larger than between the subsequent measurements. However, the total of differences was not much more than 2.0 mm Hg systolic and 0.3 mm Hg diastolic for the sphygmomanometer, and, respectively, 2.8 and 1.0 mm Hg for the Physiometrics instrument. The smallness of these differences perhaps supports the notion that basal pressure levels were approached.

For the mercury sphygmomanometer, differences between mean measurements by first and second stations (instruments) are distributed normally (Fig. 17–3).

Profile of determinants of blood pressure variability. In order to obtain a profile of determinants of blood pressure variability, we analyzed systolic and diastolic variability separately in a multiple step-

Table 17–1. Intrachild correlation coefficient of blood pressure (mercury sphygmomanometer) over a one-year interval, by age-cohort, race, and sex

Phase	Age (years) at first examination	Boys		Girls	
		White	Black	White	Black
Systolic	5	0.64 (81)[1]	0.61 (43)	0.61 (74)	0.70 (35)
	8	0.73 (90)	0.76 (60)	0.63 (88)	0.80 (52)
	11	0.61 (92)	0.68 (72)	0.68 (100)	0.71 (69)
	14	0.62 (81)	0.61 (53)	0.62 (60)	0.72 (51)
Diastolic (4th phase)	5	0.32 (81)	0.46 (43)	0.40 (74)	0.60 (35)
	8	0.61 (90)	0.48 (60)	0.60 (88)	0.15 (52)
	11	0.44 (92)	0.42 (72)	0.55 (100)	0.55 (69)
	14	0.48 (81)	0.48 (53)	0.47 (60)	0.61 (51)

[1]Sample size in brackets.

wise regression model, entering blood pressure variability as the dependent variable and all other measured characteristics as independent variables. The systolic variability was found to be negatively associated with age and positively with the index of obesity, but not with systolic level itself. The diastolic variability was found to have a negative association with body height and a weak positive one with maturation, but not with the diastolic level itself. All measured characteristics combined could explain only 1% of the variation in systolic blood pressure variability and 2% of the variation in diastolic pressure variability.

Regression of initially high blood pressure toward the mean

The pooled intra-child standard deviation as obtained monthly from the reexamined fifth graders was 4.1 mm Hg systolic and 5.1 mm Hg diastolic. Applying these results to the cross-sectional standard deviation for 11-year-olds as obtained from the initial examination of the entire population (9.2 mm Hg systolic and 7.6 mm Hg diastolic), we

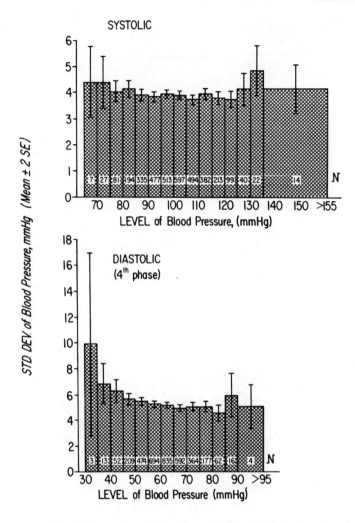

Figure 17–2. Intrachild standard deviation of systolic and diastolic (fourth phase) blood pressure (mean ±2 S.E.) within 1/2 hr by level of blood pressure. The standard deviation was ascertained for each child by six mercury sphygmomanometric measurements. The level was ascertained for each child by three Physiometrics measurements.

can compute the interchild standard deviation by taking the square root of the difference in variance. The resulting interchild standard deviations for 11-year-olds are 8.3 mm Hg systolic and 5.6 mm Hg diastolic.

Table 17–2. Mean blood pressures (mm Hg) of first, second, and third measurement in children age 5–14 years, by each instrument

Measurement	Mercury sphygmomanometer, $n = 2,362$[1]		Physiometrics $n = 1,154$[1]	
	Systolic	Diastolic (4th phase)	Systolic	Diastolic (4th phase)
First	101.7[a]	62.5	103.1[a]	62.6[a]
Second	100.8[a]	62.7	101.3[a]	62.1[ab]
Third	100.2[a]	62.6	100.3[a]	61.8[b]
All other	99.7[c]	62.4[c]	100.3[d]	61.6[d]

[1]Eight missing values excluded from above totals.
[a]Difference is significant, $p < 0.001$.
[b]Difference is significant, $p < 0.05$.
[c]Not tested; averages of three mercury sphygmomanometric and three Physiometrics measurements.
[d]Not tested; averages of six mercury sphygmomanometric measurements.

Assuming that the blood pressure values have Gaussian distributions, we can use the model of Gardner and Heady (1973) to obtain the average decrease in pressure upon reexamination as experienced by a child ranking above the 90th percentile during the first examination. This decrease is 3.1 mm Hg systolic and 6.0 mm Hg diastolic (see appendix at end of chapter). These results are based on means of six sphygmomanometer measurements on a child per examination.

Tracking of blood pressure for children originally in the extreme deciles

In the study population, with two complete examinations one year apart, children in the top and bottom deciles of blood pressures (sphygmomanometer) for the first examination were identified and their blood pressures were observed during the second examination. Also, adjusted levels from the top and bottom deciles of the original examination were calculated after taking regression toward the mean into account. The latter values were statistically adjusted by reducing the regression toward the mean to zero (Table 17–3).

After adjusting for the annual difference in mean systolic and diastolic pressure, we found that those children initially in the top ten percentiles would have had average differences in the observed and expected

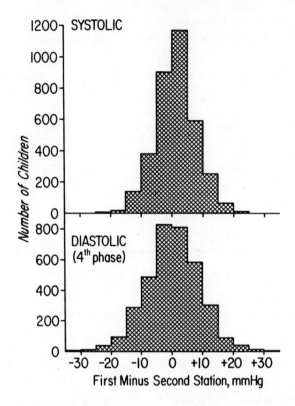

Figure 17–3. Frequency distribution of difference in mean blood pressure between first and second mercury sphygmomanometer stations.

reexamination pressures corresponding to 2.8 mm Hg systolic and 0.0 mm Hg diastolic, whereas those initially in the bottom ten percentiles would have had corresponding differences of 2.4 mm Hg systolic and 0.4 mm Hg diastolic (Fig. 17–4). These expected reexamination pressures agree very closely to those observed.

Determinants of blood pressure level

The strongest determinant of blood pressure level was the level observed one year previously (Table 17–4). In total, all measured variables could account for 39–55% of the systolic and 32–38% of the diastolic mercury sphygmomanometric pressure variations. A measure of tracking is the partial correlation coefficient of first-year with

Table 17–3. Blood pressures observed in year 2 for children from extreme deciles in year 1; expected values are adjusted for year and for regression toward the mean

	Age in year 2	Upper decile				Lower decile			
		Number of children	Observed year 1	Expected year 2[1]	Observed year 2	Number of children	Observed year 1	Expected year 2[1]	Observed year 2
Systolic	6	23	112.8 ± 2.4[2]	107.7	105.6 ± 3.3	24	84.0 ± 1.1	85.1	87.8 ± 2.6
	9	29	113.1 ± 1.7	111.8	110.1 ± 2.6	29	82.6 ± 0.9	87.5	89.4 ± 2.2
	12	32	118.1 ± 1.5	118.5	114.5 ± 2.3	33	86.3 ± 1.0	92.8	95.4 ± 2.3
	15	24	123.0 ± 1.6	122.7	119.4 ± 3.9	24	93.6 ± 1.1	99.5	101.9 ± 2.6
Diastolic (4th phase)	6	23	72.2 ± 1.1	63.2	62.6 ± 2.7	23	47.7 ± 0.9	50.7	51.2 ± 3.0
	9	25	71.1 ± 1.1	64.9	67.7 ± 2.4	29	47.5 ± 0.9	53.3	52.6 ± 3.0
	12	32	76.8 ± 0.7	72.9	72.9 ± 1.9	35	50.5 ± 1.0	58.6	59.6 ± 2.3
	15	24	78.8 ± 1.2	75.4	77.1 ± 3.2	24	54.8 ± 1.2	63.4	64.4 ± 3.1

[1]Measurements of year 1, adjusted for year and for regression toward the mean.
[2]Mean ± 2 S.E.

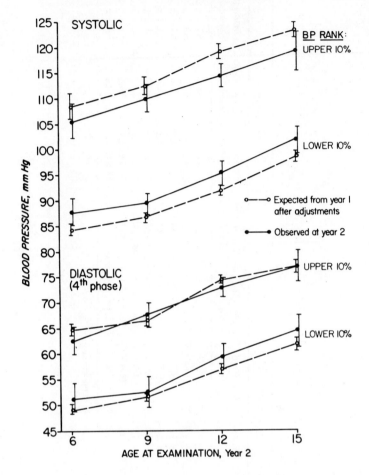

Figure 17–4. Comparison of blood pressure (mean ±2 S.E.) expected for ideal tracking with observed reexamination after one year. Systolic and diastolic (fourth phase) pressures of extreme deciles from reexamination after one year were "regressed towards the mean," resulting in pressures expected for ideal tracking. Extreme deciles from initial examination as reexamined after one year give observed values. The degree of fit is a measure of tracking.

second-year blood pressure, controlling for all other significant independent variables. This coefficient was 0.61–0.66 for systolic and 0.36–0.52 for diastolic pressure. Results for the Physiometrics instrument were quite similar.

Table 17–4. Stepwise multiple regression of blood pressure (mercury sphygmomanometer) reexamined after one year for children, ages 6, 9, 12, and 15 years

Age in year 2	Systolic			Diastolic (4th phase)		
	Source[1]	Regression coefficient	Partial correlation coefficient	Source[1]	Regression coefficient	Partial correlation coefficient
6 (n = 189)[2]	Intercept	−26.53	($R^{2(3)} = 0.47$)	Intercept	167.66	($R^{2(3)} = 0.32$)
	Systolic, yr 1	0.63[a]	0.62[a]	Diastolic, yr 1	0.39[a]	0.40[a]
	W/H[3(4)], yr 2	47.73[a]	0.31[a]	Observer 7, yr 2	4.01[b]	0.27[b]
				Observer 1, yr 2	−2.94[c]	−0.19[c]
				W/H[3(4)], yr 2	27.68[c]	0.23[c]
9 (n = 263)[2]	Intercept	−11.17	($R^{2(3)} = 0.55$)	Intercept	−9.18	($R^{2(3)} = 0.38$)
	Systolic, yr 1	0.57[a]	0.62[a]	Diastolic, yr 1	0.40[a]	0.36[a]
	W/H[3(4)], yr 2	40.57[b]	0.34[a]	Observer 2, yr 2	−4.16[a]	−0.21[b]
				Observer 1, yr 2	−3.62[a]	−0.25[a]
				W/H[3(4)], yr 2	35.05[a]	0.27[a]
12 (n = 285)[2]	Intercept	20.69	($R^{2(3)} = 0.55$)	Intercept	13.14	($R^{2(3)} = 0.37$)
	Systolic, yr 1	0.56[a]	0.66[a]	Diastolic, yr 1	0.43[a]	0.45[a]
	Observer 8, yr 2	−3.85[a]	−0.31[a]	Observer 2, yr 2	−4.38[a]	−0.23[a]
	Height, yr 2	0.17[a]	0.21[b]	Height, yr 2	0.15[c]	0.17[c]
	Maturation, yr 2	0.48[b]	0.23[a]	Maturation, yr 2	0.54[a]	0.24[a]
15 (n = 219)[2]	Intercept	40.78	($R^{2(3)} = 0.39$)	Intercept	33.66	($R^{2(3)} = 0.36$)
	Systolic, yr 1	0.65[a]	0.63[a]	Diastolic, yr 1	0.57[a]	0.52[a]
				Observer 2, yr 2	−6.11[a]	−0.29[a]
				Observer 1, yr 2	−4.19[a]	−0.26[a]

[1]All variables measured in year 2 were entered (Table 17–1, excluding hemoglobin which was not measured in year 2); in addition, blood pressure of year 1 (systolic or diastolic, corresponding to dependent variable) was entered as independent variable.

[2]A total of 16 out of 972 children fasting for examination in year 2 were not analyzed due to missing data.

[3]Multiple correlation coefficient squared.

[4]Log_{10}

[a]$p < 0.0001$

[b]$p < 0.001$

[c]$p < 0.01$

COMMENT

The measure of valid and replicable indirect blood pressure in children is fraught with pitfalls, but apparently obtainable with attention to methodology. In our study we attempted the arrangement of nearly optimal conditions under which to measure the child. Such conditions increased the predictive value of our measurements (Smirk, 1957; Harlan et al., 1973) by yielding values which approach known resting basal values for children in this age group (Chapter 16). The measurement replicability was increased by having three different observers each measure the blood pressure three times, using the fourth rather than the fifth Korotkoff phase for diastolic assessment (Voors et al., 1979b). An automatic blood pressure recorder gave independent parallel measurements. Careful selection, training, testing, and retesting of the observers was conducted according to a protocol especially designed to increase the reproducibility of the measurements (Voors et al., 1977a). Possible observer bias was further minimized by daily randomization of observers and children in the examination sequence and by a specified blind reexamination of an approximately 10% random sample of children at the end of each examination morning by the same observers (Chapter 16).

There was little difference on the average between the first measured blood pressure of an individual child and his subsequent measurements (Table 17–2). This contrasts with other studies (e.g., Diehl and Lees, 1929; Armitage and Rose, 1966) and perhaps supports our contention that basal levels were approached in our study.

In children with low diastolic levels we found increased diastolic pressure variability (Fig. 17–2). This may have been caused by more imprecise measurements at this level, since the observer effects on blood pressure were increased at lower diastolic levels (Berenson et al., 1978a). An increased nervousness of the younger children (with the lower pressure levels) is unlikely to have influenced the diastolic levels without affecting the systolic levels similarly (see Fig. 17–2).

The short-term variability of blood pressures taken under resting conditions was not increased in the children at the higher percentiles (see Fig. 17–2). No relationship is apparent between pressure level and short-term variability of the systolic pressure. The concept that increased variability of blood pressure exists in the prehypertensive phase (Goldring and Chasis, 1944; Fishberg, 1954; Pickering, 1968;

Frohlich et al., 1970; Genest, 1974) was not supported on a population basis, where basal-like pressures were determined under near optimum conditions. If blood pressure lability is operating as a part of the prehypertensive condition, we failed to detect it in this age span. This result agrees with the findings of Bagshaw et al. (1975) and of New et al. (1977).

The observation of an independent relationship between level of blood pressure and intrachild variability of blood pressure and the absence of any strong correlation with other measured characteristics enabled us to use a subsample of children from one school grade for measuring the intrachild variation during monthly reexaminations. The estimate of the latter variation allowed us to quantify the anticipated regression toward the mean from extreme percentiles at the first examination, according to Gardner-Heady model.

After taking into account this regression toward the mean, the tracking of resting blood pressures in children originally above the 90th percentile became quantifiable, and we found that their average expected–observed blood pressure difference was 3 mm Hg systolic and 1 mm Hg diastolic during the following annual reexamination. The importance of the previous year's blood pressure in determining present level was also borne out by a stepwise multiple regression analysis, where 39–55% of the systolic pressure variability was determined. From a practical standpoint three or four serial blood pressure measurements (weekly or monthly, as used in this study) appeared to approach a reproducible level for a given child.

In reexamining children with high blood pressure in the study population, we diagnosed few potential secondary hypertensives. We therefore feel that the ranking of children above the 90th percentile for blood pressure levels may well constitute a prediction of future primary hypertension.

SUMMARY

Blood pressures were taken by mercury sphygmomanometer and by an automatic recorder on 3,524 children by trained observers in a rigid, randomized design aimed at obtaining reproducible, resting blood pressure levels. The intrachild standard deviation for six sphygmomanometer pressures was computed for each child as a measure of variability during the examination. We found that children with higher pressure levels did not have increased variability. For all children, ages 5, 8, 11, and 14 years in the initial examination, age-specific systolic and diastolic (fourth phase) selected percentiles were assessed. These children were reexamined after one year. The Pearson coefficient of correlation between examination and reexamination approximated 0.7/0.5 (systolic/diastolic). Observations from a group of 35 fifth-graders examined monthly for eight months in the above manner were pooled to observe intrachild blood pressure variability and to estimate regression toward the mean. This estimate was used to reduce the regression toward the mean of the blood pressures for the after-one-year reexamined children to zero in a statistical adjustment. Upon reexamination, those children initially in the top ten percentiles had on the average expected–observed differences of 3 mm Hg systolic levels and 0 mm Hg diastolic levels. In a multiple regression analysis, the previous year's blood pressure and an index of present body size accounted for 39–55% of the systolic pressure variability, whereas the previous year's systolic pressure contributed a partial correlation coefficient of 0.6–0.7 for each age cohort. These findings, based on reliable, basal-like measurements, point to a high degree of persistence and very likely establish a background for the early diagnosis of primary hypertension.

APPENDIX TO CHAPTER 17

Regression to the Mean Blood Pressure

In Gardner and Heady's notation (1973; Armitage and Rose, 1966), assuming Gaussian distribution of blood pressure:

L = the 90th percentile pressure
μ = the mean pressure
ϵ = the cross-sectional standard deviation of pressure

Therefore $\phi\left(\dfrac{L - \mu}{\epsilon}\right) = 0.1754$ according to the normal probability density function.

Further, $\epsilon = \sqrt{\sigma^2 + \delta^2}$

where σ = the interchild standard deviation of pressure
δ = the intrachild standard deviation of pressure

A child found to be above the 90th percentile level of blood pressure during the first visit has an expected blood pressure level of X of

$$E(X \mid X > L) = \mu + \epsilon v \, [(L - \mu)/\epsilon]$$

where
$$v[(L - \mu)/\epsilon] =$$
$$\frac{\phi[(L - \mu)/\epsilon]}{0.1} = 1.754$$

After regression to the mean, the expected blood pressure level is

$$E(x \mid X > L) = \mu + (1.754) \frac{\sigma^2}{\epsilon}$$

Systolic. For the fifth-graders, who are approximately 11 years old, the following estimates were obtained:

$$\epsilon = 9.236 \text{ mm Hg } \epsilon^2 = 85.303696 \text{ mm}^2 \text{ Hg}$$
$$\delta = \sqrt{16.558389} = 4.069 \text{ mm Hg}$$
$$\sigma = \sqrt{68.745307} = 8.291 \text{ mm Hg}$$

$$E(X \mid X > L) = \mu + (1.754) \, \epsilon = \mu + 16.200 \text{ mm Hg}$$

$$E(x \mid X > L) = \mu + (1.754) \frac{68.745307}{9.236} = \mu + (1.754) \, (7.443190) =$$
$$\mu + 13.055 \text{ mm Hg}$$

The difference between these two estimates represents the estimated regression of systolic blood pressure toward the mean and amounts to 3.145 mm Hg.

Diastolic (fourth phase). For the same fifth graders, the estimates are as follows:

$$\epsilon = 7.6000 \text{ mm Hg } \epsilon^2 = 57.760000 \text{ mm}^2 \text{ Hg}$$
$$\delta = \sqrt{26.079406} = 5.107 \text{ mm Hg}$$
$$\sigma = \sqrt{31.680594} = 5.629 \text{ mm Hg}$$
$$E(X \mid X > L) = \mu + (1.754) \, \epsilon = \mu + 13.330 \text{ mm Hg}$$
$$E(x \mid X > L) = \mu + (1.754) \frac{31.680594}{7.600} = \mu + (1.754) \, (4.168499)$$
$$= \mu + 7.312 \text{ mm Hg}$$

The difference between these two estimates represents the estimated regression of the diastolic blood pressure toward the mean and is 6.018 mm Hg.

18. Relating blood pressure in children to height and weight

High blood pressure decreases life expectancy and health (Society of Actuaries, 1959; Kannel, 1974). In adulthood, it seems to be associated with the preceding blood pressure levels of adolescence (Miall and Lovell, 1967; Mathewson et al., 1972; Harlan et al., 1973; Miall and Chinn, 1973). Therefore, an assessment of the association of hypertension with potential determinants during adolescence may suggest preventive measures. What induces long-term changes in blood pressure as the body grows? What causes the blood pressure to rise during growth and development? Answers to these questions may not only delineate the criteria needed to diagnose subsequent hypertension, but may identify health determinants as well.

In analyzing the long-term correlates of human blood pressure control, we must distinguish conceptually between those blood pressure determinants for which other factors compensate within minutes or hours after their impact, resulting in negative feedback control, and those upon which the blood pressure equilibrium finally depends (Guyton et al., 1974). The latter, which determine the basal or fundamental blood pressure level, are of interest here, since in youth the basal blood pressure seems to predict future hypertension better than casual blood pressures (Harlan et al., 1973). To search for possible determinants of blood pressure in the growing child, we attempted to measure basal blood pressure in children ages $2^1/_2-14$ years by systematic avoidance of their anxiety. Age, race, sex, anthropometric measurements (height, weight, triceps skinfold thickness), measurements of external maturation, serum lipids, and blood hemoglobin were obtained. As reported previously (Voors et al., 1976), regression analysis of these variables explained approximately 40% of the variation in systolic blood pressure, and height with a combined weight and height index accounted for most of this relationship.

In a statistical analysis of population data, to assess separate influences of height and ponderosity upon blood pressure, the choice of a weight-height index will influence the amount of blood pressure variation explained separately by height and by ponderosity. Any three-dimensional structure which increases its size, while the configuration and the density remain the same, will maintain constant weight/height^3 (W/H^3), referred to as the "ponderosity index"; in contrast, W/H^2 (Quetelet index) increases proportional to H, and W/H increases proportional to H^2 according to arithmetic theorems. In other words, when an expanding hypothetical body structure maintains relative proportions of body composition, the specific gravity or density remains constant; the ponderosity index remains constant as well, but the Quetelet index and weight-relative-to-height increase. Similar reasoning applies to the human body; consequently, W/H^3 was chosen as the index of ponderosity in this population of growing children.

GENERAL METHODS

Blood pressure measurements

Although care was taken to eliminate potential sources of bias in observations with mercury sphygmomanometer (Voors, 1975; Voors et al., 1976) the results nevertheless suggested bias resulting from limitations in cuff bladder size and presumed failure to detect 10–80 Hz sound components adequately; therefore, the present analysis is limited to readings with the Physiometrics automatic recorder. In essence, the Physiometrics instrument records on a paper disk rotated by an aneroid manometer in open communication with an over-sized rubber cuff bladder. The bladder, which entirely encircles the upper arm, contains an electronic, infrasonic transducer that detects low-pitched vibrations. The means of three readings of first and fourth Korotkoff phases were used in these analyses. A multiple regression analysis was applied to the data to observe the relationship of height, ponderosity expressed as W/H^3, triceps skinfold thickness, and age with blood pressure levels. Mean blood pressures were plotted against the two major correlates, height and ponderosity, to characterize their relationship.

OBSERVATIONS

Table 18–1 gives the results of the multiple regression of blood pressure on height, ponderosity index, triceps skinfold thickness, and age. The data comprise 3,524 children, 27 of whom were omitted because one or more characteristics were unknown. The variables explain 39% and 31% of the systolic and diastolic variation, respectively. The partial correlation of blood pressure with triceps skinfold thickness is negative after controlling for these other variables. In addition, the partial correlation coefficient of age with blood pressure is low.

Figure 18–1 presents mean systolic and diastolic blood pressures on the Physiometrics instrument by age, separately for eight height groups. Clearly, there is a strong association between height and blood pressure. After maintaining height levels constant there is little or no association between age and blood pressure for this decade of life.

Figure 18–2 presents systolic and diastolic Physiometrics blood pressure by ponderosity index, separately for four height groups (for standard errors and sample sizes see Table 18–2 and 18–3). Again, there is a close correlation between height and blood pressure. In addition, however, the degree of ponderosity is positively associated with blood pressure, especially systolic pressure, when the height levels are kept constant. Both height and weight relationships are constant and proportionate over the entire ranges of height and ponderosity index except for the extremely ponderous, whose blood pressures may be higher than predicted linearly.

When the children were categorized by height into groups by 5-cm increments, the confidence intervals of the mean blood pressure (mean ± 2 S.E.) bracketed the linear regression line for the systolic and diastolic pressures in 33 out of 34 instances (Fig. 18–3). The exception, that for diastolic pressure in the tallest group, fell slightly outside of the regression line. In view of the narrowness of the confi-

Table 18–1. Multiple regression of Physiometrics blood pressure on age and selected anthropometric variables N = 3,497

Source	Systolic Regression coefficient	Systolic Partial correlation coefficient	Source	Diastolic Regression coefficient	Diastolic Partial correlation coefficient
Intercept (mm Hg)	−15.11		Intercept (mm Hg)	−3.96	
Height (cm)	0.46[2]	0.31[2]	Height (cm)	0.29[2]	0.26[2]
W/H³ (kg/m³)[1]	56.30[2]	0.26[2]	W/H³ (kg/m³)[1]	28.37[2]	0.17[2]
Triceps skinf. (mm)[1]	−10.90[2]	−0.15[2]	Triceps skinf. (mm)[1]	−7.08[2]	−0.13[2]
Age (years)	0.08[3]	0.01[3]	Age (years)	0.11[3]	0.02[3]

Systolic: Multiple correl. coeff. squared = 0.39

Diastolic: Multiple correl. coeff. squared = 0.31

[1]Log$_{10}$
[2]$P < 0.0001$
[3]$P > 0.1$

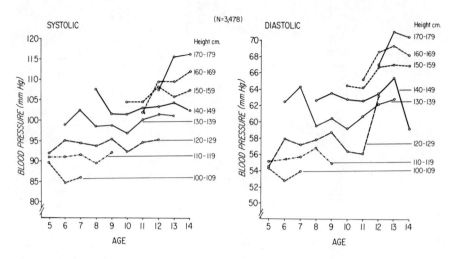

Figure 18–1. Mean blood pressures measured on school-age children by Physiometrics instrument by age for each 10 cm height interval. Similar information was obtained for blood pressures measured by mercury sphygmomanometer (Voors et al., 1976). (Sample sizes < 3 omitted.)

dence intervals, the linear fit of the regression of blood pressure on height is remarkable.

When the children were categorized by weight into groups of 5 kg, the confidence intervals of the mean blood pressure (mean ± 2 S.E., related to the logarithm of weight) also bracketed the linear regression line for the systolic and diastolic pressures in all but one interval (Fig. 18-4). One of the intervals, that for diastolic pressure in the heaviest group, fell slightly outside of the regression line, as the only exception. Again, many of the confidence intervals are narrow and the linear fit of the regression of blood pressure on the logarithm of weight is very close, although somewhat less consistent than for height.

Similar data exist for blood pressures taken with the mercury sphygmomanometer, but these data could be reported only over a shorter age-growth span because of bias in measurements with this instrument. Eliminating the ages of 5 and 6 years, where sphygmomanometer-measured blood pressures were disproportionately high due to small cuff bladder size, we found that height, ponderosity index, and skinfold thickness accounted for the same amount of variability of systolic pressure, 34%, as that measured on the Physiometrics in this age

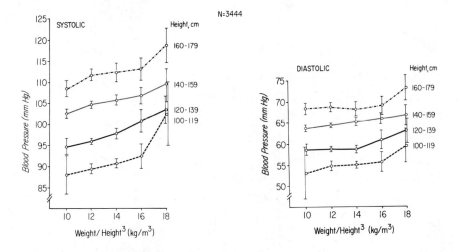

Figure 18–2. Mean (± 2 S.E.) blood pressures measured on school-age children by Physiometrics instrument by age for each 20 cm height interval. A close relationship of blood pressure and height levels is observed and, in addition, controlling for height, there is a correlation between blood pressure levels and ponderosity. (Children with ponderosity index lower than 9.0 kg/m³ or 19.kg/m³ and higher were excluded.

bracket. On either instrument, age had no association with blood pressure after adjustment for height and ponderosity.

Fit of bivariate linear regression

For school-age children, height and the logarithm of weight have a strong linear relationship with blood pressure. We compared children aged 2½–5½ years (Chapter 15) with those aged 5–14 years concerning this relation. Figure 18–3 shows means and standard errors of blood pressure for children in various height groups. The relationship is clearly linear in the school children, and, for the systolic pressure, is approximately replicated in the preschool-age children. Slight discontinuities were noted, possibly due to the effects of instruments or age. The mood score was higher at the younger age (correlation coefficient of mood score with age was −0.31), causing a spurious flattening of the systolic pressure slope in the preschool-age group. The average mood score at the Infrasonde measurement was 4.1 for height 80–89 cm, 3.9 for height 90–99 cm, 3.5 for height 100–109 cm, and

Table 18–2. Systolic blood pressure on Physiometrics instrument (mean ± 2 S.E.), by height and by ponderosity in school children

Height (cm)	Weight/height³ (kg/m^3)							Total (N)[1]
	<9.0	9.0–10.9	11.0–12.9	13.0–14.9	15.0–16.9	17.0–18.9	≥19.0	
<100	—	—	—	—	92.0 (1)[1]	—	—	(1)
100–119	—	88.1 ± 4.5 (5)	89.4 ± 1.2 (204)	90.7 ± 1.1 (273)	92.3 ± 2.9 (44)	102.4 ± 7.5 (9)	93.8 ± 9.0 (2)	(537)
120–139	—	94.7 ± 1.9 (137)	95.9 ± 0.7 (704)	97.8 ± 1.2 (281)	100.7 ± 2.7 (58)	103.4 ± 3.3 (24)	106.5 ± 6.2 (7)	(1,211)
140–159	89.3 (1)	102.5 ± 1.1 (332)	104.7 ± 0.8 (542)	105.7 ± 1.2 (229)	106.7 ± 1.9 (95)	109.5 ± 3.5 (31)	115.6 ± 3.9 (15)	(1,245)
160–179	111.2 ± 6.8 (3)	108.5 ± 1.9 (133)	111.7 ± 1.4 (218)	112.2 ± 2.3 (67)	113.0 ± 2.7 (34)	118.6 ± 4.1 (24)	116.5 ± 6.9 (11)	(490)
≥180	115.0 (1)	110.9 ± 8.5 (5)	116.9 ± 7.7 (5)	117.3 (1)	131.3 (1)	—	—	(13)
Total	(5)	(612)	(1,673)	(851)	(233)	(88)	(35)	(3,497)

[1]Sample size in parentheses.

Table 18–3. Diastolic blood pressure on Physiometrics instrument (mean ± 2 S.E.), by height and by ponderosity in school children

Height (cm)	Weight/height³ (kg/m^3)							
	<9.0	9.0–10.9	11.0–12.9	13.0–14.9	15.0–16.9	17.0–18.9	≥19.0	Total
<100	—	—	—	—	58.3 (1)[1]	—	—	— (1)
100–119	—	53.1 ± 6.1 (5)	54.8 ± 1.1 (204)	55.0 ± 0.8 (273)	55.7 ± 2.3 (44)	59.5 ± 4.0 (9)	61.0 ± 2.0 (2)	— (537)
120–139	—	58.6 ± 1.3 (137)	58.8 ± 0.6 (704)	58.7 ± 0.9 (281)	60.9 ± 2.2 (58)	63.0 ± 2.9 (24)	64.0 ± 5.9 (7)	— (1,211)
140–159	56.3 (1)	63.7 ± 0.8 (332)	64.4 ± 0.6 (542)	65.2 ± 1.0 (229)	65.9 ± 1.3 (95)	66.7 ± 2.4 (31)	69.8 ± 3.3 (15)	— (1,245)
160–179	67.8 ± 7.1 (3)	68.4 ± 1.3 (133)	68.8 ± 1.1 (218)	68.2 ± 1.7 (67)	69.0 ± 2.2 (34)	73.2 ± 3.0 (24)	71.2 ± 5.7 (11)	— (490)
≥180	63.3 (1)	69.2 ± 4.8 (5)	69.2 ± 6.2 (5)	78.0 (1)	69.0 (1)	—	—	— (13)
Total	(5)	(612)	(1,673)	(851)	(233)	(88)	(35)	(3,497)

[1]Sample size in parentheses.

281

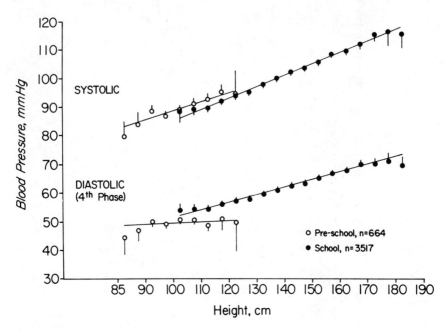

Figure 18–3. Blood pressure (mean ± 2 S.E.) measured by a low-frequency transducer in children, ages 2½–14 years, by height.

3.4 for height 110–119 cm. Thus, for height 80–89 cm, 21% of the children were hyperactive or more excited, for height 90–99 cm this percentage was 17%, for height 100–109 cm it was 7%, and for height 110–119 cm it was 3%. In contrast, the flattening of the slope of the regression of *diastolic* pressure on height cannot be explained by differences in mood alone and could be due to instrument error, although the latter conjecture remains unproven. A similar conclusion can be drawn for relations with log weight (Fig. 18–4).

COMMENT

Interpretation of observations

These studies obtained blood pressure levels approaching known basal values in children of similar age (Shock, 1944). Our observations suggest that some correlate of height and body mass, rather than age,

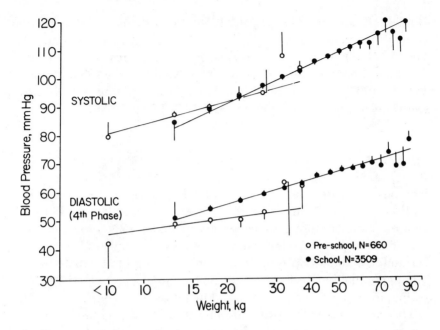

Figure 18–4. Blood pressure (mean ± 2 S.E.) measured by a low-frequency transducer in children, ages 2½–14 years, by weight.

is determining the evolution of blood pressure in children as they grow. A most parsimonious explanation in view of present knowledge is that this correlate may be the basal minute volume of intravascular blood. Such conjecture also fits current knowledge of anthropometric correlates of blood volume. Allen et al. (1956), for instance, found that blood volume (*BV*) of boys and men fits the equation

$$BV = 0.417 \, H^3 + 0.450 \, W - 0.030$$

where *BV* is expressed in liters, *H* in meters, and *W* in kilograms. Alexander et al. (1962) found that blood volume increased more with lean body weight than with increased adipose tissue.

Our data, combined with mean or median blood pressures for groups of normal children younger than those observed here (Kitterman et al., 1969; Modanlou et al., 1974; De Swiet et al., 1975), suggest a linear relationship of blood pressure with height and with the logarithm of weight. Basal blood volume as estimated from height and/or weight according to Brines et al. (1941), Morse et al. (1947),

Russell (1949), and Allen et al. (1956) could quantitatively and conceptually explain this relationship. Only well after adult stature has been attained are there new increases in blood pressure levels independent of height (Johnson et al., 1965; Nance et al., 1965; Miall and Lovell, 1967) and presumably related to a different set of causes (Moyer et al., 1958; Miall and Lovell, 1967; Tracy, 1970).

OBSERVATIONS ON THE RELATIONSHIP OF BLOOD PRESSURE AND
BODY MASS

The positive correlation between blood pressure and ponderosity is well known, and is unlikely to be explained by artifacts inherent in indirect mercury sphygmomanometry (Chiang et al., 1969). This correlation is higher in younger than in older age groups as has been described for adults (Epstein et al., 1965; Chiang et al., 1969) and for young populations in Evans County, Ga. (Johnson et al., 1975), Muscatine, Iowa (Lauer et al., 1975), and Bogalusa, La. (Voors et al., 1976).

The importance of obesity and elevated blood pressure in adolescence for the development of hypertension in adulthood is suggested by the data from Oberman et al. (1967), Paffenbarger et al. (1968), and Abraham et al. (1971), although the latter authors state that their data, which are highly suggestive (Abraham et al. 1971, Table 7) did not reach statistical significance.

Epidemiologic observations have indicated a relationship between weight gain and blood pressure. Ashley and Kannel (1974) found that changes over time in blood pressure (in the Framingham population) were more closely related to *gain* in relative weight than to actual weight. Positive correlations between weight gain and blood pressure are reported by Oberman et al. (1967), Stamler (1967), Heyden et al. (1969), Schwalb and Schimert (1970), and Johnson et al. (1973). The stronger blood pressure-relative weight correlation in younger age groups (Chiang et al. 1969) could be explained by the fact that young obese persons must have gained weight relatively recently by virtue of their limited age. Correlations between blood pressure and body weight in young populations are also shown by Levy et al. (1946), Paffenbarger et al. (1968), Londe and Goldring (1972), and Court et al. (1974). In the last-named study the rise in blood pressure lagged a number of years behind the weight increase.

Chiang et al. (1969) referred to 14 studies in which dietary weight reduction (withoug low-salt diet) in patients and volunteers was accompanied by a decrease in blood pressure. Lups and Francke (1947) observed that blood pressures in the population decreased in Holland during World War II and increased thereafter. References cited by Brozek et al. (1948) indicate that in Russia, Holland, and Germany the incidence of hypertensive cardiovascular complications declined during the hunger period of this war and rose when food conditions improved. Animal experimentation has further shown a relationship between nutritional status and blood pressure (Wood and Cash, 1939; Wilhelmj et al., 1951).

The mechanism of the causal influence, if any, of change in weight on change in blood pressure has remained a matter of conjecture. Alexander (1963), in accordance with Aygen and Braunwald (1962), surmised that the intensified force of cardiac contraction in obese patients is related to their increased blood volume as caused by increased body mass.

Guyton et al. (1973) have pointed out that oxygen demand of the tissues ultimately determines both tissue blood flow and tendency for blood to return from the systemic circulation to the heart, thereby regulating the heart minute volume. Under basal conditions, therefore, not only peripheral resistance but also blood minute volume is a function of total or lean body mass; both characteristics, blood volume and peripheral resistance, determine arterial blood pressure. The existence of a positive association between blood volume as estimated according to Allen et al. (1956) and long-term blood pressure (Borst and Borst, 1963) is supported by the cross-sectional data from this study of children.

IMPLICATIONS OF THESE OBSERVATIONS

Body height and body mass seem to be strong correlates of basal blood pressure in children. After controlling for these variables there is no association between age and blood pressure in the decade of life from 5 through 14 years of age. This finding is consistent with the hypothesis that in growing children increments in basal blood pressure are determined by increments in a quantitative tissue characteristic. Tall and heavy children have higher blood pressures than smaller children at similar ages. The practicing physician must consider this when assessing the need for close monitoring or future evaluation of a child's blood pressure.

SUMMARY

Extensive observations of blood pressure in children indicate the
need to relate blood pressure during growth to height and weight,
rather than age. Blood pressure data were obtained with an automatic
recording instrument that avoids excessive pressure readings in obese
children by the use of an over-sized arm cuff bladder with a built-in
infrasonic transducer. By reducing the anxiety of the child and by taking multiple readings, we obtained pressures that approached published basal levels. A multiple regression analysis showed that all
measured variables could account for 39% of the systolic blood pressure variation. Major determinants were weight and height. The blood
pressure levels, when related to height and to a weight-height index
(W/H^3), suggest a strong influence of height and an additional influence of W/H^3 on blood pressure, both consistent and proportionate
over the entire ranges of height and W/H^3. The total spectrum of observed correlates of blood pressure, resulting from the multiple
regression analysis, suggests that the blood pressure under basal-like
conditions increases as the child grows and is proportional to lean
body mass and total body mass. Practical criteria for evaluating abnormal blood pressure levels in children should be based on normative
values derived from body weight and body height rather than from
age.

VI. Diet

19. Dietary studies and the relationship of diet to cardiovascular disease risk-factor variables in children

The influence of diet on atherosclerosis and hypertension has been studied primarily in adults. Since pathogenetic studies suggest that these diseases begin in childhood (Strong and McGill, 1969; Voors et al., 1977a), comprehensive dietary information in early life is needed. Using an improved 24-hour dietary recall method (Frank et al., 1977a) we designed complementary dietary studies and incorporated them into the cardiovascular examinations in Bogalusa (1) to observe the diet/risk factor variable interrelationships in groups of children and (2) to describe what the pediatric population is consuming.

MATERIALS AND METHODS

Population sample

One-half of the Bogalusa children born in 1963, primarily fifth-grade students, were randomly selected and scheduled for a dietary interview. This totaled 194 students approximately 10 years old in 1973–74. Based on previous testing, the preteenage student appeared to be an attentive and reliable interviewee and perhaps less likely to fabricate responses than teenage students (Frank et al., 1977b).

In the study, 24-hour dietary recalls were obtained from 194 children; records of nine children were deleted because geographic residence requirement for participation was not met. The sample as composed of 185 children from ten schools. There were 65 black children (33 girls and 32 boys) and 120 white children (56 girls and 64 boys). Sixteen children were 9 years old; 153 children were 10; and 16 children were 11. The mean age was 10.5 years.

General preparations for dietary studies

Each child in the dietary sample rotated through the general cardiovascular examination, as has been described in Chapter 2. The 24-hour dietary recalls could not be conducted on the same day as the screening since a 12-hour fast for lipid analysis was required. Recalls were usually conducted within 10 days of the examination.

Clarification of salting procedures was an extension of the methodology described in Chapter 7. If actual foods ingested by the child included salt in preparation, then recipes which reflected the added salt were selected for nutritional analysis of the recall. Mothers were often contacted by telephone to verify the salting pattern code and ingredients in recipes. Salt acquired from the salt shaker at the table was treated as a separate food item.

Interviewers were trained periodically in the detailed protocol. Duplicate recalls inserted in intervals during the study period aided quality control and provided tests of reproducibility. Graduated food models, school lunch assessment, commercial food item research, verbal probes, and visual aids, such as a Product Identification Notebook (Chapter 7), increased the accuracy of qualitative information.

The Extended Table of Nutrients Values (ETNV) was used for analysis of the recalls for 58 dietary components (Moore et al., 1974).

Tests of reproducibility

Dietary recalls were collected by three trained nutritionists contributing 56%, 31%, and 13% of the sample. Each interviewer calculated her own recalls and checked the recalls of a co-worker. Three sets of ten children were each interviewed by two nutritionists to assess reproducibility in data collection. None of the sets showed any systematic difference between interviewers; however, the coefficients of variation for calories, polyunsaturated-to-saturated fatty acid ratio

(P/S),* and sucrose-to-starch ratio (Su/St)† implied some lack of agreement. Similar results were reported for the Franklinton pilot sample (Frank et al., 1977b).

As a means of identifying seasonal variations in nutrient intakes, the initial 15 respondents to the 24-hour dietary recalls were selected and interviewed by one nutritionist on three other occasions during the year. At ten-week intervals the 8 boys (2 black, 6 white) and 7 girls (3 black, 4 white) responded to a 24-hour recall. For the three different periods (December 1973, February 1974, April 1974), no significant difference was found between the mean intakes of 9 nutrients (calories, protein, fat, cholesterol, carbohydrate, Vitamin A, ascorbic acid, sodium, and iron).

An additional type of analysis of the 24-hour recalls included categorizing all foods into one of 17 food groups. The protein, fat, cholesterol, saturated fatty acid, carbohydrate, sucrose, starch, sodium, and caloric contents of 100 gm of each food were determined; then the percentage of these dietary components contributed by each of 17 food groups was calculated.

OBSERVATIONS

Composition of dietary intakes

Table 19–1 outlines the composition of the food consumed by the children. Protein, carbohydrate, and fat contributed 13%, 49%, and 38% of the total caloric intake, respectively. Dietary components were expressed per 1,000 kcal and per kilogram of body weight to identify the concentration of the components.

Protein and fat were mainly from animal sources. Mean fat intake

---

*Mean polyunsaturated (PUFA)-to-saturated fatty acid (SFA) ratio calculated as,

$$\frac{\sum_{i=1}^{n} PUFA/n}{\sum_{i=1}^{n} SFA/n}$$

†Mean sucrose-to-starch ratio calculated as,

$$\frac{\sum_{i=1}^{n} sucrose/n}{\sum_{i=1}^{n} starch/n}$$

Table 19–1. Mean intake and range of dietary components expressed as actual, per 1,000 kcal and per kilogram of body weight and the percentage of total calories from dietary components in 24-hour dietary recalls, $N = 185$.

Nutrient	Mean intake				
	Total (range) (N = 185)		Per 1,000 kcal (N = 185)	Per kg body weight (N = 184)	% of total calories
Calories (kcal)	2,141	(412–6,440)	—	66	—
Protein (gm)[1]	69	(4–227)	33	2.1	13
animal	47		22	1.4	9
vegetable	22		10	0.7	4
Carbohydrate (gm)[2]	262	(65–793)	124	8.1	49
starch	88		42	2.7	17
sugar[3]	144		68	4.5	27
sucrose	98		46	3.0	18
Su/St ratio	1.1		—	—	—
Fat (gm)[4]	93	(17–325)	43	2.8	38
animal	59		27	1.8	25
vegetable[5]	25		11	0.8	10
saturated[5]	38		18	1.2	16
polyunsaturated	12		5	0.4	5
P/S ratio[6]	0.3		—	—	—
Cholesterol (mg)	324	(0–1,536)	150	10.0	—
Sodium (gm)	3.33	(0.26–11.13)	1.57	0.1	—
Fiber (gm)	2.5	(0–16)	—	—	—

[1]Protein = sum of amino acid values.
[2]Carbohydrate = sum of starch, fructose, glucose, lactose, maltose, sucrose, pectic substance, other known, and unknown.
[3]Sugar = sum of fructose, glucose, lactose, maltose, and sucrose.
[4]Fat × .95 = total fatty acids; total fatty acids = saturated + unsaturated + unknown (within 0.1 gm).
[5]Saturated = myristic + palmitic + stearic + other known + unknown saturated fatty acids.
[6]Polyunsaturated = linoleic + linolenic + arachidonic.

included 8 gm of known hydrogenated fat. Saturated fat intake was high and produced a P/S ratio of less than 0.4. Carbohydrate intake indicated a sucrose-to-starch proportion of 1.1 and supplied a major source of calories. Sodium intake was quite variable.

The percentages of nine dietary components as determined by food group analysis are shown in Table 19–2. A quick survey of this table shows the food groups that are the major sources for each of the dietary components. Although eggs were the main source of cholesterol, milk was the prime source of saturated fatty acids and protein and

Table 19-2. Percentage of dietary components contributed by food groups appearing in 24-hour dietary recalls of 185 children

				Dietary component					
Food group	Calories	Protein	Fat	Saturated fatty acids	Cholesterol	Carbohydrate	Sucrose	Starch	Sodium
Beef	6	15	10	9	13	1	0	1	7
Beverages	7	0	0	0	0	14	37	0	0
Breads[1]	18	14	6	6	5	26	4	60	31
Candy	8	1	4	5	0	13	25	1	1
Cheese[2]	1	2	1	2	1	1	0	3	2
Condiments	—	—	0	—	—	0	1	0	7
Desserts[3]	12	6	13	13	11	14	19	13	6
Egg	2	3	4	4	26	0	0	0	1
Fats	5	3	11	7	0	1	1	1	5
Fruits	3	1	0	0	0	6	7	0	0
Milk	15	23	18	26	16	10	3	0	7
Mixed meat[4]	3	4	5	5	5	1	0	1	6
Pork	5	7	10	9	6	0	0	1	5
Poultry	2	7	3	2	7	0	0	1	2
Seafood	0	1	0	0	1	0	0	0	1
Snack[5]	3	1	4	3	0	2	0	6	3
Vegetables, soups	8	9	9	7	4	8	1	14	17

[1]Includes biscuits, cereals, pancakes, plain pastas.
[2]Includes cheese with pasta dishes, cheese spreads, and sauces.
[3]Includes cookies, cakes, pies, cobblers, puddings, donuts, and ice cream.
[4]Includes food products containing more than one type of meat, e.g., sausage, weiners, casseroles.
[5]Includes chips, crackers, popcorn, pretzels, and similar items.

milk contributed sizeable amounts of cholesterol and calories. Beef, breads, and vegetable dishes also added appreciably to the protein intake. Desserts represented more saturated fatty acids and cholesterol than pork, poultry, or seafood. Breads and desserts, candy and vegetable dishes contributed significantly to the total calories. Breads also contributed the most carbohydrate, chiefly as starch, but vegetable and dessert groups provided much of the starch intake. Beverages ranked higher than candy and desserts as a sucrose contributor. Sodium had two primary sources, breads and vegetables.

Sex-race differences

The white girls ingested fewer calories and less protein, fat, cholesterol, carbohydrate, and sodium than the other three sex-race groups. Interestingly, the mean protein intake for white and black girls was approximately 10 gm lower than that of their male counterparts. White boys had a greater fat and total caloric intake than the other three groups, but the black boys ingested more cholesterol-rich protein sources. When comparing geometric means for select nutrients, significant differences among the four sex-race groups were noted for starch and sodium. Both the white boys and the black girls had significantly greater intakes of starch than the white girls ($p < 0.01$). Figure 19–1 outlines the frequency distribution of sodium by sex. Black girls had a significantly greater sodium intake than white girls ($p < 0.01$), and both black and white boys ($p < 0.05$). No significant differences were noted between the four sex-race groups for cholesterol or fat intakes.

Interviewers categorized respondents for salting procedures by reviewing qualitative information in the recall and combining these data with the child's description of usual salting technique at the table. All black girls reported that salt was added to their food at some point of preparation or ingestion; 22% of white boys reported salting their food before tasting as compared to 7% of the white girls, 6% of the black boys, and 12% of the black girls. Approximately one-fourth of the children received salt only during the cooking process. Salting during cooking and after tasting was the most common procedure for white boys (47%), white girls (63%), and black girls (67%). A small percentage reported no salting of food.

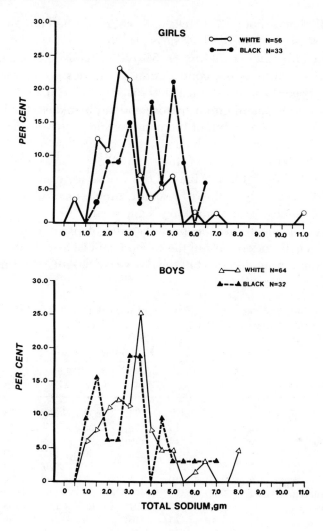

Figure 19–1. Frequency distribution of 24-hour sodium intake in 10-year-old children.

Meal pattern

For the total sample, 92% ate breakfast; 99%, lunch; 96%, dinner; and 98%, snacks. Fewer blacks (81% boys and 88% girls) than whites (97% boys and 95% girls) ate breakfast, which may be related to socioeconomic differences noted in blacks and whites in the community. Of the three sex-race groups, black boys ate dinner and snacks less frequently, i.e., 9% did not eat dinner; 6% did not consume snacks.

Table 19–3 outlines the contribution of calories, cholesterol, and other dietary components by meal and snack periods. Snacks provided the most calories; mainly from sucrose and fat; breakfast, the least calories. A closer examination of the contribution of total calories from snacks for the 182 children who ate snacks shows that snacks contributed from 40–50% of the total calories for 30 children and 50–70% of the calories for 25 children. Many of the snacks were small meals eaten between a clearly defined breakfast, lunch, or dinner; for some children, an almost hourly snacking is apparent.

The evening meal was the prime source of protein, niacin, and starch. Lunch provided most of the calcium and lactose intake. Breakfast and dinner provided most of the day's cholesterol, vitamin A, and

Table 19–3. Mean intake and percentage of total daily intake of dietary components from meals and snacks

Nutrient	Mean intake (%)							
	Breakfast N = 170		Lunch N = 184		Dinner N = 177		Snacks N = 182	
Calories, kcal	360	(17)	497	(23)	632	(29)	723	(34)
Protein, gm	12	(17)	19	(28)	26	(37)	14	(21)
animal, gm	9	(18)	14	(29)	18	(38)	8	(17)
Fat, gm	16	(17)	21	(23)	30	(31)	29	(31)
SFA, gm	7	(17)	10	(26)	11	(29)	12	(30)
USFA, gm	8	(17)	10	(21)	17	(33)	16	(32)
cholesterol, mg	101	(30)	73	(23)	98	(29)	60	(19)
Carbohydrate, gm	43	(16)	56	(21)	66	(25)	105	(40)
sucrose, gm	10	(10)	13	(13)	19	(19)	59	(59)
starch, gm	14	(16)	26	(29)	32	(35)	20	(23)
lactose, gm	7	(29)	9	(36)	2	(10)	7	(28)
Vitamin A, gm	1300	(35)	924	(25)	1026	(28)	590	(16)
Thiamine, mg	0.45	(30)	0.28	(19)	0.38	(26)	0.23	(16)
Niacin, mg	7.17	(22)	7.06	(27)	9.83	(32)	5.98	(19)
Riboflavin, mg	0.63	(30)	0.51	(25)	0.39	(19)	0.42	(20)
Ascorbic acid, mg	30	(43)	8.8	(13)	13	(20)	18	(27)
Calcium, mg	210	(25)	278	(33)	140	(17)	238	(28)
Iron, mg	2.4	(19)	2.9	(23)	4.2	(33)	2.4	(19)
Sodium, mg	487	(14)	994	(30)	1276	(37)	660	(20)

thiamine. Snacks were high in sucrose and fat. Breakfast and snacks provided rich sources of ascorbic acid.

Comparison of intake with recommended dietary allowances (RDA)

The daily intakes of nine dietary components were compared with RDA (Food and Nutrition Board, 1974) and are presented in Figure 19–2 as the percentage of boys and girls achieving various levels. Bogalusa boys generally had slightly higher intakes than girls of nine select components except for vitamin A and ascorbic acid. For boys, more blacks than whites appeared in the lower quartiles for calories, protein, vitamin A, iron, calcium, and thiamine. The reverse was true for females, as more white girls than black girls were in the lower quartiles for most dietary components. Interestingly, only 9% of the black girls but 16% of the white girls reported taking vitamin supplements regularly, which were usually multiple vitamin preparations (84%).

Nineteen percent of the boys and 25% of the girls achieved less than two-thirds the RDA for calories. A more than adequate daily protein intake (greater than 100% of the RDA) was noted for most children in each sex-race group. This is easily seen when a vertical line

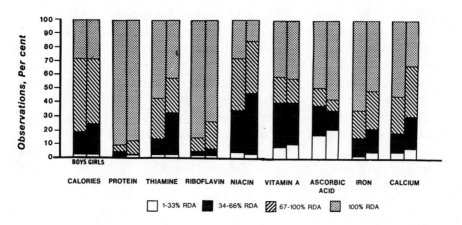

Figure 19–2. Comparison of nutrient intakes of 10-year-old children with recommended dietary allowances.

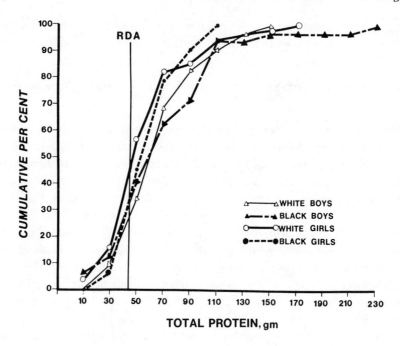

Figure 19–3. Cumulative frequency distribution of 24-hour protein intake in 10-year-old children.

indicating the protein RDA of 44 gm for 10-year-old children is inserted on a cumulative frequency distribution of protein (Fig. 19–3). Riboflavin and iron intakes were similar to protein, but niacin intake which included tryptophan conversion (60 mg tryptophan = 1 mg niacin) did not reflect this trend. At least one-third of all children did not achieve two-thirds of the RDA for vitamin A, ascorbic acid, and niacin. Calcium intakes were lower for girls than for boys with mean intakes of 748 mg and 920 mg, respectively. Diets of Bogalusa children reflected greater intakes of iron, calcium, thiamine, and riboflavin than those of the pilot sample (Frank et al., 1977b), thereby placing fewer Bogalusa children at lower levels.

Eating span

The eating span, or the number of hours from the first food or beverage until the last food or beverage, was determined for each child.

Nineteen children had an eating span of less than 10 hr (Group A); 95 children 10–13 hr (Group B); and 71 children more than 13 hr (Group C). The sex distribution amoung the three groups was approximately the same. The groups were compared for differences in, (a) risk-factor variables of triglyceride, serum cholesterol, skinfold average, Quetelet obesity index (weight/height^2), and systolic blood pressure; (b) 9 dietary components each expressed as actual intake and per 1,000 kcal; and (c) percentage of calories from carbohydrate, fat, and protein.

Group C had significantly greater intakes of calories, protein, fat, carbohydrate, and sodium than either Group A and Group B. The amount of difference was consistent for all components; in other words, Group C had 40% greater intakes of the component than Group A and 20% greater than Group B. When risk-factor variables were compared for each eating span, only total serum cholesterol for Group C was significantly greater than that for Group A ($p < 0.05$) and Group B ($p < 0.05$), with the difference being roughly 20% and 10% higher per time interval, respectively.

Eating frequency

Eating frequency, or the number of different times a day a student ingested food or beverage, was identified for each child. The students were divided into three groups. Group 1 ($N = 49$ students), had 5 or fewer times in which food or beverage was eaten; Group 2, ($N = 105$ students) had an eating frequency of 6–8; Group 3, ($N = 31$ students) had 9–12 eating times.

Group 3 had significantly greater dietary intakes than Groups 1 and 2 for calories, protein, carbohydrate, sucrose, starch, fat, saturated and polyunsaturated fatty acids, cholesterol, sodium, iron, and calcium. The average caloric intake of Group 3 was 1.8 times that of Group 1 ($\bar{x}$ of Group 3 = 3,100 kcal, $\bar{x}$ of Group 1 = 1,700 kcal).

The comparison of risk-factor variables showed that children in Group 2 had significantly greater values than those of Groups 1 and 3 for W/H^2, triglyceride, and pre-β-lipoproteins; and Group 2 had significantly greater β-lipoprotein values than did Group 1. Group 1 had significantly higher α-lipoprotein values than both Groups 2 and 3. There were no differences among the three groups in cholesterol, blood pressure, or skinfold measurements.

Risk-factor levels

The mean levels of risk-factor variables for the randomly selected 185 children were compared with those values for the 10-year-old population not selected for diet study. None of the differences noted in risk-factor levels in the two groups were significant, indicating that the randomly selected sample was representative of this age of children in the community.

Mean levels of anthropometric measurements of the dietary subsample were (a) skinfold average: 11.3 mm for boys, 13.3 mm for girls; (b) weight: 34 kg for boys and girls; (c) height: 139 cm for boys, 141 cm for girls; and (d) Quetelet index: 17.4 kg/m² for boys and 17.0 for girls. Total serum cholesterol averaged 164 mg/100 ml for boys and 168 mg/100 ml for girls. The β- and pre-β-lipoprotein cholesterol fractions were slightly higher for girls with triglyceride levels averaging 65 mg and 69 mg/100 ml for boys and girls, respectively. Systolic blood pressure averaged 98 mm Hg for boys and 99 mm Hg for girls and diastolic blood pressure (fourth phase) was 61 mm Hg for both sexes. Mean hemoglobin level was 12.9 gm/100 ml.

Interrelationship of dietary components and other variables

Twenty dietary components provided by the ETNV were expressed as total intake and intake per 1,000 kcal for each child and analyzed for possible correlation with blood hemoglobin, blood pressure, skinfold average, Quetelet obesity index, and fasting serum lipids (total cholesterol and α-, pre-β-, and β-lipoproteins). Positive correlations significant at the 5% level were noted for only a few variables, such as β-LP (lipoprotein) and arachidonic acid expressed as actual intake and per 1,000 kcal (Table 19–4). Triglyceride and vegetable fat were negatively correlated for both total and per 1,000 kcal intake. Dietary cholesterol had only a weak postive correlation with β-LP. An association of starch per 1,000 kcal with α-LP and sucrose per 1,000 kcal with serum cholesterol, triglyceride, and α-LP is suggested. None of the dietary components, however, accounted for more than 4% of the variability in the risk-factor parameter, leaving 96% of the variability unexplained. In other studies based on this approach to data analysis, a similar lack of relationship of diet to serum lipids has been observed (Keys et al., 1956; Kannel et al., 1971b).

Table 19–4. Pearson correlation coefficients[1] for risk-factor variables and dietary components as expressed per se and per 1,000 calories for 185 10-year-olds

Dietary component	Risk-factor variable							
	Total cholesterol	Triglyceride	Systolic blood pressure (Baum)	β-LP	pre-β	α-LP	Wt/Ht²	Skinfold
Vegetable fat	—[2]	-0.159³	—	—	—	—	—	—
Arachidonic acid	0.154³	—	—	0.176³	—	—	—	—
Cholesterol	—	—	—	0.171³	—	—	—	—
Dietary component per 1,000 kcal			Risk factor variable					
Protein	0.151³	—	—	—	—	—	0.145³	—
Fat	—	—	—	—	—	—	0.146³	—
vegetable	—	-0.194⁴	—	—	—	—	—	—
polyunsaturated fatty acids	—	-0.156³	—	—	—	—	—	—
saturated fatty acids	—	—	—	—	—	—	—	0.154³
arachidonic acid	—	—	—	0.152³	—	—	—	—
linoleic acid	—	-0.160³	—	—	—	—	-0.143³	—
Carbohydrate	-0.151³	—	—	—	—	—	-0.176³	—
starch	—	—	—	—	—	0.149³	—	—
sucrose	-0.165³	0.148³	—	—	—	-0.189³	—	—
Sodium	—	—	0.143³	—	—	—	—	—

[1]Only statistically significant correlation coefficients shown.
[2]—designates not significant.
³$p < 0.05$
⁴$p < 0.01$

A further comparison of the data included grouping children according to high or low intakes of select nutrients, and, again, no observable differences were noted in any risk-factor levels. Children were then grouped according to risk-factor variable levels, that is, below the 25th percentile, between 25th and 75th percentiles, and equal to or greater than 75th percentile for nine risk-factor variables. The mean intakes of 22 dietary components expressed as both actual intake and per 1,000 kcal were compared for the three groups for each risk factor.

Results of the comparison of mean intakes of the dietary components for children grouped according to serum cholesterol level were most interesting. Even when the fat intake was expressed several ways, as shown in Table 19–5, the children with the middle (between 25th and 75th percentiles) and high (greater than 75th percentile) serum cholesterol values showed significantly greater fat intakes than those with the lowest serum cholesterol levels. The reverse relation

Table 19–5. Mean intake of dietary components for children grouped according to serum cholesterol level percentile[1]

| | Serum cholesterol level percentile | | |
| | Group 1 (< 25th) | Group 2 (25th ≤ x < 75th) | Group 3 (≥ 75th) |
Dietary component	n = 49	n = 81	n = 49
		gm	
Total fat (TF)	75.3	100.6[3]	101.4[3]
TF/1,000 kcal	38.1	44.8[4]	44.3[4]
Animal fat (AF)	44.9	65.6[2]	65.5[2]
AF/1,000 kcal	23.1	29.4[2]	28.5[2]
Saturated fatty acid (SFA)	30.7	41.0[2]	42.3[2]
SFA/1,000 kcal	15.6	18.4[4]	18.5[2]
Unsaturated fatty acid (USFA)	40.1	53.4[2]	52.4[2]
USFA/1,000 kcal	20.2	23.6[3]	22.9[2]
Carbohydrate/1,000 kcal	133.3[6]	119.5	120.2
Sucrose/1,000 kcal	53.1[5]	43.5	43.1
Iron/1,000 kcal	6.6[7]	5.8	5.3
Sodium	2.9	3.5[2]	3.6[2]

[1]Other variables compared but not found significant
[2]Mean greater than mean for group 1 ($p < 0.05$)
[3]Mean greater than mean for group 1 ($p < 0.01$)
[4]Mean greater than mean for group 1 ($p < 0.001$)
[5]Mean greater than mean for group 2 ($p < 0.05$) and group 3 ($p < 0.05$)
[6]Mean greater than mean for group 2 ($p < 0.01$) and group 3 ($p < 0.01$)
[7]Mean greater than mean for group 3 ($p < 0.05$)

was true for carbohydrate and sucrose intakes. No significant relationship was observed for exogenous cholesterol.

Other significant correlations resulting from this type of grouping suggested these trends: highest ($\geq$ 75th percentile) systolic blood pressure group had diets with lowest sucrose; highest diastolic blood pressure group matched with highest potassium intake; lowest ($<$ 25th percentile) α-LP levels found for children with highest cholesterol intakes; lowest serum triglyceride group had highest vegetable fat intakes; and children in the highest group for obesity index had significantly larger protein intakes.

COMMENT

The purpose of this study was to determine the dietary factors that might account for elevated levels of blood pressure and serum lipids present in children. Understanding such relationships and determining them in early life would offer directions for modifying dietary patterns in an effort to forestall coronary artery disease and hypertension. Unfortunately, to collect detailed quantitative data on food consumption of the total 3,524 children examined during the first cross-sectional survey would have been expensive and difficult. We chose a subsample and a method that seemed most promising for our resources. Despite these limitations certain useful information was obtained.

A random sample of the children in the fifth grade would serve only indirectly to reflect the dietary intake of all school children of all ages. Obviously certain changes occur across the age spectrum, for instance in milk and snack food consumption. Snacking patterns certainly change as children become older and more independent.

It was most obvious that the percentage of calories from total fat and saturated fat in the children's dietary intakes exceeded the American Heart Association (1970) recommendation of less than 35% and 10% of the total calories from total and saturated fat, respectively. The mean exogenous cholesterol intake was roughly half of the 600 mg thought to be ingested in the average daily diets of adults. The P/S ratio reflects a high saturated fat intake for the children, and an almost equal proportion of sucrose-to-starch is obvious.

In general, the composition of the diets was not vastly different from a general composition of diets of the majority of persons in the United

States (American Heart Association, 1968; Connor and Connor, 1972). No significant seasonal variations were observed in the food intakes. Although food substitutions occur with seasons, the composition of the diet remains basically the same. Obviously, throughout the year basic food groups supply the major portion of calories and dietary components in food intakes of Bogalusa children, a pattern also observed in food intakes of U.S. households (U.S. Dept. of Agriculture, 1974).

The mean protein intake of these children was lower than values reported for both sex groups studied in the Ten State Nutrition Survey (U.S. Dept. of H.E.W., 1972), and the U.S. Department of Agriculture Survey in 1965 (1969). According to the recommendation of optimal protein intake for adolescents by Johnston (1957) of 15% of caloric intake, that of the Bogalusa children was low. However, when using the National Research Council's RDA for protein, a more than adequate intake is noted. Bogalusa boys generally had higher intakes of protein and other components than did girls; this has been noted for children in other populations (Burke et al., 1959; Hodges and Krehl, 1965).

Limited data are available from studies that include both dietary and risk-factor variable assessment. Although the Bogalusa study examined a younger age group and collected data more than a decade later than the Framingham Study (Kannel and Gordon, 1970), it is similar to the cardiovascular survey of Framingham adults, which examined diet and risk-factor variables.

Average caloric intake of the Bogalusa children was identical to the mean value reported for Framingham adult females. Likewise, the percentage of calories from fat compares with the 39–40% reported for individuals in Framingham. Sixty-three percent of the fat was from animal sources in the children's diets, P/S of 0.32; whereas 71% was noted in the Framingham population, P/S of 0.42. Exogenous cholesterol for the children was less than for adult females ($\bar{X} = 492$ mg) and less than half the intake of adult males ($\bar{X} = 704$ mg).

When protein, fat, carbohydrate, and cholesterol intake were expressed per kilogram of body weight, Bogalusa children had higher intakes than the Framingham adults as shown in Figure 19–4. On the other hand, Framingham adults exhibited higher intakes of protein, fat, and cholesterol per 1,000 kcal than the children.

The noted difference in sodium intake, especially for the black fe-

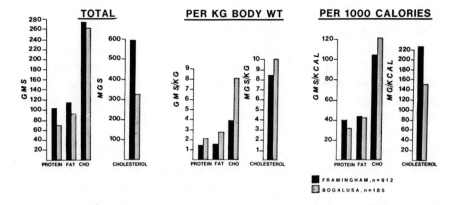

Figure 19–4. Comparison of daily dietary intakes of Framingham adults with Bogalusa children.

male, is striking. Already by age 10 or 11, the black female, known in adulthood to be at high risk for hypertension (Langford et al., 1968; Gordon, 1973), exhibits a higher sodium intake than other sex-race groups. It is unknown whether exposure to high sodium intake continues. Some children are already salting foods before tasting; Louisiana cookery includes use of salted meats in vegetable preparation; and a high intake of starches which are high in sodium was noted for the black girls and white boys.

Hemoglobin levels of the children were compared with the National Nutrition Survey recommendations (O'Neal et al., 1970); 9.7% of the black and 3.5% of the white children were ranked as "low" (10.0–11.4 gm/100 ml), but no significant correlation was noted between iron intake and hemoglobin level in the 185 children. The overall evaluation of the total Bogalusa pediatric population noted that white children exhibit greater hemoglobin levels than black children (Frerichs et al., 1977).

The lack of a correlation of risk-factor levels and dietary components noted in our population and in others requires a closer examination. It is known that significant dietary differences and risk-factor levels can be found by comparing populations on an international basis (Hartog et al., 1968), and we know that dietary changes can alter levels in a given individual (Connor, 1970). Yet, within a given population significant interrelationships are difficult to observe. Studies of experimental dietary manipulations of serum cholesterol and lipoproteins over a broad range of dietary cholesterol, in several species of nonhuman primates, including chimpanzee, indicate a low order of responses; and, interestingly, the low levels of exogenous cholesterol administered (0.05–0.2%) (Srinivasan et al., 1976b) encompass the total international range of human dietary exposure. Much larger doses are used experimentally (usually up to 2%). Most striking is the marked individual variability of the primates at all levels of intake.

Extrapolated to studies of humans, the individual variability of serum lipids seems to be so great within a given population consuming a relatively narrow range of dietary cholesterol that correlations cannot be observed. Further, in most populations the variability in dietary intake on a day-to-day basis, coupled with the differences of serum lipid levels from one individual to the next on similar dietary intakes, negates the possibility of close correlations. As shown in these studies, however, comparison of groups based on risk-factor variable levels detects some of the influence of diet within a population study, even when the sample size is limited. The observations from this study of children as might be expected, essentially point to a relationship of saturated fat and sucrose intake with serum lipids. Patterns of dietary habits are also important since long eating spans and snack foods contribute to the excessive intake of calories, fat, protein, and sodium. Food intake may be only one factor or may play a small role in the development of arteriosclerosis.

SUMMARY

A dietary study was planned to complement a longitudinal investigation of arteriosclerosis risk-factor variables in children. Fifty percent of the 10-year-old age group, 185 children, each responded to an improved 24-hour dietary recall. The method, containing quality controls to increase the accuracy of the data, provided a detailed group description of meal patterns, including quantitation of select dietary components.

Significant sex-race differences were noted for sodium and starch intakes; none for cholesterol or fat intakes. The black female was identified in this age group as ingesting large amounts of sodium. The bread group contributed the most calories, starch, and sodium; eggs were the prime source of cholesterol; milk contributed appreciably to the protein, fat, and cholesterol intakes.

Caloric adequacy was almost identical for boys and girls; but differences were noted between sexes for intakes of protein, B-vitamins, iron, and calcium. Protein intake was more than adequate for most children. Black boys, who reported eating fewer meals than the other sex-race groups; and white girls generally had the lowest nutrient intakes. As eating span and eating frequency increased, an increase was noted for most dietary components. The serum cholesterol level was significantly higher for students with the longest eating span. Differences in mean intakes of dietary components, when expressed per 1,000 kcal and per kilogram of body weight, were noted between Bogalusa children and Framingham adults.

In the clinical setting, diet has been shown to influence risk-factor levels for individuals. Population studies are needed to support these findings. A lack of correlation was observed in large correlation matrices of dietary components and risk-factor variables for our population. However, group comparisons of dietary intakes for children at high and low risk-factor levels did yield interesting relationships as might be predicted. Food may well be one environmental determinant of risk-factor levels, but its definite influence remains to be clarified.

VII. Multiple risk factors

20. Occurrence of multiple risk-factor variables for cardiovascular disease in children

Early lesions of coronary artery disease (CAD) and initiation of essential hypertension probably begin in children (Holman et al., 1958; Strong et al., 1972; Voors et al., 1977a), hence recent interest has focused on the presence in pediatric populations (Kannel and Dawber, 1972; Lauer et al., 1975) of risk factors known to occur in adults. Although the association of obesity with blood pressure (Kannel et al., 1967a) and hyperlipidemia (Montoye et al., 1966; Keys et al., 1972; Ashley and Kannel, 1974) is established in adults, comparable information has not yet been found in children. In adults these risk factors have been shown to act independently in determining risk of CAD, however, the subsequent rise in risk is greatly increased if any two or more risk factors are present at high levels (Cornfield, 1962). Although the factors at risk in children are not clearly defined at this time, it is possible to describe similar variables in children. The distributions of serum lipids and lipoproteins, blood pressure, and growth characteristics have been discussed in detail, but do these risk-factor variables occur independently in children or do they cluster? By identifying those children who have elevations of multiple risk-factor variables, we can focus on primary prevention in the population with the greatest risk. This chapter examines the internal relationships of blood pressure, serum lipids and lipoproteins, and a measure of obesity.

METHODS

Population

These studies include 3,524 school children ages 5–14 years and 676 preschool children ages 2½–5½ years. For 101 school children and 35 preschool children, either no blood was drawn or anthropometric or blood pressure data were missing. Since fasting serum is needed to assess serum lipoproteins, 294 additional nonfasting children were excluded, yielding a total of 3,770 children for lipoprotein analysis.

Examination

Details of the screening flow, methods of measurement including observation of indirect blood pressure, and serum lipids are described in Chapters 8–12 and 15–16; Frerichs et al., 1976; Srinivasan et al., 1976a; Voors et al., 1976; Foster et al., 1977. The fourth-phase mercury sphygmomanometer readings, which we found to be more reliable as the diastolic pressure, were used (see Chapter 6). In addition to the sphygmomanometer, the Infrasonde 3000 recorder (La Barge, Inc., St. Louis, Mo.) and the Arteriosonde 1010 (Roche Medical Electronics, Inc., Cranberry, N.J.) were used for the preschool children (Berenson et al., 1978a). The systolic pressure obtained on the Infrasonde, which coincided more closely with measurements obtained on the school children, was used for analysis of data on the preschool children. All readings were taken to the nearest 2 mm Hg.

Obesity

Several weight-for-height *(W-H)* indices were examined as measures of body fat. We selected for this analysis an index that was independent of height and highly correlated with another index of obesity obtained during the screening process, the triceps skinfold. Using the formula devised by Benn (1971), we found that weight/height$^{2.77}$ *(W/H$^{2.77}$)* fits our data best for the school children while *W/H$^{2.00}$* was best for the preschool children. Skinfold measurements could also have been used directly as a measure of body fat, but they are correlated in children with age and height.

Statistical analysis

Age-, race-, and sex-specific percentiles were obtained for each of the risk-factor variables. A chi-square statistic was used to compare the number of children observed to be above the 75th percentile with the number expected under a model of no association.

OBSERVATIONS

School children

There were 114 (3.3%) school children at or above the age-, race-, and sex-specific 75th percentiles for $W/H^{2.77}$, total serum cholesterol, and diastolic blood pressure (Table 20–1). Under a null hypothesis of no association only 53 (1.56%) would have been expected. This difference is statistically significant ($p < 0.001$) when comparing the number observed to the number expected. Although more school children were at high risk in each race-sex group than were expected, there seemed to be a greater clustering among white males (3.8%) and black

Table 20–1. Children with multiple risk factors at or above the 75th percentile by race and sex

	N	High risk[1] n (%)
School children		
white boys	1,133	43 (3.8)
white girls	1,025	29 (2.8)
black boys	661	18 (2.7)
black girls	604	24 (4.0)
	N	High risk[2] n (%)
Preschool children		
white boys	218	3 (1.4)
white girls	214	3 (1.4)
black boys	96	2 (2.1)
black girls	113	2 (1.8)

[1] ≥75th percentile for diastolic blood pressure, total cholesterol, and weight/height$^{2.77}$
[2] ≥75th percentile for systolic blood pressure, total cholesterol, and weight/height^2

females (4.0%) than among white females (2.8%) and black males (2.7%). If we define the risk ratio as the number children observed divided by the number expected, the risk ratio is 2.4 for white boys and 2.5 for black girls, but only 1.8 for white girls and 1.7 for black boys (see Fig. 20–1).

Table 20–2 identifies the school children who are at high risk by age, race, and sex. For both white boys and black boys, the percentage at high risk increases with age (2.1–4.6% for white boys and 1.1–4.3% for black boys). This age trend is less obvious for white girls and black girls.

When examining these risk factor variables two at a time, the greatest association is between $W/H^{2.77}$ and diastolic blood pressure. About 10% of those children who were at or above the 75th percentile for $W/H^{2.77}$ were also high on diastolic blood pressure. Under the null hypothesis of no association only 6.25% would have been expected

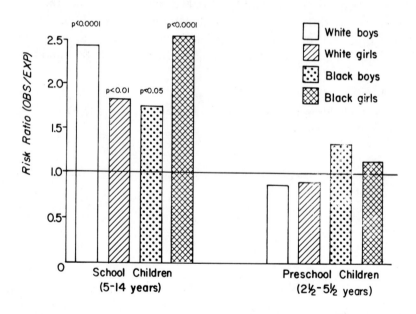

Figure 20–1. Risk ratios for children with levels at or above the 75th percentile for three factors (blood pressure, cholesterol, and obesity) by race, sex, and age. For school children for each race and sex the number observed is greater than the number expected under a null hypothesis of no association (white boys, $p < 0.0001$; white girls, $p < 0.001$; black boys, $p < 0.005$; black girls, $p < 0.0001$).

Table 20–2. School children with two or more risk factor variables at or above the 75th percentile by age, race, sex

Age	N	Blood pressure and cholesterol		$W/H^{2.77}$ and cholesterol		$W/H^{2.77}$ and blood pressure		$W/H^{2.77}$, cholesterol and blood pressure	
		n	(%)[1]	n	(%)[1]	n	(%)[1]	n	(%)[2]
White boys									
5–6	188	13	(6.9)	13	(6.9)	19	(10.1)	4	(2.1)
7–8	210	15	(7.1)	15	(7.1)	21	(10.0)	8	(3.8)
9–10	232	15	(6.5)	19	(8.2)	25	(10.8)	8	(3.4)
11–12	263	19	(7.2)	24	(9.1)	29	(11.0)	12	(4.6)
13–14	240	18	(7.5)	29	(12.1)	18	(7.5)	11	(4.6)
Black boys									
5–6	93	2	(2.2)	4	(4.3)	9	(9.7)	1	(1.1)
7–8	118	7	(5.9)	6	(5.1)	13	(11.0)	3	(2.5)
9–10	154	8	(5.2)	10	(6.5)	15	(9.7)	3	(1.9)
11–12	156	12	(7.7)	12	(7.7)	12	(7.7)	5	(3.2)
13–14	140	8	(5.7)	15	(10.7)	16	(11.4)	6	(4.3)
White girls									
5–6	177	11	(6.2)	12	(6.8)	16	(9.0)	4	(2.3)
7–8	191	15	(7.9)	14	(7.3)	17	(8.9)	6	(3.1)
9–10	209	11	(5.3)	12	(5.7)	21	(10.0)	4	(1.9)
11–12	240	20	(8.3)	18	(7.5)	24	(10.0)	8	(3.3)
13–14	208	18	(8.7)	15	(7.2)	19	(9.1)	7	(3.4)
Black girls									
5–6	93	6	(6.5)	8	(8.6)	8	(8.6)	3	(3.2)
7–8	111	11	(9.9)	8	(7.2)	10	(9.0)	7	(6.3)
9–10	119	8	(6.7)	9	(7.6)	10	(8.4)	4	(3.4)
11–12	146	11	(7.5)	15	(10.3)	13	(8.9)	6	(4.1)
13–14	135	8	(5.9)	9	(6.7)	13	(9.6)	4	(3.0)

[1] If no association, then 6.25% expected   [2] If no association, then 1.56% expected

for each race-sex group ($p < 0.0001$ for white boys and girls, $p < 0.001$ for black girls, and $p < 0.01$ for black boys). About 8% were high on both $W/H^{2.77}$ and serum cholesterol ($p < 0.001$ for white boys) and about 7% on both diastolic blood pressure and serum cholesterol ($p > 0.05$ for all four race-sex groups). Altogether 206 white boys (18.2%), 185 white girls (18.0%), 113 black boys (17.1%), and 99 black girls (16.4%) were high on *at least* two risk-factor variables. We would expect 15.6% under a no-association hypothesis.

Preschool children

For preschool children only 10 (1.56%) were at or above the age-, race-, and sex-specific 75th percentile for W/H^2, for total serum cholesterol, and systolic blood pressure (Infrasonde). This was no different than what would be expected under a hypothesis of no association. (see Table 20–1).

Other variables

If we substitute β-lipoprotein, perhaps a better indicator of risk, for total cholesterol and restrict the analysis to fasting children only, we have essentially the same results as we found with total cholesterol for both preschool-age and school-age children. There were 115 (3.6%) school children and 8 (1.3%) preschool children who would be considered at high risk. Similarly, the clustering of blood pressure, obesity, and serum triglycerides was examined in fasting children. Above the 75th percentile for each were 122 (3.9%) school children and 19 (3.1%) preschool children. For the school children, there was little change in the number of white males (3.9%) at high risk but an increase in the number of white females (4.2%) and black males (3.5%), and a slight decrease in the black females (3.6%) at high risk. In preschool children the increase was principally due to a greater aggregation in white females (4.4%) and black females (3.7%).

Low risk

The tendency for risk factors in children to cluster was also examined for lower levels of the risk-factor variables. There were 132 (4.2%) school-age children with diastolic blood pressure, β-lipoprotein, and

$W/H^{2.77}$ below their age-, race-, and sex-specific 50th percentile and α-lipoprotein above the 75th percentile (Table 20–3). Under a null hypothesis of no association, only 99 (3.1%) would be expected. This aggregation was most evident for white boys (5.3%, $p < 0.0001$) and black girls (4.3%) but was only exhibited by 3.4% of the white girls and 3.5% of the black boys. The percentiles are chosen arbitrarily to study this size population. We selected those at presumably normal or low risk to examine clustering with α-lipoprotein at high levels.

None of the race-sex groups showed any age trends when all four variables were considered. In examining these variables two at a time, we see a statistically significant association between diastolic blood pressure and $W/H^{2.77}$ (white boys, $p < 0.01$ and white girls, $p < 0.01$) and between β-lipoprotein and $W/H^{2.77}$ (white boys, $p < 0.05$).

Similar results for preschool children were noted in eleven white boys (5.3%) and eight black girls (7.4%) who were at or below the 50th percentile for systolic blood pressure, β-lipoprotein, and W/H^2 and above the 75th percentile for α-lipoprotein. Only three (1.5%) white

Table 20–3. Children[1] with low levels of several risk-factor variables by age, race and sex

| | N | Low risk[2] | |
		n	(%)
School children			
white boys	1,026	54	(5.3)
white girls	970	33	(3.4)
black boys	601	21	(3.5)
black girls	564	24	(4.3)
	N	Low risk[3]	
		n	(%)
Preschool children			
white boys	209	11	(5.3)
white girls	201	3	(1.5)
black boys	91	0	(0.0)
black girls	108	8	(7.4)

[1]Fasting only.
[2]<50th percentile for diastolic blood pressure, β-lipoprotein, and weight/height$^{2.77}$, and ≥75th percentile for α-lipoprotein
[3]<50th percentile for systolic blood pressure, β-lipoprotein and weight/height^2, and ≥75th percentile for α-lipoprotein

girls and no black boys showed this aggregation. Overall 22(3.7%) pre-school children were in this group.

DISCUSSION

Although in children, absolute risk-factor variable levels have not been adequately defined, they do seem to cluster at high levels much as in adults. Cornfield (1962) has shown in Framingham adults that high blood pressure and high serum cholesterol act as independent risk factors for heart disease. A rise in both, however, will have a mul-tiplicative effect on the rise in risk for coronary heart disease.

In Bogalusa this clustering at high levels of blood pressure, serum cholesterol, and a weight-height index occurred in all four race-sex groups. The greatest clustering was among white boys and black girls. We have shown previously that whites have greater skinfolds than blacks, (Chapter 8), that black boys tend to be leaner than white boys, that black boys have slightly higher blood pressure than whites (Chapter 16 and Voors et al., 1976), and that blacks have higher serum cholesterol than whites (Chapter 12 and Frerichs et al., 1976). The latter finding is due to the fact that blacks have higher α-lipoproteins, but there is no detectable racial difference in β-lipoproteins (Chapter 13 and Srinivasan et al., 1976a).

We have shown in our Bogalusa population that height, weight, and age will explain some 39% of the variability in blood pressure levels in school-aged children (Voors et al., 1976). However, only about 4% of the variability in serum cholesterol can be explained by such vari-ables as age, race, sex, triceps skinfold, maturation (Tanner scale), and weight-for-height index. This can be explained by the fact that in our population as obesity levels increase, β-lipoprotein increases but α-lipoprotein decreases. We have shown that more obese children, both blacks and whites, tend to have significantly elevated levels of triglyc-erides and pre-β-lipoproteins (Frerichs et al., 1978b). White obese children tend to have higher levels of cholesterol and β-lipoprotein also. On the other hand, α-lipoprotein levels are significantly lower in the more obese children. Of particular interest is that the presence of two factors increases the likelihood that three factors will occur, a clustering for increased risk for CAD. While the association of high diastolic blood pressure and elevated serum cholesterol is no greater than expected, we did find that children with high levels of both diastolic blood pressure and a weight-for-height index had elevated cholesterol.

Restricting our population to those in the top 25 percentiles for a weight-height index, we found a tendency for these variables to aggregate more than expected. A similar finding was noted by Lauer et al. (1975), in a survey of children in Muscatine, Iowa. Of the children who were in the top decile for relative weight, some 18% were also in the top decile for serum cholesterol and some 29% in the top decile for blood pressure. Wilmore and McNamara (1974) also noted in their study of 95 boys 8–12 years of age, that CAD risk factors could be identified and that the percentage of boys with one or more risk factors is high.

In an effort to study the early evidence of factors related to risk for coronary artery disease or hypertension, many programs are focusing on school-age children. But it is as important to extend observations into the preschool years to broaden our information on the early natural history of arteriosclerosis. Numerous studies have characterized growth patterns from infancy onward, but there are few studies of child populations where anthropometric, blood pressure, lipid, and nutritional data are collected simultaneously.

Perhaps one of the most interesting observations is this apparent low correlation between the risk-factor variables, that is, less interrelationship in preschool-age children. For example, a ponderosity index did not relate to blood pressure levels, and the multiple independent variables could explain only about 20% of blood pressure variability and 5% of the lipid variability. These values are about one-half of those observed for school-age children. Garn and Clark (1976) have observed that a positive skewness of weight distribution relative to height becomes more manifest after 9 years of age. Therefore, observations of these young children become more important since they show less of the compounding environmental effects on the risk-factor variables that occur at older ages. Further, if young children remain fixed at age-specific percentile levels (tracking), which is likely, then it is important to observe the risk factors at young ages. Current studies are testing the tracking hypothesis by determining trends over time for the risk-factor variables from birth to young adulthood.

School children, particularly those 10 years of age and older, showed more clustering of the risk-factor variables than did preschool children. It is interesting to note that aggregation in children of these variables that put adults at risk increases as the children become older. One implication is that environmental factors begin to show more and more of an impact, and probably increase even more into adulthood.

SUMMARY

The aggregation of risk-factor variables for coronary artery disease (CAD) at high levels was studied in 4,064 Bogalusa children. There were 114 (3.33%) school children above the age-, race- and sex-specific 75th percentiles for serum cholesterol, blood pressure, and a weight-height index. This was greater than expected ($p < 0.001$) under a null hypothesis of no association. The relationship was stronger in white males (3.8%) and black females (4.0%) than in white females (2.8%) and black males (2.7%). This aggregation tended to increase with age. For preschool children only minimal aggregation was observed. Data from these and future observations may enable us to identify a cohort of children who persistently exhibit multiple risk-factor variables at high levels. This identification would be essential should prevention efforts for CAD be initiated.

The capability of detecting a child with multiple risk-factors occurring at a high level is probably the most important accomplishment of these studies and indicates the need for considering all of the clinical factors in the early development of arteriosclerosis.

21. Childhood sibling aggregation of cardiovascular risk-factor variables

Among the classic cardiovascular risk factors are hypertension and elevated serum cholesterol. Recent evidence has also suggested an inverse relationship between α-lipoprotein and the risk of CAD (Rhoads et al., 1976; Berg et al., 1976). Investigators have shown that certain risk factors tend to aggregate in households (Deutscher et al., 1966; Miall et al., 1967; Hayes et al., 1971; Zinner et al., 1971; Blumenthal et al., 1975; Gerson and Fodor, 1975; Beaglehold et al., 1976; Hennekens et al., 1976; Lee et al., 1976). While the presence of familial aggregation is important from a public health standpoint (Kohn et al., 1969; Carter, 1974), the cause of aggregation can be primarily genetic, environmental, or an interaction of both.

The purpose of this chapter is to determine if aggregation of risk factors and related variables exist within full siblings participating in the Bogalusa Heart Study.

Study population

Our study population included 4,538 children, 2–18 years old, screened between September 1973 and September 1974. Chapter 2 describes the population in detail.

The authors express appreciation to Charles L. Shear for his work while a graduate student in the Tulane University School of Public Health and Tropical Medicine, and Roger Weinberg, Ph.D., Associate Professor, Department of Biometry, LSU Medical Center.

To determine the genetic relationships among the children screened, we abstracted school records that contained a listing of the children belonging to a set of parents. All records were abstracted without prior knowledge of the results of the screening.

Using this method of determining parentage, we identified 4,181 (92%) of the children screened. The majority of those children not identified by the records were preschool-age and had no older siblings in the school system. Of the children identified by the school records, the 2,535 included in this chapter were members of households in which at least one other sibling was screened. We included data only on full siblings so that the assessment of the aggregation could be based on the largest sample of children with the same genetic relationship. In all, 720 white full sibships and 255 black full sibships were identified. On the average, a white full sibship contained 2.46 children, while a black full sibship contained 2.99 children (Table 21–1).

In an attempt to validate the parental data obtained from the school records, we used two other sources. The first was the Louisiana Bureau of Vital Statistics Birth-Death Index. In a random sample of 106 children, only five inconsistencies between the two sources of data were noted (95% agreement). The second source of information was a mailed questionnaire administered three years later which asked for the "true" parents of the children residing in the household. In the

Table 21–1. Number (N) and percent of full sibships and children identified through Bogalusa school records by sibship size and race

| | Sibships | | | | Children | | | |
| | White | | Black | | White | | Black | |
Number in sibship	N	(%)	N	(%)	N	(%)	N	(%)
2	475	(66)	116	(45)	950	(54)	232	(30)
3	180	(25)	78	(31)	540	(30)	234	(31)
4	46	(6)	26	(10)	184	(10)	104	(14)
5	16	(2)	21	(8)	80	(5)	105	(14)
6	3	(1)	11	(4)	18	(1)	66	(9)
7	—	—	2	(1)	—	—	14	(2)
8	—	—	1	(1)	—	—	8	(1)
Total	720	(100)	255	(100)	1,772	(100)	763	(100)

610 households for which there were school record data, inconsistencies were found in 26 households, resulting in a 96% agreement between these two sources of data. Due to the smaller number of inconsistencies, no further comparison was made of reliability within race.

Examination procedures

Height, weight, and the right triceps skinfold were measured on each child as described earlier (Foster et al., 1977).

All serum samples were analyzed for total cholesterol, triglycerides, and lipoprotein levels (α-, β-, pre-β) (Frerichs et al., 1976; Srinivasan et al., 1976a) in the SCOR-A Core Lipid Laboratory in New Orleans. Only full sibs who were reported as fasting for 12–14 hr were used for the lipid and lipoprotein analyses.

Blood pressure

Nine blood pressures were taken on the preschool and school-age children with both automatic instruments and standard mercury sphygmomanometers (Voors et al., 1976; Berenson et al., 1978a). For the purpose of this chapter, only blood pressures taken with the mercury sphygmomanometer were included in the analysis (mean of six readings at two stations for the school-age children; mean of three readings at one station for the preschool children). First and fourth Korotkoff phases are reported as systolic and diastolic blood pressures, respectively.

Statistical analysis

Before measuring the degree of aggregation of all variables, we used multiple regression to remove the race-specific linear effects of age and sex from serum triglycerides, β-lipoproteins, and pre-β-lipoproteins; and the race-specific curvilinear effects of age, age^2, and sex from height, weight, triceps skinfold, systolic and diastolic blood pressure, serum total cholesterol, and α-lipoproteins. These regression analyses included all children in our sample and provided residual values (difference between predicted and observed) for each full sibling. These residuals were then log-transformed in order to normalize the data, and they served as the input for a one-way analysis of variance with unequal class sizes (Barr et al., 1976).

From the analyses of variance, two measures of aggregation were computed:

(1) variance ratio (F-ratio) $= \dfrac{MS_a}{MS_w}$

MS_a = mean square among full-sibling households
MS_w = mean square within full-sibling households

(2) intraclass correlation coefficient (r_f) defined as:

$$r_f = \frac{s_a^2}{s_a^2 + s_w^2}$$

s_a^2 = sample estimate of σ_a^2, the component of variance among full sibling households

s_w^2 = sample estimate of σ_w^2, the component of variance within full sibling households

Standard methods were used to test the significance of the F-ratio's departure from unity (Barr et al., 1976). Using the Z-transform of the intraclass correlation coefficient (Fisher, 1954), we tested the differences between the correlation coefficients for blacks and for whites. For these tests, the distributions of the differences between the transformed intraclass correlation coefficients were assumed to be approximately normal. The intraclass correlation coefficient permitted utilization of data on full sibships with more than two sibs.

OBSERVATIONS

The F-ratios and intraclass correlation coefficients for height, weight, triceps skinfold, systolic blood pressure, and diastolic blood pressure are shown in Table 21–2. All F-ratios were highly significant ($p < 0.0001$), with height in each race showing the highest correlation and diastolic blood pressure the lowest correlation. No statistically significant difference was found in the degree of correlation between blacks and whites for any of these five variables. By squaring the intraclass correlation coefficient and multiplying by 100, we estimate the per-

Table 21–2. F-ratios and intraclass correlation coefficients for selected anthropometric and blood pressure measurements in white and black full siblings

Measurement[1]	Race	Degrees of freedom[2]	$\dfrac{MS_a}{MS_w}$	F-ratio[3]	Intraclass correlation coefficient (r_I)
Height	White	(719, 1,044)	$\dfrac{0.00069}{0.00025}$	2.76	.42
	Black	(254, 503)	$\dfrac{0.00085}{0.00026}$	3.27	.44
Weight	White	(719, 1,044)	$\dfrac{0.01326}{0.00554}$	2.39	.36
	Black	(254, 503)	$\dfrac{0.01573}{0.00617}$	2.55	.34
Triceps skinfold	White	(719, 1,044)	$\dfrac{0.03794}{0.01706}$	2.22	.33
	Black	(254, 503)	$\dfrac{0.05760}{0.02735}$	2.11	.27
Systolic blood pressure	White	(719, 1,044)	$\dfrac{0.00190}{0.00110}$	1.73	.23
	Black	(254, 503)	$\dfrac{0.00225}{0.00109}$	2.06	.26
Diastolic blood pressure	White	(719, 1,044)	$\dfrac{0.00348}{0.00232}$	1.50	.17
	Black	(254, 503)	$\dfrac{0.00409}{0.00259}$	1.58	.16

[1]Excludes eight white children and five black children from whom data were not obtained for all five variables

[2]Degrees of freedom $= \left(k - 1, \sum_{i=1}^{k} (n_i - 1)\right)$ where: k = number of full sibships and n_i = number of full sibs in the ith sibship.

[3]$p < 0.0001$

centage of the variance among children which is "explained" by (i.e., associated with) the values of a child's siblings. For example, among white children, 5.3% of the interchild variability in systolic blood pressure is explained by knowledge of the blood pressure of the respective siblings.

For lipids and lipoproteins (Table 21–3), all F-ratios were signifi-

Table 21–3. *F*-ratios and intraclass correlation coefficients for lipid and lipoprotein fractions in white and black full siblings

Measurement	*Race*	*Degrees of freedom*[3]	$\dfrac{MS_a}{MS_w}$	*F-ratio*	*Intraclass correlation coefficient* (r_l)
Cholesterol[1]	White	(709, 876)	$\dfrac{0.00677}{0.00361}$	1.88[4]	.28
	Black	(251, 422)	$\dfrac{0.00799}{0.00425}$	1.88[4]	.25
Triglycerides[2]	White	(707, 878)	$\dfrac{0.03603}{0.02326}$	1.55[4]	.20
	Black	(251, 418)	$\dfrac{0.02920}{0.02158}$	1.35[4]	.12
β-lipoprotein[2]	White	(707, 878)	$\dfrac{0.01556}{0.00701}$	2.22[4]	.35
	Black	(251, 418)	$\dfrac{0.01671}{0.00874}$	1.91[4]	.26
Pre-β-lipoprotein[2]	White	(707, 878)	$\dfrac{0.18127}{0.12412}$	1.46[4]	.17
	Black	(251, 418)	$\dfrac{0.17044}{0.14109}$	1.21[5]	.07
α-lipoprotein[1]	White	(709, 876)	$\dfrac{0.04586}{0.03501}$	1.31[4]	.12
	Black	(251, 422)	$\dfrac{0.03083}{0.02774}$	1.11[6]	.04

[1]Excludes 186 white children and 89 black children who were reported as nonfasting or from whom data were not obtained.
[2]Excludes 186 white children and 93 black children who were reported as nonfasting
[3]Degrees of freedom $= \left(k - 1, \sum\limits_{i=1}^{k} (n_i - 1)\right)$ where: k = number of full sibships and n_i = number of full sibs in the ith sibship.
[4]$p < 0.01$
[5]$p < 0.05$
[6]Not statistically significant

cant except for the α-lipoprotein of black children. The intraclass correlations for total cholesterol (and its major carrier in children, β-lipoprotein) were of a greater magnitude than those for triglycerides (and its major carrier pre-β-lipoprotein). For α-lipoprotein, the correlations were lower than for cholesterol or β-lipoprotein. For all five lipids and lipoproteins, the intraclass correlations were lower than those previously noted for the three anthropometric variables but of the same order of magnitude as for blood pressure. While the correlations for the lipids and lipoproteins in blacks tended to be lower than for whites, none of the racial differences were statistically significant.

COMMENT

The results for height, weight, and blood pressure agree with those of previous population-based studies (Johnson et al., 1965; Deutscher et al., 1966; Hayes et al., 1971; Zinner et al., 1971; Gerson and Fodor, 1975; Rao et al., 1975; Beaglehole et al., 1976). For example, Hayes et al. (1971) cite product moment correlations for white and black adult sib pairs, respectively, of 0.41 and 0.34 for height, 0.20 and 0.14 for systolic blood pressure, and 0.17 and 0.19 for diastolic blood pressure. It is interesting to note that the correlations found in the children of our study are of the same order of magnitude as those found in the Evans County (Ga.) population of adults.

Aggregation of lipids and lipoproteins has also been studied previously (Johnson et al., 1965; Deutscher et al., 1966; Feldman et al., 1973; Blumenthal et al., 1975; Glueck et al., 1975; Hennekens et al., 1976). While we show significant aggregation of most of these risk-factor variables during childhood, the correlations for the lipids and lipoproteins tend to be lower than in other studies on adult populations. This observation could imply that levels of lipids and lipoproteins (in contrast to height and weight) are more responsive during childhood than during adulthood to environmental factors.

For no variable did we find significantly different aggregation between blacks and whites. Apparently, whatever mechanisms produce the black-white differences in levels of risk-factor variables and in CAD rates either do not affect the degree of sibling aggregation or are not evident in childhood.

Preliminary evidence suggests that children "track" with respect to levels of risk-factor variables (Frerichs et al., 1979). Therefore, the screening of first-degree relatives, namely parents and sibs, for these factors would seem in order from the viewpoint of both the physician and the epidemiologist (Falconer, 1965; Kohn et al., 1969; Carter, 1974; Epstein, 1976).

Aggregation may result from common genes or common environment. Our analyses do not separate those influences since all full sibs in a family resided in the same household. However, previous investigators have attempted to separate these two influences. Comparison of monozygotic and dizygotic twins has been the classic method of determining genetic variations. Using this method, the National Heart and Lung Institute Twin Study (U.S. Dept. of H.E.W., 1976b) found significant genetic variability in height, weight, systolic blood pressure, diastolic blood pressure, and plasma triglycerides. No significant genetic variability was found for total cholesterol or cholesterol fractions in the lipoproteins. These results are in general agreement with the literature (Feinleib et al., 1975; Rao et al., 1975; Weinberg et al., 1976).

With respect to the lipids and lipoproteins in twins, Christian et al. (1976) have reported differences in the sources of variation for free and esterified cholesterol. Significant genetic variance was found in plasma for the free fraction of total cholesterol, high-density lipoprotein (α-lipoprotein) cholesterol, and low-density lipoprotein (β-lipoprotein) cholesterol, while the esterified fractions of the same macromolecules appeared to be influenced by environmental factors.

Supporting the view of environmental determination of lipids is the report by Brunner et al. (1971) of the absence of familial aggregation in an Israeli collective settlement in which all residents ate the same foods prepared in a single kitchen. Levels of total cholesterol and triglycerides and the percentage of total cholesterol in β-lipoproteins were not significantly less variable within families than between families.

Spouse concordance studies also help to elucidate the role of the common environment; these studies deal with environments shared by marital partners. For example, spouse concordance seems to be significant for blood pressure, indicating an environmental effect (Winkelstein et al., 1969; Hayes et al., 1971), although Sackett (1975) suggests that assortative mating is the more plausible explanation.

Although the relative importance of heredity and environment in these risk-factor variables is an unsettled issue, it is an important area of research which can lead to a greater understanding of the etiology of the disease process and also to eventual control and prevention. We are now attempting to separate the environmental and genetic components of aggregation by using a one-generation model which includes data on full sibs, half sibs, and cousins.

SUMMARY

Cardiovascular risk-factor variables on 4,538 Bogalusa children were analyzed to observe sibling aggregation. Of these children, 2–18 years old, 2,535 had at least one sibling, permitting the calculation of F-ratios and intraclass correlation coefficients. Those calculations revealed statistically significant F-ratios for all anthropometric, blood pressure, and lipid variables studied. Of the lipoprotein variables studied, only α-lipoprotein showed no statistically significant aggregation (for black children). The analysis failed to reveal any significant differences in intraclass correlations between black and white children.

22. Relation of serum lipids and lipoproteins to obesity and sexual maturity in white and black children

In earlier chapters, we described the distributions of blood lipids (cholesterol, triglycerides), lipoproteins (β-, pre-β-, α-), blood pressure, and anthropometric measurements for children, ages 5–14 years (Frerichs et al., 1976; Srinivasan et al., 1976a; Voors et al., 1976; Foster et al., 1977). The relation of levels of blood lipids and lipoproteins with maturation and selected anthropometric variables in black and white children is further explored in this chapter.

GENERAL METHODS

Population

Of the 3,524 children ages 5–14 years who were examined as part of the Bogalusa Heart Study, no blood was obtained from 78. An additional 295 children were excluded from the present analysis because they reported nonfasting (less than 12–14 hr) or had missing anthropometric or maturation values. The remaining 3,151 children yielded the data in this chapter.

Physical examination

Details of the examination are presented in Chapter 8. Included was a physical examination by a physician, part of which was to determine external maturation by visual assessment using the photographs of Tanner (Tanner, 1962). The ratings ranged from 1 (no development) to 5 (complete development) according to the maturation levels of the child's pubic hair.

Serum lipid and lipoprotein analysis

All serum samples were analyzed as described in Chapter 3. Measurement of serum total cholesterol, triglycerides, and lipoprotein levels are detailed in that chapter.

Obesity indices

Besides the triceps skinfold thickness, numerous weight-for-height (W/H) indices were considered as measures of body fat. The criterion for an ideal index was that it should be independent of height and highly correlated with another index of adiposity, namely the triceps skinfold. Using the formula derived by Benn (Benn, 1971), we found weight/height$^{2.77}$ $(W/H^{2.77})$ to be the index which best fit our data. In the total population, the correlation coefficients of $W/H^{2.77}$ with height and with triceps skinfold are 0.03 and 0.74, respectively.

Statistical analyses

Various statistical methods were used to examine the relationship of obesity to the lipids and lipoproteins. The population was divided into four groups based on values of $W/H^{2.77}$. A one-way analysis of variance was run separately for each age-race-sex group to test for differences in lipids, lipoproteins, and triceps skinfold values among the four $W/H^{2.77}$ groups. A *posteriori* comparisons among the means were tested by the Student-Newman-Keuls test (Sokal and Rohlf, 1969). A one-way analysis of variance was run for each age-race-sex group to see if there were any differences in the mean levels of $W/H^{2.77}$ for children whose lipids or lipoproteins were either at or above the 90th percentile, the 10th–90th percentile, or at or below the 10th percentile. Weighted individual degrees of freedom contrasts were employed (Sokal and Rohlf, 1969). The combined effect of age, race, sex, $W/H^{2.77}$, triceps skinfold, and maturation on levels of the serum variables was determined by multiple linear regression.

OBSERVATIONS

Mean values of measured variables

All children were divided by race and sex into age groups: 5–9 and 10–14 years. The number of children in each of eight race-age-sex-groups as well as the means and standard deviations for the lipid, lipoprotein, anthropometric, and maturation variables, which for the total population of 3,524 children have been presented elsewhere (Frerichs et al., 1976; Srinivasan et al., 1976a; Foster et al., 1977), are summarized in Table 22–1. In general, males had smaller triceps skinfold measurements than females, with blacks having lower values than whites. Only minor differences in $W/H^{2.77}$ are observed among the four race-sex groups. Maturation scores increased with age with blacks tending to have greater scores than whites and females greater than males. Cholesterol values were lower in whites than in blacks while triglycerides and pre-β-lipoprotein values were higher in whites. In addition, triglyceride levels in females were higher than those of males. For β-lipoprotein, girls had slighly higher values than boys in both racial groups. Both race and sex differences are observed in the α-lipoprotein concentrations with blacks exhibiting much higher levels than whites and boys having greater values than girls.

Interrelationship among serum lipids, lipoproteins, obesity, and maturation

Simple correlation coefficients between the lipids and lipoproteins and four other variables (age, triceps skinfold, $W/H^{2.77}$, and maturation stage) are seen in Table 22–2 by age group, race, and sex. For the most part, the correlations in the 10- to 14-year-olds are slightly greater than for the 5- to 9-year-olds. In general, both anthropometric variables (triceps skinfold and $W/H^{2.77}$) were positively correlated in all children with triglycerides, β-lipoprotein, and pre-β-lipoprotein

Table 22–1. Means and Standard deviations for serum lipids, lipoproteins and other variables in children, by age group, race and sex

Variables	Ages 5–9 years				Ages 10–14 years			
	White males N = 456	White females N = 439	Black males N = 262	Black females N = 234	White males N = 572	White females N = 520	Black males N = 342	Black females N = 326
Age (years)	7.6 ± 1.4	7.6 ± 1.4	7.9 ± 1.4	7.7 ± 1.4	12.4 ± 1.4	12.4 ± 1.4	12.4 ± 1.4	12.5 ± 1.4
Height (cm)	124.8 ± 9.8	123.2 ± 10.0	126.9 ± 9.3	125.7 ± 9.5	151.2 ± 12.1	151.9 ± 10.3	152.0 ± 11.6	153.9 ± 10.1
Weight (kg)	25.7 ± 6.2	24.6 ± 6.6	26.5 ± 6.7	25.6 ± 6.4	43.4 ± 12.9	44.3 ± 11.9	42.5 ± 12.2	46.5 ± 13.7
Triceps skinfold (mm)	10.7 ± 4.1	12.5 ± 4.3	8.3 ± 4.1	10.3 ± 4.2	13.0 ± 6.0	16.1 ± 5.7	9.6 ± 5.2	14.1 ± 6.4
W/H$^{2.77}$ (kg/m)	13.7 ± 1.7	13.6 ± 1.7	13.5 ± 1.7	13.4 ± 1.7	13.6 ± 2.3	13.7 ± 2.3	13.1 ± 2.1	13.8 ± 2.6
Maturation[1]	1.0 ± 0.0	1.0 ± 0.2	1.0 ± 0.2	1.1 ± 0.5	2.0 ± 1.3	2.9 ± 1.3	2.3 ± 1.3	3.5 ± 1.3
Total cholesterol (mg/dl)	163.7 ± 30.7	164.2 ± 27.7	171.6 ± 35.2	173.2 ± 31.1	159.9 ± 27.4	162.6 ± 25.7	168.4 ± 28.7	168.6 ± 28.8
Triglycerides (mg/dl)	64.6 ± 29.5	69.5 ± 29.7	57.5 ± 25.5	61.4 ± 22.7	72.4 ± 36.0	83.6 ± 42.1	60.6 ± 24.4	64.9 ± 25.1
β-lipoprotein (mg/dl)[2]	192.1 ± 51.3	194.9 ± 47.1	194.0 ± 53.1[3]	199.3 ± 49.2	181.8 ± 48.2	189.2 ± 46.1[3]	181.6 ± 46.7	188.6 ± 47.7
Pre-β-lipoprotein (mg/dl)[2]	30.4 ± 29.2	33.1 ± 29.4	27.3 ± 22.9[3]	30.1 ± 23.4	41.0 ± 33.5	51.3 ± 38.5[3]	34.0 ± 28.2	36.8 ± 26.6
α-lipoprotein (mg/dl)[2]	394.2 ± 133.3	386.0 ± 128.2	439.5 ± 139.8[3]	431.2 ± 131.3	387.0 ± 122.5	368.4 ± 119.8	446.6 ± 135.4	424.8 ± 126.4

[1] Tanner maturation scale (pubic hair, 1–5)
[2] Multiplying by following factors converted lipoproteins into corresponding lipoprotein cholesterol: β-lipoprotein × 0.469; pre-β-lipoprotein × 0.222; α-lipoprotein × 0.17 (see chapter 3).
[3] One missing value

Table 22–2. Simple correlation coefficients between serum lipids, lipoproteins, and other variables in children, by age groups, race, and sex

Serum Variables	Ages 5–9 years				Ages 10–14 years			
	AGE	TSF	W/H$^{2.77}$	MAT	AGE	TSF	W/H$^{2.77}$	MAT
Total cholesterol								
white males	0.06	0.16[1]	0.10[3]	0.01	−0.14[2]	0.26[1]	0.21[1]	−0.23[1]
white females	0.13[2]	0.09	0.05	0.00	−0.04	0.04	0.10[3]	−0.07
black males	0.04	0.09	0.10	0.05	−0.07	−0.01	−0.05	−0.11[3]
black females	0.02	0.00	−0.05	−0.11	−0.09	0.08	0.06	−0.08
Triglycerides								
white males	−0.03	0.19[1]	0.18[1]	0.01	0.07	0.32[1]	0.35[1]	0.07
white females	0.10[3]	0.19[1]	0.18[1]	0.10[3]	0.00	0.19[1]	0.28[1]	0.04
black males	0.07	0.09	0.09	0.10	0.10	0.16[2]	0.17[2]	0.05
black females	−0.02	0.10	0.17[2]	−0.01	−0.02	0.16[2]	0.25[1]	0.01
β-lipoprotein								
white males	0.04	0.21[1]	0.20[1]	−0.01	−0.09[1]	0.30[1]	0.27[1]	−0.15[1]
white females	0.13[2]	0.13[2]	0.09	0.00	−0.14[2]	0.13[2]	0.21[1]	−0.14[2]
black males	−0.03	0.10	0.16[3]	0.08	−0.03	0.11[3]	0.08	−0.10
black females	−0.06	−0.00	−0.01	−0.15[3]	−0.13[3]	0.14[2]	0.17[2]	−0.14[2]
Pre-β-lipoprotein								
white males	0.05	0.20[1]	0.19[1]	0.02	0.10[3]	0.30[1]	0.31[1]	0.10[3]
white females	0.14[2]	0.17[1]	0.11[3]	0.13[2]	0.06	0.18[1]	0.27[1]	0.12[2]
black males	0.18[2]	0.09	0.09	0.20[2]	0.08	0.20[1]	0.21[1]	0.08
black females	0.08	0.14[3]	0.17[2]	0.09	0.04	0.16[2]	0.20[1]	0.05
α-lipoprotein								
white males	0.01	−0.06	0.12[2]	0.01	−0.12[2]	−0.09[3]	−0.14[2]	−0.17[1]
white females	−0.01	−0.08	−0.06	−0.04	0.07	−0.16[1]	−0.22[1]	0.00
black males	0.05	−0.00	−0.03	−0.05	−0.08	−0.17[2]	−0.19[1]	−0.06
black females	0.07	−0.03	−0.10	−0.02	−0.00	−0.08	−0.15[2]	0.02

Levels of significance (t-test):
[1]$p < 0.001$
[2]$p < 0.01$
[3]$p < 0.05$

TSF = triceps skinfold; W/H$^{2.77}$ = weight/height$^{2.77}$; MAT = Tanner maturation scale (pubic hair, grades 1–5)

and were negatively correlated with α-lipoprotein. The highest correlation ($r = 0.35$) was observed in the oldest group of white boys between triglycerides and W/H$^{2.77}$. For cholesterol, only white boys exhibited significant correlations with both anthropometric variables. In the older children, age and maturation stages were both negatively correlated with total cholesterol and β-lipoprotein, although these findings were not statistically significant in all race-sex groups. In

Table 22–3. Multiple linear regression for serum lipids, lipoproteins, and other selected variables in children, ages 5–14 years

Serum variables (mg/dl)	Number of children	Constant	Coefficients for multiple linear regression equation						Multiple R^2
			Age (years)	Race (W = 1, B = 2)	Sex (M = 1, F = 2)	TSF (mm)	$W/H^{2.77}$ (W = kg, H = m)	MAT (Tanner)	
Total cholesterol	3,151	139.7	0.4	10.1[1]	2.1	0.5[2]	0.4	-3.6[1]	0.04
Triglycerides	3,151	11.3	1.6[1]	-10.8[1]	6.2[1]	0.2	3.4[1]	-0.5	0.11
β-lipoprotein	3,149	133.4	0.1	5.3[2]	7.3[1]	0.7[3]	3.0[1]	-6.5[2]	0.06
pre-β-lipoprotein	3,149	-22.1	2.1[1]	-6.5[1]	4.0[2]	0.3	2.7[1]	0.3	0.11
α-lipoprotein	3,150	483.9	-0.6	53.6[1]	-13.0[3]	0.8	-9.7[1]	-3.8	0.06

Levels of significance (t-test):
[1] $p < 0.001$
[2] $p < 0.01$
[3] $p < 0.05$

W = whites, B = blacks; M = males, F = females; TSF = triceps skinfold; W = weight; H = height; MAT = Tanner maturation scale (pubic hair, grades 1–5).

most instances, the relationships were more apparent in whites than in blacks, with the highest correlations observed in white boys.

All 3,151 children were included in a multiple linear regression with the serum lipids and lipoproteins as dependent variables and age, race, sex, and $W/H^{2.77}$, triceps skinfold, and maturation as independent variables. The results, shown in Table 22–3, indicate that in the total population, knowledge of the six independent variables only explains between 4 and 11% of the variability in the levels of the various serum categories. Both triglycerides and pre-β-lipoprotein show a significant independent increase with age. The coefficients for race were statistically significant for all five serum categories and coefficients for·sex were significant for all serum variables except total cholesterol. With the exception of total cholesterol, all coefficients of the serum variables showed greater statistical signficiance with $W/H^{2.77}$ than with the triceps skinfold. The coefficients for maturation stage were significant only with total cholesterol and β-lipoprotein, indicating that both of these serum variables decrease with increasing maturation.

Lipid and lipoprotein levels in children in four weight/height divisions

The population was divided into four groups based on *a priori* selected values of $W/H^{2.77}$. In previous analyses we observed that blacks tend to be leaner than whites and boys leaner than girls. Consequently, a division of the population based on race-sex percentile cutpoints would have resulted in black children from the most ponderous group being less obese than white children in the same group. Instead, we selected arbitrary cutpoints based on values of $W/H^{2.77}$ so that approximately 10% of the population would be in the high and low groups and 80% in the middle two groups. The numbers of children that were in each of the four $W/H^{2.77}$ groups are shown in Table 22–4.

The groups vary in size between 15 (< 11.50, ages 5–9, black females) and 305 (11.50–13.75, ages 10–14, white males) with a greater percentage of the older children, when compared to the younger group, in the most extreme obese and lean categories.

The mean age and triceps skinfold thickness of children in each of the four $W/H^{2.77}$ categories is seen in Figure 22–1. As expected, the

Table 22–4. Number of children, by age group, race, and sex, included in the analysis of four weight/height categories

	Obesity index $(W/H^{2.77})$[1]									
	< 11.50		11.50–13.75		13.75–16.00		≥ 16.00		Total	
Population	N	(%)	N	(%)	N	(%)	N	(%)	N	(%)
Ages 5–9 years										
white males	23	(5)	248	(54)	142	(31)	43	(9)	456	(100)
females	24	(5)	245	(56)	131	(30)	39	(9)	439	(100)
black males	17	(6)	153	(58)	76	(29)	16	(6)	262	(100)
females	15	(6)	137	(59)	66	(28)	16	(7)	234	(100)
Ages 10–14 years										
white males	73	(13)	305	(53)	110	(19)	84	(15)	572	(100)
females	54	(10)	270	(52)	125	(24)	71	(14)	520	(100)
black males	59	(17)	189	(55)	72	(21)	22	(6)	342	(100)
females	41	(13)	150	(46)	82	(25)	53	(16)	326	(100)
All children	306	(10)	1,697	(54)	804	(26)	344	(11)	3,151	(100)

[1] W = weight (kg); H = height (m)

337

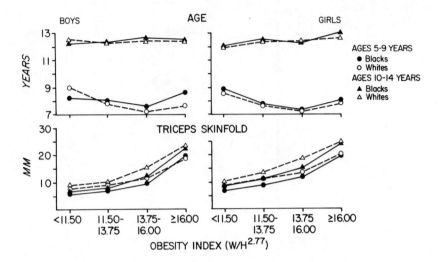

Figure 22–1. Relationship of age and triceps skinfold with the obesity index, $W/H^{2.77}$, in children by race and sex. The mean levels of age and triceps skinfold thickness are plotted for each of four $W/H^{2.77}$ categories for black and white children ages 5–9 and 10–14 years.

average triceps skinfold thickness increases with increasing body mass in all eight race, sex, and age groups. It is interesting to note that within the most obese groups (≥ 16.00), the mean triceps skinfold is comparable in both black and white children and that in all groups, the skinfold is consistently greater in the older children. The mean ages of the four $W/H^{2.77}$ groups vary except among older boys. For example, in the 5- to 9-year-olds, the lean and obese extremes are slightly older than children in the remaining population. Among the 10- to 14-year-old girls of both races, those in the obese groups are older than children in the leanest category while in the older boys, the mean ages among all four $W/H^{2.77}$ categories are equivalent.

The average serum lipid and lipoprotein levels of children within the four $W/H^{2.77}$ categories are shown in Figure 22–2. In general, the more obese children had elevated levels of triglycerides, β-lipoproteins, and pre-β-lipoproteins, and lower levels of α-lipoproteins. No consistent association of cholesterol with body habitus was observed in girls or in 10- to 14-year-old white boys; mean cholesterol levels tended to be higher among the more obese groups.

In order to determine if these changes were statistically significant

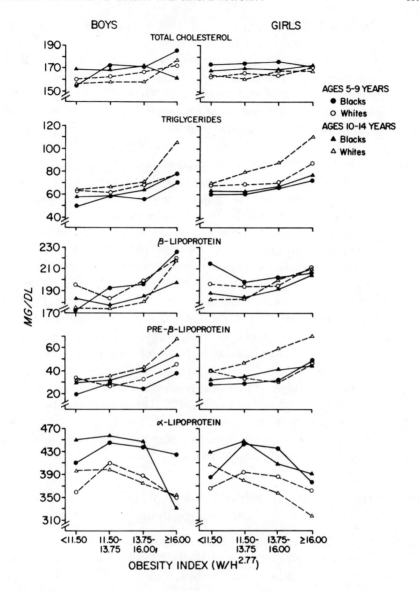

Figure 22–2. Relationship of serum lipids and lipoproteins with the obesity index, $W/H^{2.77}$, in children by age, race, and sex. The mean levels of serum total cholesterol, triglycerides, and lipoproteins (β, pre-β, α) are plotted for each of four $W/H^{2.77}$ categories for black and white children ages 5–9 and 10–14 years.

among the four $W/H^{2.77}$ categories, an analysis of variance was performed for each of the eight race-sex groups. For total cholesterol,
none of the F-ratios were significantly different among the four
$W/H^{2.77}$ categories. In the older children (ages 10–14), the F-ratios
were significant only for the whites ($p < 0.0001$, white boys; $p < 0.05$,
white girls), with greater levels of cholesterol present in the most
obese groups. The F-ratios in the triglyceride analyses were significant ($p < 0.01$) within all race-sex-age groups except the younger
black boys and girls. The most obese groups consistently had greater
triglyceride levels than the remaining population. For β-lipoproteins,
the F-ratios were significant for white boys in both age groups and for
the older white girls ($p < 0.001$). The mean levels of β-lipoprotein did
not differ significantly among the four $W/H^{2.77}$ groups in either older
or younger black children or in the younger white girls. As expected,
the pre-β-lipoprotein analyses were similar to those of triglycerides
with all race-sex-age groups having F-ratios significantly different
from 1.0 ($p < 0.05$). In each group of children, the most obese ($W/H^{2.77}$
≥ 16.00) had significantly greater pre-β-lipoprotein levels than the remaining population. The trend for α-lipoprotein was the opposite of
that observed for the other lipid and lipoprotein categories. The most
obese groups generally had the lowest level of α-lipoprotein with F-
ratios significant in all four race-sex groups of older children and in
the younger group of white boys ($p < 0.05$). The changes in the levels
of lipoproteins (lipoprotein cholesterol) account for the inconsistent
relationships among the eight age-race-sex groups between the serum
cholesterol and the weight/height index.

Weight/height levels in children with high, medium, and low percentiles of serum lipids and lipoproteins

In order to study further the relationships between the serum variables and the weight/height index, $W/H^{2.77}$ levels were compared for
children who had high, medium, or low lipid and lipoprotein levels.
Figure 22–3 shows by race, sex, and age group, the mean values of
$W/H^{2.77}$ for children with levels of serum variables greater or equal to
the 90th percentile, levels between the 10th and 90th percentiles, and
levels equal to and below the 10th percentile. Among the 10- to 14-
year-old white boys and girls, those with cholesterol values at or
above the 90th percentile were significantly more obese than either

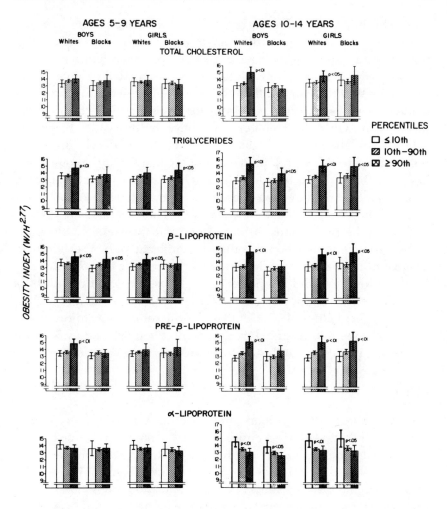

Figure 22–3. Mean values (± 2 standard errors) of the obesity index, $W/H^{2.77}$, in the children with high (≥ 90th percentile), medium (10th–90th percentiles), or low (≤ 10th percentile) levels of total cholesterol, triglycerides, and lipoproteins (β, pre-β, α) by age, race, and sex. The significance level at which one lipid or lipoprotein group differs statistically from the remaining two is indicated.

the middle group (10th–90th percentile) or the low group (≤ 10th percentile). Neither the black children nor the younger group of white children exhibited any statistically significant differences in $W/H^{2.77}$ among the three cholesterol percentile groups. For triglycerides, those children with values at or above the 90th percentile were significantly more obese than the remaining children. The only exceptions were in the younger (ages 5–9) black boys and white girls. The children with high levels of β-lipoprotein also tended to have greater values for $W/H^{2.77}$ than did the other children. This finding was most evident in white children, while in black children the results were inconsistent. Only the younger black boys and the older black girls exhibited relationships similar to those of the white children. The results for pre-β-lipoprotein were similar (especially among white boys) to those of triglycerides and β-lipoprotein. The group with serum values at or above the 90th percentile tended to be more obese than did those children with lower values. The exceptions to this pattern were the two groups of black boys and the younger black and white girls, none of whom exhibited significant $W/H^{2.77}$ differences. The patterns for α-lipoprotein were exactly opposite to those observed for the other lipid and lipoprotein categories. The children with the lowest levels of α-lipoprotein (at or below the 10th percentile) tended to have higher values of $W/H^{2.77}$ than did the remaining children. This difference was not observed in the younger children (ages 5–9) but was observed in most of the 10- to 14-year-olds.

COMMENT

If efforts aimed at the primary prevention of coronary artery disease are to be initiated during childhood, it becomes essential to learn what factors influence lipid and lipoprotein concentrations in a pediatric population. Based on our analyses of both black and white children, we found that measures of obesity or maturation within the context of a total population explain very little of the interchild variability in lipid and lipoprotein levels. Weak to nonexistent associations between measures of obesity and levels of total cholesterol and triglycerides were also observed in other pediatric studies (Montoye et al., 1966; Hickie et al., 1974; Wilmore and McNamara, 1974; Court and Dunlop, 1975; Lauer et al., 1975). In general, the obesity indices were more strongly correlated with blood triglyceride levels than with concentrations of serum total cholesterol. The weak cholesterol-obesity association is readily explained by our observations that with increased obesity, levels of β-lipoprotein cholesterol tend to increase while levels of α-lipoprotein cholesterol tend to decrease. Lauer et al. (1975) reported that the correlations of relative weight and triceps skinfold in over 4,000 Muscatine, Iowa, children (almost all white) with serum cholesterol were 0.09 and 0.17, respectively while the correlations with serum triglycerides were 0.20 and 0.25, respectively. These correlations are comparable to those found among the white Bogalusa children (Table 22–2).

Limited information is available comparing the associations of body habitus and maturation with the serum lipids and lipoproteins in both black and white children from a total community. In general, the association of obesity with the serum variables was most apparent in white boys, of intermediate strength in both black and white girls, and least evident in black boys. These differences may be genetic or reflect physiologic, hormonal, or dietary interactions within the four race-sex groups. We have previously noted that there are significant differences between the races and sexes with respect to the absolute levels of both the anthropometric and serum variables. For example, white Bogalusa children have thicker triceps skinfolds and greater levels of both triglycerides and pre-β-lipoprotein than do black children, while blacks tend to mature earlier (as measured by the visual method of Tanner) and have greater levels of serum total cholesterol and α-lipoprotein. No differences were observed between the races in levels of β-lipoprotein. Within each race, girls have thicker triceps skinfolds and greater levels of triglycerides, pre-β-lipoprotein, and β-lipoprotein when compared to boys (Frerichs et al., 1976; Srinivasan et al., 1976a; Foster et al., 1977). Based on our analyses it appears that there are also internal race and sex differences with respect to the influence that maturation and body habitus have on the serum variables.

The lower levels of both cholesterol and β-lipoprotein which were observed during the early adolescent years have been previously noted in Bogalusa children as well as in other pediatric studies (McGandy, 1971; Frerichs et al., 1976; Hennekens et al., 1976; Srinivasan et al., 1976a). Based on our cross-sectional data (Table 22–3), we see that this decline is associated with changes in the level of maturation independent of changes in age, triceps skinfold, or $W/H^{2.77}$, reflecting possible hormonal influences.

The exact physiologic mechanisms which link obesity and the serum lipids and lipoproteins is unknown, although there is evidence that the level of insulin may play a role in the association (Olefsky et al., 1974). Hyperinsulinism is a common finding in obese children when compared to normal-weight children (Chiumello et al., 1969;

Martin and Martin, 1973; Drash, 1973; Brook and Lloyd, 1973; Deschamps et al., 1977). Olefsky and co-workers (1974) have shown that elevations in insulin levels lead to an increase in plasma triglycerides (and pre-β-lipoproteins). The hypothesized mechanism is that insulin resistance leads to a compensatory increase in plasma insulin levels which in turn acts on the liver to accelerate triglyceride (pre-β-lipoprotein) production, thereby causing increased levels of blood triglycerides and pre-β-lipoprotein. Hypertriglyceridemia, however, need not always be associated with high insulin levels or obesity since dietary as well as hormonal and genetic factors are known to affect serum triglyceride levels (Harlan et al., 1967; Goldstein et al., 1973b; Fujita et al., 1975; Pykalisto et al., 1975).

Indirect evidence for the lipid- and lipoprotein-elevating role of insulin is derived from the Westland-Holland study of children ages 9–12 (Florey et al., 1976b). Florey and his associates reported age and sex trends for insulin levels which closely resemble the trends observed in Bogalusa children with respect to triglycerides and pre-β-lipoprotein. Girls in Westland had greater insulin levels than boys and in both sexes the insulin levels increased with age. In Bogalusa, girls had greater triglyceride and pre-β-lipoprotein levels than boys, and concentrations of both serum variables tended to increase with age (Frerichs et al., 1976; Srinivasan et al., 1976a). In addition, measures of body habitus were positively correlated with insulin levels in the Westland study, as they were with the serum lipids in Bogalusa.

The association of total cholesterol (and possibly β- and α-lipoprotein) with the measures of obesity may be due to a common relationship with serum triglycerides (Rifkind et al., 1968). For example, in Bogalusa children both cholesterol and β-lipoprotein are positively correlated with triglycerides in blacks ($r = 0.13$, cholesterol; $r = 0.28$, β-lipoprotein) and in whites ($r = 0.25$, cholesterol; $r = 0.44$, β-lipoprotein). In addition, there is a negative correlation of triglycerides with α-lipoprotein ($r = -0.29$, blacks; $r = -0.42$, whites). Metabolic studies of obese subjects have shown that the weak but positive association between cholesterol and excess body weight is most likely due to increased internal cholesterol synthesis, although the exact mechanism is unknown (Miettinen, 1971; Nestel et al., 1973).

The negative relationship between obesity and levels of α-lipoprotein was most apparent in our older group of children (10–14 years). The correlations of α-lipoprotein and triceps skinfold ranged from

−0.14 to −0.22 and are similar (but slightly lower) than those observed in Honolulu adults of Japanese origin ($r = -0.30$, α-lipoprotein cholesterol and sum of two skinfolds) (Rhoads et al., 1976).

Since α-lipoprotein levels have been shown in two major prospective studies to be negatively related to coronary disease (Rhoads et al., 1976; Gordon et al., 1977), the finding that children with high levels of α-lipoprotein tend to be leaner than their peers may have considerable importance.

All of the analyses which have been presented were derived from a single cross-sectional study. Consequently, we can only observe the internal relationships at a single point in time. In adults, the Framingham and other data showed that a change over time in relative weight related more strongly to the risk-factor variables than did the general level of adiposity at any single examination (Keys et al., 1972; Ashley and Kannel, 1974). The data from subsequent examinations in Bogalusa should enable us to focus on similar longitudinal relationships as observed in Framingham but at a much earlier age of the examinee.

SUMMARY

The interrelationships of serum lipids and lipoproteins with measures of body habitus and maturation stages were analyzed in 3,151 school-age children. In general, triglycerides, pre-β-lipoprotein, and β-lipoprotein were positively correlated with body habitus and maturation, while α-lipoprotein was negatively correlated. The relationships in most instances were more apparent in white children, with the highest correlations observed in white boys. No significant correlations were observed between serum cholesterol and the anthropometric variables except in white boys. However, the most obese children tended to have higher levels of triglycerides, pre-β-lipoprotein, and β-lipoprotein, and lower levels of α-lipoprotein than the remaining population. And children with high levels ($\geq$ 90th percentile) of triglycerides, pre-β-lipoprotein, and β-lipoprotein, and low levels, ($\leq$ 10th percentile) of α-lipoprotein, also tended to be more obese than their race-, sex-, and age-specific peers. In the total population the squared multiple correlation coefficients, with the children's age, race, sex, weight/height index, triceps skinfold, and maturation stage as the independent variables and the different serum variables as the dependent variables, ranged from 0.04 to 0.11.

VIII. Implications for clinical practice

23. Abnormalities on physical examination of a community of children

The prevalence of abnormalities in children has been the subject of numerous reports, but the populations studied usually were narrowly selected for age or socioeconomic status or to identify specific medical problems (Sundelin and Vuille, 1975; Richardson and Walker, 1975; Brooks, 1976; Dodge et al., 1976; Kirk et al., 1976). Other studies, such as the Health Examination Survey (HES), have been part of national health surveys (National Center for Health Statistics, 1973b). In contrast, this report is concerned with the prevalence of physical abnormalities in noninstitutionalized black and white children who were examined by primary physicians during a survey of a total community.

The physical examination was included in the survey primarily to provide medical service to the participating children and to obtain health data that might be correlated with the other findings of the research program (see Chapter 2).

The findings are of interest because abnormalities detected by physical examination of growing children may predict future clinical disease in adults that might be ameliorated or prevented by early therapeutic intervention. Determination of the prevalence of physical abnormalities should also be of value to planners of health delivery systems for estimating the health care needs of children.

METHODS

Study population

During the school year 1973–74, 1,840 boys and 1,684 girls (93% participation) were examined, and in the summer 714 preschool age children 2½–5½ years were examined. One-third of the children were black and two-thirds were white.

General examination procedures

Chapter 2 describes the general examination procedure. The physicians performed routine physical examinations. Although no attempt was made to standardize the specific examination techniques, a written protocol outlined the examination of each part of the body and included criteria for graded estimations of acne severity (Pillsbury et al., 1956) and sexual maturity by the Tanner Scale (Tanner, 1962). Visual acuity, and audiometric and psychological examinations were not included. Severity of dental caries (none, minimal, moderate, or severe) was graded according to the physician's visual examination. The physician also classified nutritional status by visual appraisal—noting if the child was undernourished, normal, or obese by a subjective estimate of percent of the norm. Specific criteria were based on distribution of an obesity index, weight/height$^{2.77}$, calculated by the Benn formula (Benn, 1971).

Based on the results of the screening procedures and the information on the health history form, the physician judged each system examined as normal, suspicious, abnormal, or unknown and decided whether to identify the chart for review by the pediatrician, who was responsible for notifying the parents of children with abnormal physical or laboratory findings. For follow-up, the children were referred to the private physician designated by the parents on the health history form or to the Washington-St. Tammany Charity Hospital.

Blood pressure. For the purposes of this chapter, a mean systolic blood pressure recording of at least 130 mm Hg or a mean diastolic reading of at least 85 mm Hg was considered abnormally high. This blood pressure level was arbitrarily chosen to reflect currently accepted medical practices, and it is not meant to be a recommendation for any age (Loggie, 1971). Detailed analyses and recommendations for evaluation of blood pressure levels in children are presented in chapters 14, 15, and 16. (Voors et al., 1976; Voors et al., 1977a; Voors et al., 1977b; Berenson et al., 1978b). The children were randomly rotated through three stations, and three blood pressure recordings were made at each station.

The examinations were performed by eleven physicians on a rotation basis; 2 physicians examined children each day. More than 80% of the children were examined by three of the eleven physicians. Al-

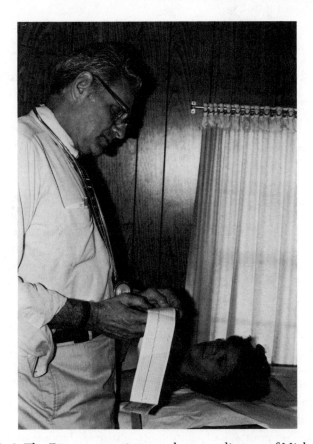

Figure 23–1. The Director examines an electrocardiogram of Michael Degen, a participant in a murmur study. Children who had been examined during the general screening and were found to have murmurs were studied more intensively.

though all the physicians received orientation and followed a written protocol, no strict attempts were made to standardize the examinations except as noted above. The only diagnostic instruments used were a stethoscope and an otoscope.

The examiners measuring blood pressures (usually a registered nurse or a licensed practical nurse) were trained according to written protocols with specific criteria for definition of a "trained examiner." Throughout the entire data collection period there were frequent review sessions, as well as scheduled and unannounced observations and oral examinations.

Rescreening

On each screening day, four children of the same sex were randomly chosen to be screened a second time (including the physical examination) except for venipuncture. A total of 535 children (12.6% of the total screening population) were reexamined the same day by a physician whom they had not previously seen.

Statistical analysis

A chi-square analysis was used to compare the number of children with abnormalities in the four race-sex groups, within race and within sex. These analyses were performed for all children and also for the preschool and school children separately. The Yates correction was applied when the frequency of abnormalities was compared within race and within sex (Maxwell, 1961).

RESULTS

On examination, 9.9% of the preschool children and 11.9% of the school-age children were found to have some physical abnormality that, in the physician's clinical judgment, needed further medical attention either for diagnostic or treatment purposes (Table 23–1). Although the percentage of school-age children having abnormalities was higher than the preschool-age children, abnormalities did not consistently increase with age for the entire population.

Black children were significantly more likely to have abnormalities than white children during both preschool (13.6% versus 8.2%, $p <$

Table 23–1. Percent of children by age, race, and sex with at least one physical abnormality (N = 4,238)

Age (years)	White Male (%)*	White Female (%)	Black Male (%)	Black Female (%)	Total (%)
	Preschool children				
2	2.7	15.2	16.7	5.3	8.9
3	11.2	2.6	12.5	13.2	8.8
4	7.9	5.8	12.5	5.3	7.5
5	9.8	16.7	25.0	24.0	17.4
Preschool subtotal	8.5	7.9	15.7	11.7	9.9
	School-age children				
5	8.7	6.1	20.0	23.7	11.7
6	8.6	9.2	16.7	15.5	11.6
7	15.0	4.2	8.9	13.1	10.2
8	12.5	5.8	18.5	16.1	12.2
9	15.9	8.6	7.3	15.2	11.6
10	14.7	7.2	6.7	12.9	10.6
11	10.1	11.3	16.0	12.8	12.1
12	21.6	10.2	12.6	17.3	11.0
13	14.1	13.3	14.7	16.2	14.4
14	12.9	7.8	17.6	17.5	13.4
School-age subtotal	11.9	8.6	13.5	15.8	11.9
Totals	11.3	8.4	13.8	15.1	11.6

*percent of age- race-, and sex-specific population

0.05) and school-age years (14.6% versus 10.3%, p < 0.005). Black girls were more likely to have abnormalities than white girls (15.1% versus 8.5%, p < 0.005), but for boys the difference between the racial groups was not significant (13.8% versus 11.3%). Boys were more likely than girls to have abnormalities (12.2% versus 10.9%) but the differences were not statistically significant.

A total of 562 abnormalities were found in 490 children: 1 in 428 children, 2 in 55 children, and 3 or more in 7 children. Only 1.4% of the school-age and 1.3% of the preschool-age children had more than one abnormality. Most of the children with more than one abnormality had either all abnormalities in the same organ system (for example, enlarged heart and heart murmur) or one that was nutritional or dental.

Table 23–2 shows the categories of abnormal conditions for each race-sex group, and Table 23–3 details the specific abnormalities found within each of these categories. The most common abnormalities were obesity, undernutrition, and severe dental caries. The next most common abnormalities involved the cardiovascular system. Primarily, these were grade 3 or greater systolic murmurs (scale 1–6) or diastolic murmurs. Functional or innocent murmurs, for which consultation was not suggested, were not included. Of 60 murmurs identified, the physicians classified (on physical examination alone) 26.7% as congenital and 8.3% as rheumatic lesions.

The abnormalities detected varied among race and sex groups. Blacks were more likely than whites to be undernourished ($p <$ 0.005), and obesity was most common among black girls and white boys. Blacks also had significantly more cardiovascular ($p < 0.05$) and abdominal abnormalities (hernias, either inguinal or umbilical) ($p <$ 0.005) than whites. Blood pressure recordings in excess of 130/85 mm Hg were also more common among black children ($p < 0.025$). Although boys were slightly more likely than girls to have abnormalities of the heart, eye, skin, and genitalia or to be undernourished, the differences were not statistically significant.

The reliability of the examination in detecting abnormalities was assessed for both the preschool and school-age children by rescreening a selected sample of 535 children. A comparison of the two diagnostic impressions (excluding blood pressure examinations) showed that 82.2% were considered normal and 3.6% were considered abnormal on both examinations. An abnormality was found in 8.4% of the children only on the first examination and in 5.8% only during the second examination. The overall agreement between the two physicians was 85.8%. However, if an abnormality was found by one of the physicians, only 20% of the time did both physicians agree that an abnormality was present.

COMMENT

Individual medical judgment based on interpretation of health history and physical findings is the primary method by which physicians determine if an asymptomatic patient has a medical problem requiring

Table 23–2. Children ages 2½–14 years with at least one physical abnormality by race, sex, and category of abnormality (N = 4,238)

Race and sex	Skin Abnormal	P per 1,000[1]	Eyes Abnormal	P per 1,000[1]	Ear, Nose & Throat Abnormal	P per 1,000[1]	Dental Abnormal	P per 1,000[1]	Neck Abnormal	P per 1,000[1]
White										
boys N = 1,405[2]	17	12.1	8	5.7	5	3.6	37	26.3	0	—
girls N = 1,301[2]	8	6.2	5	3.8	6	4.6	30	23.1	1	0.8
Black										
boys N = 790[2]	14	17.7	5	6.3	4	5.1	21	26.6	1	1.3
girls N = 742[2]	11	14.8	2	2.7	2	2.7	23	31.0	0	—
Total	50	11.8	20	4.7	17	4.0	111	26.2	2	0.5

Race and sex	Pulmonary Abnormal	P per 1,000[1]	Cardiovascular Abnormal	P per 1,000[1]	Abdomen Abnormal	P per 1,000[1]	Nodes Abnormal	P per 1,000[1]	Extremities Abnormal	P per 1,000[1]
White										
boys	2	1.4	19	13.5	0	—	0	—	0	—
girls	2	1.5	13	10.0	0	—	0	—	1	0.8
Black										
boys	4	5.1	17	21.5	8	10.1	2	2.5	1	1.3
girls	1	1.3	15	20.2	4	5.4	0	—	3	4.0
Total	9	2.1	64	15.1	12	2.8	2	0.5	5	1.2

Race and sex	Breast & Genital Abnormal	P per 1,000[1]	Obesity Abnormal	P per 1,000[1]	Undernourished Abnormal	P per 1,000[1]	Blood Pressure[3] Abnormal	P per 1,000[1]
White								
boys	3	2.1	49	34.9	27	19.2	5	3.6
girls	0	—	35	26.9	14	10.8	5	3.9
Black								
boys	2	2.5	14	17.7	32	40.5	10	12.7
girls	0	—	25	33.7	29	39.1	6	8.1
Total	5	1.2	123	29.0	102	24.1	26	6.5

[1] Prevalence of conditions per 1,000 children
[2] Three or fewer children are missing data for various stages of the examination.
[3] Thirteen children are missing blood pressure data.

Table 23–3. Abnormal physical conditions found in 4,238 children, ages 2½–14 years

Category/diagnosis	Number of cases	Percent of all conditions	Category/diagnosis	Number of cases	Percent of all conditions
Skin			Cardiovascular		
impetigo	19		suspicious murmur (tentative diagnosis)		
fungal infections	10		congenital lesions	16	
eczema	2		rheumatic lesions	5	
other rashes	9		unknown origin	39	
other lesions	10		enlarged heart	3	
Total	50	8.9	abnormal heart sounds	3	
			abnormal rhythm	2	
Eye			Total	68	12.1
strabismus	12				
inflammation	4		Abdomen		
blindness	1		umbilical hernias	11	
other conditions	3		inquinal hernias	1	
Total	20	3.6	Total	12	2.1

Condition	Number	Percent		Condition	Number	Percent
Ear				**Nodes**		
otitis	9			abnormally enlarged	2	0.4
perforated or deformed tympanic membrane	6			**Extremities**		
foreign body	1			osseous deformity	3	
Total	16	2.8		muscular atrophy	1	
Other Ear, Nose, and Throat				cerebral palsy	1	
Total	4	0.7		Total	5	0.9
Dental				**Breast & Genital**		
severe decay	111	19.8		undescended testes	4	
Neck				paraphimosis	1	
enlarged thyroid	1			Total	5	0.9
webbing	1			**Nutritional**[1]		
Total	2	0.4		obesity	123	21.9
Pulmonary				undernourished	102	18.1
asthma	2			**Blood Pressure**		
chest wall deformity	3			(systolic ≥ 130 mm Hg and/or diastolic ≥ 85 mm Hg)	33	5.9
other conditions	4					
Total	9	1.6			562	100

[1]Physicians subjective appraisal by observation only (>20% above or below ideal body weight)

357

further examinations or elaborate laboratory testing. As a result of this approach in our study, nearly one-tenth of all Bogalusa children age 2½–14 years were judged to have an abnormality that required medical attention, including referral for dental care. The latter was based on the presence of severe caries.

A comparison of our prevalence rates with those of other studies is difficult because of differences in populations studied, study goals, methodology, and definitions of abnormalities. For example, our prevalence of total abnormalities in children age 6 years was 11.6%, far less than the 21% found by Yankauer and Lawrence (1955) in Rochester, N.Y. (even though that study excluded dental abnormalities), but it was close to the 11% found in the HES for this age (National Center for Health Statistics, 1973b).

Overall rates for abnormalities in the Bogalusa and HES children age 6–11 years were also similar—Bogalusa, 11.8% for boys and 10.3% for girls; HES, 12.2% for boys and 10.2% for girls. As in the HES, the rate of total abnormalities was higher in the older age groups, but neither study revealed a consistent increase of abnormalities with age.

For children age 12–14 years, the abnormality rate in Bogalusa was 12.8%, whereas in the HES it was 19–25%. This difference may be due to the different examination data gathered from the older (12–17 years) than the younger (6–11 years) children in the HES. For example, in the HES, severe ear abnormalities were included in the overall diagnostic impression of the older, but not the younger, children. Also, most of the increase in abnormalities in the older group was due to conditions associated with the onset of puberty. In contrast, in Bogalusa the same examination data were gathered for all age groups, and few cases of severe acne or other conditions related to maturation were noted.

In a 1967–70 study of school children in El Paso (Grant et al., 1973), 13.4% were found to have significant abnormalities previously undetected or inadequately followed. The examination included a tuberculin test, urinalysis, and hearing and vision screening (producing the most common abnormality), but it excluded dermatologic conditions and dental problems. In the Head Start Project in California (Gilbert et al., 1967), 51.3% of the preschool-age children examined were found to have abnormalities that, in the judgment of the examining physician, needed referral; one-third of these were classified as "major" abnormalities. As in Bogalusa, dental findings (severe caries) were the most common abnormalities, contributing 39% of the total abnormalities (compared to 25% for Bogalusa preschool children).

A comparison of the prevalence of cardiovascular abnormalities reveals a rate of 0.9% in Rochester first-grade children, 0.6% for all ages in the El Paso study, and 1.5% for all ages in our study.

Although none of the studies clearly define obesity, the stated prevalence of obesity among the various studies was similar: 1.1% of the boys and 1.6% of the girls in El Paso compared to 1.3% for each sex in Bogalusa school children and approximately 1.2% of the study children in Rochester. An equal number (1.2%) were unclassified "below-par" in the Rochester study compared to 1.8% in Bogalusa who were considered to be undernourished.

Abnormal ear, nose, and throat findings (0.4%) among Bogalusa children may appear unusually low for a pediatric group when compared to the Health Examination Survey where 1.6% of the children had otitis media alone. This low percentage may have been related to the lack of audiometry screening or to the possibility that an acute illness (tonsilitis, earache, or other) might have been a reason for a Bogalusa parent to postpone a child's screening.

Blood pressures above 130/85 mm Hg were recorded for 0.6% of the older and 0.9% of preschool children in Bogalusa. These percentages are comparable to the 0.3% of the children in the El Paso study ("established norms for the child's age" as the criteria) and to the 0.6% who had "persistent hypertension" in the Muscatine, Iowa study (pressure $\geq$ 140/90 or the 95th percentile) (Von Behren and Lauer, 1977). The overall rates in Bogalusa are somewhat misleading, especially the comparisons of blacks and whites in the older and younger groups. Elevated blood pressure was detected in 0.3% of the white school-age children of both sexes compared to 0.8% of the black girls and 1.3% of the black boys of school age. For the preschool group the rates for all race-sex groups were between 0.8% and 0.9%. This finding may reflect the gradual emergence with increasing age of differences in hypertension rates between blacks and whites similar to those commonly seen in studies of adults.

Since the criteria for defining abnormal conditions were not rigidly standardized (a situation similar to clinical practice), reliability of the clinical diagnosis was ascertained by randomly selecting nearly 13% of the children for a second examination by another physician. Although the overall agreement was relatively high (85.8%) due to the large number of normal children, when an abnormality was discovered the physicians agreed only 20% of the time. This small percentage of agreement reflects both the variation in the examinations performed by the different physicians and the subjectivity of the physicians' judgment in their definition of abnormality, particularly when the abnormalities were relatively minor. Low inter-observer agreement appears to be a common occurrence, as summarized by Koran for other studies with physician examiners (Koran, 1975).

It is interesting that the three most prevalent abnormalities seen in the Bogalusa Study—obesity, undernutrition, and dental caries—could, at least to some extent, be preventable by such traditional public health measures as health education, dietary counseling and intervention, and fluoridation of water supplies. Diet intervention by controlling weight and salt intake may be an important modification measure among children already exhibiting abnormally high blood pressures.

For other communities similar to Bogalusa in which medical needs are at least partially defined by physicians, the findings of this study should also be of general interest to persons responsible for planning the allocation of medical care resources or personnel.

24. A consideration of essential hypertension in children

Since the prevalence of essential hypertension is recognized as high as 30% in the adult population, the disease constitutes a major health problem. It is generally recognized that the current high incidence of coronary heart disease and cerebrovascular accidents in the United States is in part caused by essential hypertension. When hypertension is controlled, a reduction of morbid events can ocur (V. A. Cooperative Study Group, 1970). We can assume, then, that these serious complications would be more successfully prevented if hypertension could be controlled in its earlier phases. Some studies have even suggested that a control of early hypertension may not require continued drug management (Perry and Schroeder, 1955; Page and Dustan, 1962).

Current concepts about the nature of hypertension in children are changing. Earlier reports held that most hypertension in childhood is secondary, with essential hypertension occurring rarely (Loggie, 1975; Dustan, 1976). Other recent studies indicate that hypertensive children often do not show an underlying cause (Londe et al., 1971) and that children ranking high in blood pressure among their peers are likely to continue this high ranking (Zinner et al., 1974). Further studies indicate that the level of blood pressure in adolescence is closely related to hypertension in adulthood (Londe, 1968; Harlan et al., 1973; Miall and Chinn, 1973; Sneiderman et al., 1976). These observations, along with our current studies indicating a high degree of

tracking of blood pressure in children (Webber et al., 1979b), indicate
that essential hypertension likely begins in childhood.

In the general population, blood pressure levels during childhood
rise with age until adult stature is reached (18–20 years). Blood pressures then level off, but systolic pressure exponentially increases in
later years (Robinson and Brucer, 1939; Hamilton et al., 1954; Comstock, 1957; Johnson et al. 1965; Nance et al., 1965; Miall and Lovell,
1967; Roberts and Maurer, 1976).

In childhood, large body mass and height are strong correlates of
blood pressure levels (Levy et al., 1946; Lovell, 1967; Chiang et al.,
1969; Londe and Goldring, 1972; Court et al., 1974; Johnson et al.,
1975; Lauer et al., 1975; Voors et al., 1977b). But what are the determinants of early hypertension? High protein intake, which is also a
determinant of serum albumin level, correlates with blood pressure
levels (Fraser et al., 1974; Stine et al., 1975), as do extreme levels of
sodium intake (Joossens et al., 1970; Gleiberman, 1973; Oliver et al.,
1975). Blood sugar and diabetes, furthermore, seem to relate to hypertension (Moss, 1962; Florey, et al., 1976a). Although the precise contribution is not clear, a genetic tendency obviously plays a strong role.

If one wants to diagnose not only secondary hypertension, but also
incipient essential hypertension in children, then the criterion of
what constitutes hypertension needs clarification. In contrast to most
bedside physical examination procedures which are qualitative or
semi-quantitative, the diagnosis of early essential hypertension has a
dominant quantitative component and needs to be approached accordingly for observing blood pressure in children.

The decision to study the trends of blood pressure over time seems
fundamental to us. At this point we still do not know the early natural
history of hypertension, clinically or anatomically. Figure 24–1 shows
the incidence of hypertension measured by the current practice of diagnosis in surveys of school-age children, university students, and
adults. This practice does not take into consideration the possibility
that blood pressure already "tracks" in childhood to a much higher
degree than was believed until recently. Regression to the mean is a
function of the intrachild variability of the measured blood pressure
and decreases in magnitude as our methodology improves. With care
in obtaining measurements and with serial measurements, it will become possible to predict essential hypertension even better; and,

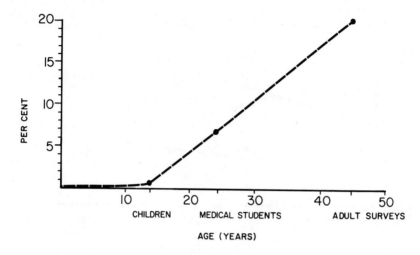

Figure 24–1. Currently recognized incidence of hypertension at different ages.

moreover, it will be easier to observe the possible instances where the child may shift tracks (Fig. 24–2) because of pathobiologic mechanisms.

OBSERVATIONS FROM STUDIES OF CHILDREN

Blood pressure norms based on studies of a large population of children

The distribution of blood pressure levels for the Bogalusa children are shown in Figures 24–3 to 24–5. The data, which may be used as a reference for sitting, right-arm measurements are presented in several ways for convenience and are simplified by not indicating slight differences due to race and sex. In a population of many children, small differences between boys and girls are detectable, particularly at age groups starting around 12 years. Slightly higher values in black children can also be detected beginning around the age of 10 years with the sphygmomanometer.

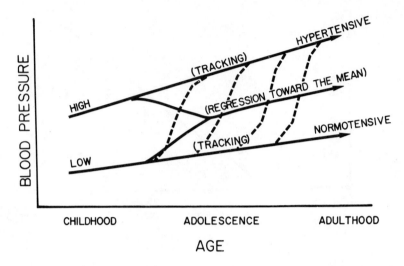

Figure 24–2. A highly schematic presentation of the time-course of blood pressure levels consistent with the tracking hypothesis and the onset of essential hypertension at an early age. Those children at the high percentile tend to remain high; those low tend to remain low. Variation of blood pressure occurs over time and regression toward the mean occurs. We also recognize that blood pressure levels may be clinically translocated to higher levels within short periods of time.

Relationship of blood pressure to age, weight, and height

Blood pressure levels are usually presented relative to age (Fig. 24–3), indicating a progressive increase with age. Because of technical limitations described earlier, it is difficult to obtain valid blood pressures below the age of 6 or 7 years, although these data may be replicable. In smaller children, automatic instruments will improve these measurments. Unfortunately, data obtained in our study resulted in suspected artifactually low values for diastolic pressures from children under 7 years of age. From cross-sectional studies, blood pressure levels show an increment of 1.2–1.7 mm Hg per year for the systolic pressure and approximately 1.0 mm Hg for the diastolic fourth-phase blood pressures. Such small increments of blood pressure are not apt to be detected on a single child but again can be noted in a epidemiologic survey. We also observed that after adjusting for the effects of height and weight on the blood pressure levels, age appears to have no relationship. Approximately 40% of the variability

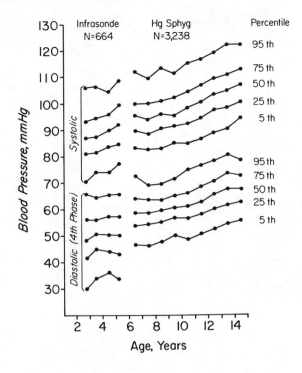

Figure 24–3. Selected percentiles of blood pressure as measured by Infrasonde and mercury sphygmomanometer, by age, in children ages 2–14.

of blood pressure levels seems to be explained by a combination of factors like height, weight, triceps skinfold thickness, or arm circumference (Voors et al., 1977b). The relation of blood pressure with height and log weight is remarkably linear (Chapter 18). Therefore, sets of reference values for blood pressure levels are shown in Figures 24–4 and 24–5 which can be related either to the child's height or weight.

Use of reference standards from several population studies

Customarily, percentile charts used to compare individuals to a described population are shown only related to age and are given separately for boys and girls (Blumenthal et al., 1977). Since heights and weights are the strongest determinants of blood pressure in children, correction for race and sex, except perhaps for the top five per-

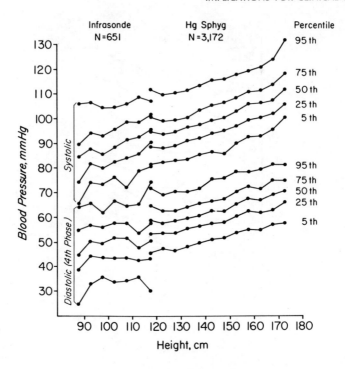

Figure 24–4. Selected percentiles of blood pressure as measured by Infrasonde and mercury sphygmomanometer, by height, in children ages 2–14.

centiles, is not needed in this age group so that the data shown in Figures 24–4 and 24–5 can be used. Since weight is such a strong correlate and more variable among children than height, as a standard reference blood pressure levels for a growing child should be related to height. Weight, as a standard reference, would imply the acceptance of certain high weights for our population of children and thus the corresponding blood pressure levels.

Obviously, information used as a reference standard for a given child should be obtained from a population comparable to the origin of that child. For practical purposes, the Bogalusa Heart Study population (Voors et al., 1976; Berenson et al., 1978a) would appear to qualify as a standard population when children in the United States are examined, because age-specific heights, weights, skinfold measurements, and dietary habits of the Bogalusa children were practically indistinguishable from those of a sample representative of the United States in general (Foster et al., 1977; Frank et al., 1978). It cannot be

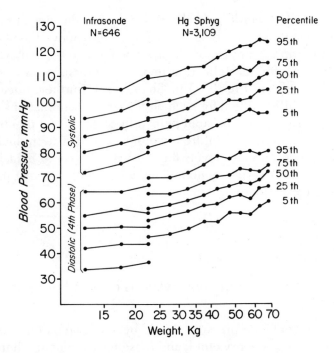

Figure 24–5. Selected percentiles of blood pressure as measured by Infrasonde and mercury sphygmomanometer, by weight, in children ages 2–14.

emphasized too strongly that in deciding to investigate or treat a patient, percentile charts should be used only when the methods of measuring blood pressure are comparable. Measurements in the Bogalusa Heart Study were made strictly according to the guidelines given in this book and are representative of relaxed, sitting, right-arm blood pressure.

Need for repeat (serial) examinations of children for blood pressure levels

Since the blood pressure varies widely from moment to moment, it is also apt to vary from examination to examination. Blood pressure is so variable that the phenomenon of a "regression toward the mean" is observed in an epidemiologic study. This variation may cause a pressure, found to lie in the top percentiles during a first observation, to decrease during a second examination. On the average this decrease will be larger the more the child's pressure varies from one examination to the next. According to observations from the Bogalusa Heart Study, the blood pressure of an 11-year-old child above the 90th percentile will drop 2.2 mm Hg on the average for systolic, and even less on the average for diastolic (fourth phase) pressure on a second examination (refer to Fig. 17–4 in Chapter 17). Further, since blood pressure variability differs for each child, repeat examinations are required to determine a consistent percentile status. From monthly observations on a group of children, we observed that reproducible or consistent blood pressure levels for a given child could be achieved after three to four serial examinations, when replicate readings are made at each examination.

COMMENTS

Physicians' role in routine observations of blood pressure in children

The recording of blood pressure should be a routine part of the physical examinations of every child, and these measurements should become a basic part of the child's medical record. Although it is important to understand the distributions of blood pressures in a cross-section of free-living and presumably healthy population of children, it is equally important to follow children over time in an effort to understand the early natural history of essential hypertension. A number of large-scale studies, which can be used as reference standards, have been conducted around the United States under a variety of circumstances; some levels have been recorded under such casual conditions as might exist in a physician's office (Blumenthal et al., 1977), while others have been recorded with greater care to obtain resting and basal-like readings on children (which is also possible in a physician's office setting). As pointed out earlier, the basal level appears to more likely predict subsequent levels of blood pressure or the occurrence of hypertension later (Smirk, 1957; Harlan et al., 1973).

There remains a great need to follow the changes of blood pressure in individual children over time to observe how "tracking" or trends over time occur. The subsequent high levels of blood pressure observed in adulthood need to be documented from youth, yielding information on how blood pressure levels change with time. Until these changes are understood, our clinical definition of early hypertension remains incomplete. It appears that the practicing physician is in a good position to obtain such information by charting the time course of blood pressure in the children being observed. Repeat observations for a given child serve to indicate the course of blood pressure on that child and can be compared against a background of data already obtained in cross-sectional studies. Such observations would yield invaluable information for the development of new criteria of abnormal levels. Recognition of persistent high levels and their course could be used to indicate the need for further diagnostic studies, intervention for prevention, or even treatment to reduce existing levels.

Subtle biologic differences in children

A large-scale study of children can detect subtle biologic differences, for example, the effect of age, race, sex, or height and weight. For research purposes it is important to understand biologic control which eventually will influence our ability to prevent and manage hypertension. One example has already emerged. The strong relationship of weight to blood pressure that has been found in adults is now noted in children. An important preventive measure would seem to be the control of weight in growing children, especially in those with a family history of hypertension. Further, the detection of higher levels of blood pressure in black children is relevant to the high incidence of hypertension in black adults. And current studies of hormonal changes suggest that essential hypertension is a complex syndrome of more than one etiology (Laragh, 1973). The detection of other differences in large numbers of children can be extrapolated to the systematic search for and evaluation of differences both in whole populations and individuals.

Observations primarily on young adults now indicate that some characterization of blood pressure levels can be shown. Tracking does occur. Those with higher levels of blood pressure noted in adolescence have been found to have hypertension in adulthood (Paffenbarger et al., 1968; Harlan et al., 1973). Similar observations of tracking have been made over a sixteen-year period in the Evans County (Ga.) study (Sneiderman et al., 1976). Observations in our study from one year to the next (Chapter 17) suggest that children, at least within higher blood pressure ranks, are apt to maintain their rank in subsequent years; more recently we note a remarkable tracking to occur over three years (Webber et al., 1979b). The occurrence of blood pressure levels in children at consistently high percentiles should be suspect. External conditioning factors in addition to heredity determine hypertension. From a conjectural standpoint, conditioning and perpetuating factors are shown in Figure 24–6. It is possible that children enter adulthood with certain characteristics or predisposing mecha-

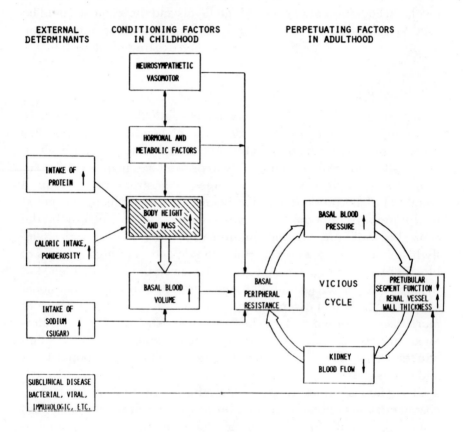

Figure 24–6. A conjectural role of body mass in determining diastolic blood pressure in early life is schematically shown. During adulthood, increased peripheral resistance leads to increased blood pressure and ensuing renal-vascular changes; and to decreased kidney blood flow, which in turn activates the Goldblatt mechanism causing increased basal peripheral resistance, thus closing the vicious cycle. Children can enter adulthood with characteristics predisposing to this vicious cycle.

nisms that perpetuate hypertension in adulthood. Our studies (Chapter 18) suggest that body mass and perhaps basal blood volumes may play a role in this predisposition to hypertension later in life.

A lack of satisfactory criteria for definition of hypertension in children

At this time we can hardly arrive at a precise or even clinically satisfactory definition of essential hypertension in youth. By what criteria should hypertension levels be defined? Should an arbitrary level based on experience in adulthood be used? A level of 130/85 has been suggested for children below age 10 (Loggie, 1975); in our total population study, the criterion would designate only a few children as hypertensive, but such a value is arbitrary. In contrast to adults, in children there are no correlates of blood pressure levels with morbidity, cerebrovascular accidents, congestive heart failure, cardiomegaly, or renal dysfunction; nor are there any anatomic correlates of vascular changes (Heptinstall, 1976), even eye-ground changes, that can be detected in the early stages. Yet, if similar criteria were applied in children as in adults 45 to 54 years of age—two standard deviations from the mean or approximately 180/110 (Roberts and Maurer, 1976)—this would be equivalent to a level of 124/75 for a 14-year-old child. Specific criteria cannot be given at present, although such deliberations are important.

An approach to intervention on high levels of blood pressure in a general population of children

Eventually, decisions will have to be made on when to begin intervention, prevention, or treatment. Unfortunately, no rules or guidelines can be established now. The observations on tracking and predictability of basal blood pressures suggest that essential hypertension originates in youth and may already exist in a significant number of presumably healthy children. These considerations show the importance of further understanding the early natural history of essential hypertension. For the present, only the simplest modifications of life style, such as prevention of obesity, regular exercise, and a general reduction of salt intake, are warranted. More vigorous therapeutic measures to reduce the blood pressure levels for the higher percentiles, except at the highest one or two percentiles, in the general population of this age should not be instituted at this time. However, essential hypertension clearly exists in youth, and the continued study of blood pressure in children should receive a high priority in an effort to prevent the devastating cardiovascular disease in adults. Measurement of blood pressure in children is practical, and in fact necessary, at least by school age. The simple but basic measures of weight control, reduction of dietary salt, and routine exercise, which help in the prevention of hypertension, are not in themselves harmful.

SUMMARY

Essential hypertension, a highly prevalent and devastating disease, likely begins in childhood, a stage at which it would respond to general preventive measures. The problems encountered in the recording of reproducible blood pressure levels are largely quantitative and involve instrument validity, observer (examiner) training, and the interaction between child and the physician's office environment. The problems of early diagnosis of hypertension are related to lack of long-term observations on children. Population percentiles of normal blood pressure values could aid in the early diagnosis of hypertension, but for this purpose the method of measuring blood pressure in the physician's office has to be strictly comparable to methods employed in accumulating the percentiles or reference observations. For accuracy, repeated measurements under basal-like, resting, or relaxed conditions are advised; for standardization, the weight or height of the child is more important than his age.

25. A consideration of hyperlipoproteinemia in children

A great deal of attention has focused on hyperlipoproteinemia as a risk factor in coronary artery disease and on the management of patients with abnormal lipoprotein levels, but at present very little is known about the management of hyperlipoproteinemia in the general population, especially in children. The lack of unequivocal evidence that end-stage disease, i.e., coronary insufficiency or morbid events such as myocardial infarction, may be prevented by reducing serum lipids is frustrating and has stirred considerable controversy over the value of dietary changes in the general public. Most attempts to prevent atherosclerosis by modifying lipid levels have involved adults with established evidence of disease. Only recently has attention been directed toward younger persons as a general means of reducing the high morbidity of coronary heart disease in this country (Kannel and Dawber, 1972; Mitchell and Jesse, 1973; Blumenthal, 1973). Scattered efforts have been made to treat children, but only those with extremely high lipid levels suspected to be familial (Levy and Rifkind, 1973), and clear recommendations for all children have not yet been made.

In 1954, Gofman and co-workers called attention to the different classes of serum lipoproteins that could be separated using flotation techniques and the ultracentrifuge. These authors emphasized that hyperlipidemia should be dealt with in terms of hyperlipoproteinemia. The serum lipoprotein classification system subsequently developed by Fredrickson and colleagues (1967) significantly advanced that concept and demonstrated the need to search for abnormal levels of lipoproteins and relate them to genetic, metabolic, or other causes.

The development of simplified methods to study serum lipoproteins by electrophoresis and other laboratory techniques now enables clinicians to probe for levels in their patients, relate them to distributions in entire populations, and observe disorders associated with hyperlipoproteinemia.

We feel, however, that the cut points used to separate normal from elevated lipoprotein levels, as defined by the 95th percentile criterion established by Fredrickson and colleagues (1967), are far too high for children (Table 25–1). From our observations of young adult medical students (Berenson et al., 1971b) and a large number of children from one community (Frerichs et al., 1976; Srinivasan et al., 1976a), only a very small number of presumably healthy, free-living individuals would be categorized as having hyperlipoproteinemia according to these criteria (Table 25–2). When individuals with secondary hyperlipoproteinemia are excluded, the remaining persons might be found to have abnormal lipoprotein levels of a genetic nature.

Goldstein and co-workers (1973b) have recently suggested that the genetic etiology for hyperlipoproteinemia is more complex than was originally suggested by a rigid typing system. The more current consideration suggests that classification by phenotype is a descriptive pattern to guide further clinical study as well as dietary and other therapeutic management.

Table 25–1. Mean and 95th percentile levels (mg/dl) of serum lipid and lipoprotein cholesterol in Bogalusa children (5–14 years) as compared to the suggested levels for children (0–19 years)

Serum lipids and lipoprotein cholesterol	Suggested levels [1] (0–19 yrs)			Bogalusa children (5–14 yrs)		
	N	Mean	95th percentile	N	Mean	95th percentile
Total cholesterol	81	176	230	3,446	165	216
Triglycerides	81	67	140	3,183	69	125
LDL cholesterol	81	108	170	3,181	89	131
VLDL cholesterol	81	10	25	3,181	8	22

[1]Established by Fredrickson et al. (1967).

Table 25–2. Frequency of hyperlipoproteinemia in children 5–14 years of age as defined by the 95th percentile of upper normal limits [1]

	Number of children (%)	
Lipoprotein elevation	Black	White
β-lipoprotein > 170 mg/dl	6 (0.5)	9 (0.5)
Pre-β-lipoprotein > 25 mg/dl	20 (1.7)	94 (4.7)
β-lipoprotein and pre-β-lipoprotein > 170 and 25 mg/dl, respectively	1 (0.1)	3 (0.1)

[1]Fredrickson et al. (1967)

In contrast to the 5% of the population judged to have abnormal levels of serum lipoproteins by the 95th percentile cut point, a much broader segment of the population should be considered to be affected by atherosclerosis (Gertler and White, 1954). Unfortunately, our inability to relate specific lipid and lipoprotein abnormalities to the extent and progression of atherosclerosis by noninvasive means limits our precision regarding specific levels of abnormality.

Defining hyperlipoproteinemia

The specific typing of serum lipoproteins, although serving to stimulate interest in the study of these entities and drawing attention to metabolic and genetic disorders associated with them, aids little in the diagnosis of lipid disorders in the general population subject to the development of coronary artery disease. The distribution of serum lipid and lipoprotein levels in the general population is skewed somewhat toward high values but is not clearly bimodal, and any definition of the upper limits of normal becomes arbitrary.

Should one use specific cutpoints, percentiles, or standard deviations as criteria for abnormality? For example, in Figure 25–1 three different levels have been recommended for evaluating total serum cholesterol in children. By each of these criteria the approximate percentage of Bogalusa school-age children that could be designated as abnormal can be seen.

Our preschool studies (Berenson et al., 1978a) show that by the age of 3 children have serum lipid and lipoprotein levels approaching those found in young adults; that average lipid levels in young school-

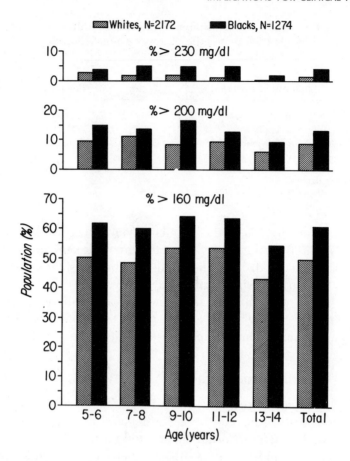

Figure 25-1. Prevalence of serum total cholesterol levels in school children, ages 5-14, by race.

age children are as high as those in young adults; and that there is a broad range for the mean values.

The difficulties associated with and some of the considerations arriving at a clinical classification of primary hyperlipoproteinemias have been outlined by Carlson (1973). He suggests that definitions of hyperlipidemia may be made from a statistical or a clinical viewpoint as well as a biologic one. At this time it may be premature to arrive at any firm classification of abnormality for children in the general population, except for those at the extremes. But from a practical stand-

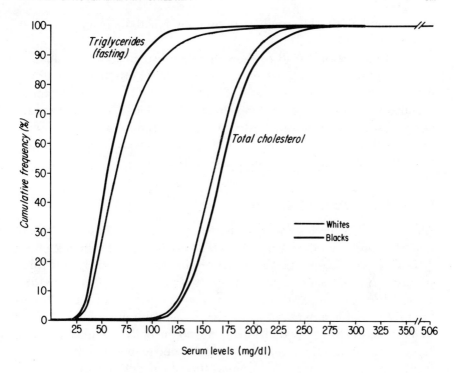

Figure 25–2. Cumulative frequency for levels of serum cholesterol and tri-glycerides in white and black children, 5–14 years of age.

point, the higher the percentile of serum lipid levels (Fig. 25–2), the more crucial the need for aggressive intervention.

Significance of distribution of cholesterol in serum lipoproteins

Although most clinical judgments or recommendations at present are based on total serum cholesterol, we must again emphasize that this determination reflects the cholesterol transported in α-, β, and pre-β-lipoproteins. (See Chapter 9 for details on lipoprotein levels). We have pointed out that children have higher α-lipoprotein levels than adults, a greater proportion of the total cholesterol occurs as α-lipoprotein in children, and pre-β-lipoprotein tends to be low in children. The significance of the latter as an independent variable related to coronary heart disease remains debatable, but its interrelationship with obesity and with abnormal carbohydrate metabolism occurs as in adults.

Our cross-sectional studies show that there can be dramatic changes in lipoprotein distributions with age. Consequently, some children may have high total serum cholesterol because of high α-lipoproteins. We also know that HDL fractions may be protective against coronary artery disease (Miller and Miller, 1975). Therefore, a serum cholesterol level known to be high after repeated analysis needs to be further evaluated as to the lipoprotein distributions.

Feasibility of early detection

Although it has been suggested that specific genetic abnormalities of hyperlipoproteinemia can be detected in cord blood (Glueck et al., 1971; Kwiterovich et al., 1973), data from the Bogalusa Heart Study indicate that dramatic changes occur within the first 6 months to 1 year of life, and suggest that observations predictive of future levels are more reliable at 6 months to 1 year of age (Berenson et al., 1979 c) than at birth. Since pediatricians do not usually obtain lipid and lipoprotein determinations, it might be recommended that serum lipids be routinely included among the blood determinations made on children, at least by school age. Practical laboratory methods have now been refined for obtaining serum cholesterol and triglycerides as well as abbreviated lipoprotein quantitations on children as a routine part of an examination. An improved laboratory method for cholesterol determinations is now available on capillary blood (Bhandaru et al., 1977). Such determinations are important in the general population of children, especially when an overall examination shows a family history of coronary heart disease and the presence of other potential risk-factor variables. The prevalence of coronary artery disease in the United States and other industrially advanced countries certainly warrants studies at an early age.

Treatment

Intensive therapy is obviously warranted in individuals with β-lipoprotein levels at the highest percentiles, although at this time specific recommendations for children in the general population may be premature. A distinction should first be made between primary hyperlipoproteinemia and a condition that is secondary to other disorders. The prevalence of specific forms of hyperlipoproteinemia as suggested by the World Health Organization classifications would imply 0.5–5.0% of all children might fall into a primary or clear genetic type of hyperlipoproteinemia. (Beaumont et al., 1970) In the remaining population less identifiable genetic factors interact with environmental conditions and appear to have a greater influence on the variability of lipid abnormalities. A finding of primary hyperlipoproteinemia would necessitate a complete family screening, with repeated evaluations, as a preventive measure. High serum total cholesterol due to α-lipoprotein would, of course, have to be distinguished.

The presence of certain metabolic or genetic disorders leading to hyperlipoproteinemia would call for aggressive treatment by dietary changes, selected drug therapy, and then surgical therapy. Unfortunately, drug therapy for hyperlipoproteinemia has not yet been evaluated clinically in terms of its influence on vascular lesions. Although the initial clinical trials of some drugs have been disappointing (Stamler et al., 1978), regression of lesions has been accomplished in nonhuman primates by dietary changes and selected drugs that reduce serum cholesterol levels after the induction of experimental atherosclerosis (Armstrong, 1976; Wissler and Vesselinovitch, 1977).

Mild hyperlipoproteinemia (which is rampant in the United States) is being related to dietary indiscretion and sedentary habits. Although it has not yet been proved that coronary artery disease can be prevented by reducing dietary cholesterol content or by exercise, evidence from clinical and epidemiologic studies, as well as from experimentation, justifies a modification of diet for the entire population. As a minimum, recommendations by the American Heart Association (1972) for a prudent diet seem justifiable.

Although precise relationships of diet to serum lipid levels within a given population fail to specify the dietary components at fault, we recognize in our pediatric populations excessively high intakes of total calories, fat, saturated fatty acids, cholesterol, sucrose, and NaCl. Modification of these levels, then, may be a basic recommendation. The prudent diet of the American Heart Association can be advised as a beginning. In a prudent diet, the amounts of animal (saturated) fat, cholesterol, and refined sugar should be reduced, the relative amount of polyunsaturated fat should be increased, and the total caloric intake should not exceed individual requirements. If the risk of development of coronary artery disease is low in a population like the Japanese, which has lipid levels far below any suggested as "normal" in the United States, it should be considered prudent to strive for the lower levels in this country.

The prudent diet is not difficult to follow, nor is it more expensive. Diet per se could be greatly improved by proper selection of ingredients and food products. As a beginning, dietary management coupled with regular and dynamic exercise regimens seems to be a realistic approach to the problem of mild hyperlipoproteinemia and the epidemic of heart disease. In the future, dietary and behavior patterns, which can be modified by better understanding the problem, may be introduced through appropriate educational programs for children. The task now at hand is to learn more about nutrition in children in relationship to atherosclerosis and hypertension and how nutrition and modified life styles can be presented effectively in school educational programs. The last chapter considers this area further.

If correction of serum lipids to desired levels fails, especially in children with persistence of levels in the high percentiles and with family histories of early coronary heart diseases (below the age of 50 years), more stringent methods, which may include lipid-lowering drugs, are advocated. (Beaumont et al., 1970; Fallat et al., 1974).

SUMMARY

Observations on a large number of free-living children now indicate the need for practicing physicians to incorporate studies on serum lipids at a young age. There is a dramatic transition of lipid and lipoproteins from birth to 2 or 3 years of age which may reflect future levels in childhood, perhaps even in adulthood. Since serum cholesterol level is considered to be a continuum of risk for the probability of developing coronary artery disease, it is prudent to strive for the lowest serum lipid levels possible without creating any biologic ill effects. Methods for quantitating serum lipoproteins have now been adapted for practical use. These determinations should be included among the lipid observations on children for a better appreciation of lipids as a risk-factor variable. Since serum lipid levels represent only one risk-factor variable in the context of arteriosclerosis, the child should be observed in view of his or her family history as well as the other factors producing risk for adult cardiovascular disease.

26. A summing up

Train a child in the way he should go—and walk there yourself
once in a while.

In the course of our study we have been asked many questions about
risk factors in children by both scientists and laypersons. This chapter
attempts to answer some of these questions and provides an overview
of the application of current information.

IS THERE REASON TO BE CONCERNED ABOUT
ARTERIOSCLEROSIS IN CHILDREN?

To understand risk-factor variables in children, the study of life patterns and lifestyles that may influence the early natural history of atherosclerosis and essential hypertension is critical to prevention of our
major cardiovascular diseases and premature causes of death.

Observe the prevalence of cardiovascular disease in any general
hospital. Hypertension, diabetes, myocardial infarction, cerebrovascular accidents, and congestive heart failure are the most common
problems. They form the bulk of serious health problems in internal
medicine and cardiology and pervade all other branches of medicine.
Our cardiology service at Charity Hospital of New Orleans answers
almost half of the total consultations to all subspecialty services of the
department of medicine. Consider the number of these disease states
in persons under the age of 65, even in patients in their middle or late
40s. In many private hospitals and medical centers, coronary artery

surgery has become one of the most common surgical procedures; economically it rates highest. Obviously, surgery is not the long-term solution.

Nevertheless, it is frustrating that we have little hard data to show that longevity can be extended or morbid events reduced by controlling risk-factor levels at an early age or in "healthy" populations. The evidence is clear for controlling moderate to severe hypertension (Veterans Administration Cooperative Study Group, 1967); lowering blood pressure with drugs reduces cerebrovascular accidents and congestive heart failure secondary to hypertension. Evidence is now being provided for treating mild hypertension (Veterans Administration Cooperative Study Group, 1970; Smith, 1978), but long-term effects of treatment are not yet known. The effects of altered lipid levels and weight reduction are less apparent and no data are available on young people over long periods of time. The North Karelia Project in Finland where the highest morbidity and mortality exists for coronary heart disease (Puska et al., 1978) has indicated significant reduction in disease incidence by dietary and risk-factor reduction. Although primary intervention or dietary modification is not being recommended for children generally, except at extremely high levels of both lipids (American Academy of Pediatrics Committee on Nutrition, 1972) and blood pressure (Blumenthal et al., 1977; Berenson et al., 1978b), substantial evidence is accumulating to support intervention in children who would be ranked at mild to moderate risk. Deciding when these children are truly at risk of developing cardiovascular disease and developing appropriate intervention are major public health problems in the United States.

If today's children grow up like their parents, 20–30% of them will have hypertension as adults. Ninety percent will develop significant atherosclerotic lesions (Holman et al., 1958), and over 50% will die from hypertension and atherosclerosis (Gordon and Devine, 1966).

WHAT HAVE WE REALLY ACCOMPLISHED?

This question is usually asked by someone who impatiently awaits a quick answer as to why we have not solved the problems of heart disease. To that person, our answer may not be exciting, but to us the accomplishments represent real advances toward health care for much of our population. The major accomplishment is simple: we now have a pretty good idea of how to study a population of children, or a single child, for risk-factor variables known to be related to coronary artery disease and essential hypertension. This is the beginning of prevention of the major cardiovascular diseases in our population.

We have developed models—in a sense, know-how applicable by the primary physician when examining children, as in measuring blood pressure. We have learned how to take indirect blood pressure in children as young as age five; we can recommend proper cuff sizes. We appreciate the value and limitations of automatic blood pressure recording instruments for mass screening, and we can identify blood pressure levels in relaxed children, a significant step for making observations over time. Further, we know the limitations in measuring indirect blood pressure, whether by physicians, nurses, or multiple observers. We have learned that serial observations over three to four visits are required to obtain reproducible levels of a child's blood pressure. We have provided tables showing the normative distribution of blood pressure in a large sample of free-living children. In this text, blood pressure measurements are described at one point in time, but in the future they can be obtained at intervals and under a variety of conditions, just as we now record heart rates and rhythms by electrocardiography.

Similarly, we know how to measure serum lipids and lipoproteins and relate them to levels in a total population of children under risk for cardiovascular disease. We have learned the importance of measuring serum lipoproteins, not just serum lipids. We know the potential for error in obtaining laboratory determinations, especially for a single sample, and we have developed techniques for quantitating serum lipids and lipoproteins, even on small samples of sera.

Simply, we have developed models, protocols,* normative grids (See Appendix), and detailed tables (National Heart, Lung and Blood Institute, 1978) that are available to the practicing physician and the epidemiologist. Comparative studies of dietary intakes of infants to children and adults have been obtained (Frank et al., Table 26-1).

The study has gone a step further: important interrelationships of the risk-factor variables are observed.

The risk factors tend to aggregate or cluster, and we can now identify a group or a single child in Bogalusa with one, two, or three risk-

*Detailed protocols, unpublished

Table 26–1. A comparison of mean intakes of infants, children and adults

Dietary component per kg body weight	6 mo.[1] N = 125	12 mo.[1] N = 99	10 yr.[2] N = 185	Adult[3]
Kcal	126	141	66	39
Protein, g	3.9	4.7	2.1	1.2
Carbohydrate, g	17.3	17.2	8.1	4.4
Fat, g	4.9	6.1	2.8	1.8
Cholesterol, mg	14.4	25.2	10.0	10.0
Sodium, mg	116	191	102	57

[1]Frank et al. (1979b).   [2]Frank et al. (1978).
[3]National Academy of Sciences—National Research Council reference adult male: 70 kg, 2700 Kcal (46% carbohydrate, 42% fat, 12% protein), 700 mg cholesterol, 10g NaCl.

factor variables at high levels (Webber et al., 1979a)—smoking should be included as a fourth variable. The studies indicate a tendency for the variables to persist at high levels in a larger percentage of children than if there was no association of the factors (see Chapter 20). Clustering already begins in childhood! These variables increase in association with each other with age, suggesting the increasing environmental impact. Further, our studies show that white boys, already targeted for coronary artery disease by their tendency for the highest aggregation of risk-factor variables, show a marked decrease of HDL around puberty and during adolescence (Berenson et al., 1979b; Cresanta et al., 1979) (Fig. 26–1). And, of course, white male adults have the highest incidence of myocardial infarction.

The high incidence of hypertension in blacks, on the other hand, is now a well-recognized problem (Gordon, 1973; Gordon and Devine, 1966). Higher blood pressure levels have been found in black children; early obesity and its association with hypertension, in black girls. Other studies are beginning to show lower renin levels in black children with higher blood pressure levels and certain differences in urinary sodium and potassium excretion, suggesting greater susceptibility of blacks to the high sodium chloride content of our diets (Table 26–2) (Berenson et al., 1979a; Voors et al., 1979b; Berenson et al., 1979d).

We have come a long way toward answering the questions: What are the distribution and prevalence of risk-factor variables and what are their interrelationships? What levels constitute risk still remain uncertain. It will remain for future observations to relate levels of risk-factor variables in children to early coronary vascular lesions and early essential hypertension.

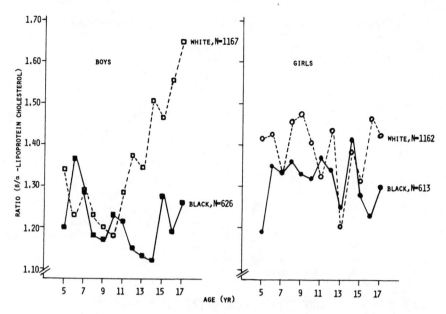

Figure 26–1. Dramatic changes occur in the ratios of mean β-LP cholesterol/mean α-LP cholesterol in children with age. Around puberty there is a decrease in serum total cholesterol. This decrease is due to serum lipoprotein changes and it can be noted that the ratios of β-LP cholesterol/α-LP cholesterol (LDL cholesterol/HDL cholesterol) are about the same in girls and black boys. However, there appears to be an inordinate decrease of HDL in white boys which is reflected by a precipitous increase in the ratio with age or sexual maturation. LDL begins to rise around age 17, especially in white boys. These changes may well relate to the greater incidence of coronary heart disease in white men at a younger age than in women and black men.

Further, our studies are documenting that in childhood these risk-factor variables already "track," that is, the rank of a child with respect to the levels of his peers remains constant over time (Fig. 26–2). A single measurement of blood pressure or serum cholesterol is highly predictive of future measurements (see Table 26–3). Several serial measurements provide even stronger predictions of future levels. Multiple risk factors will probably be found to track at a given level and a child with several risk factors at high values is apt to have a specially high risk of developing clinical disease as an adult. The capability of identifying such a child is the most important accomplishment of our program. Here is where prevention can now begin.

Table 26–2. Racial differences related to blood pressure of children[1]

Higher values noted in:	
Whites	Blacks
All blood pressure strata	
Percent body fat	
Plasma renin activity	
Serum dopamine β-hydroxylase (DβH)	
24-hr urine K^+	
Fasting serum glucose	
High blood pressure strata	
Resting heart rate	Sitting blood pressure levels
Renin activity and DβH combined	Pos. association 24-hr urine Na^+
1-hr serum glucose	versus sitting blood pressure
	Neg. association of plasma renin
	versus systolic blood pressures
	(black boys only)

[1]Berenson *et al.* (1979a, 1979d); *Voors et al.* (1979b).

HOW MANY CHILDREN HAVE BEEN DETECTED WITH HYPERTENSION?

One objective of a pediatric research program concerned with hypertension is to describe reliable blood pressure levels and develop methods for determining such levels in children. One of the most common questions that we are asked is: What is the prevalence of hypertension in children? It would be easy to say "five percent" and evade the underlying problem. A similar question could be posed and answer given for lipids—hyperlipoproteinemia, specific genetic types or phenotypes—or obesity. For each of the risk variables, however, specific criteria have to be examined. The question of "normality" or ideal levels has to be considered (Carlson, 1973; Berenson et al., 1976). For this reason we refer to risk-factor *variables* rather than risk-factors. We are only examining parameters that have been correlated with morbid events in adult studies (Kannel, 1972).

Take blood pressure, for example. Deciding what specific blood pressure levels are abnormal in children has inhibited an understanding of the onset of early hypertension. For practical considerations, Loggie (1971) uses a cut-off point of 130/85. The NIH Task Force Report on Blood Pressure (Blumenthal et al., 1977) suggests monitoring at the 95th percentile, which is stated as 130/100 for a 13-year-old child. But this is much higher than we observed in the Bogalusa Heart

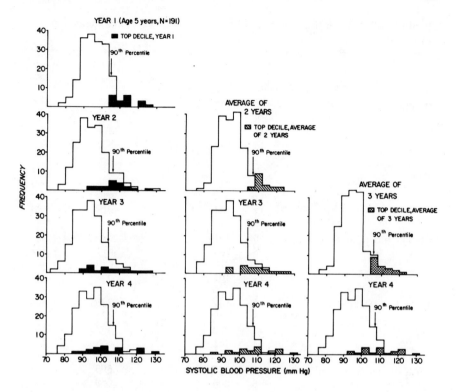

Figure 26–2. Systolic blood pressure readings for 5-year-old children (1973) screened annually over three successive years. The readings for those children who were in the upper decile according to various criteria are shaded. These children tended to have readings in the upper 2 deciles at all subsequent times.

Study, and is not an acceptable diastolic level, even for adults (Berenson et al., 1978b). Other criteria for the definition of hypertension use two and three standard deviations from the mean for the population. Yet, means for risk-factor variables may differ from study to study or from country to country, and in the latter case risk for disease may be known to vary.

Blood pressure levels in a large population follow what is essentially a continuous unimodal distribution. This is so for all the risk-factor variables under consideration, though perhaps they show a slight skewing to the right. The selection of criteria of abnormality remains arbitrary. We might conclude because of the tracking phe-

Table 26–3. Correlation coefficients for risk factor variables measured 1, 2 and 3 years apart

	Age	N	Year 1 vs. year 2	Year 1 vs. year 3	Year 1 vs. year 4
Height	5	192	.981	.964	.925
	8	246	.977	.921	.876
	11	270	.961	.877	.682
	14	164	.931	.832	.765
Weight	5	181	.825	.845	.804
	8	246	.983	.954	.899
	11	268	.963	.926	.854
	14	164	.956	.918	.880
Systolic blood pressure	5	191	.645	.595	.576
	8	246	.729	.674	.621
	11	270	.678	.640	.629
	14	161	.624	.596	.519
Diastolic blood pressure	5	191	.413	.366	.397
	8	246	.481	.421	.422
	11	270	.515	.439	.424
	14	161	.537	.388	.271[2]
Total serum cholesterol	5	175	.674	.695	.687
	8	235	.749	.689	.751
	11	260	.690	.699	.614
	14	162	.705	.745	.659
Triglycerides[1]	5	113	.387	.258[3]	.385
	8	183	.492	.423	.418
	11	174	.502	.593	.569
	14	92	.415	.403	.492
α-lipoprotein cholesterol[1]	5	113	.369	.212[4]	.311[2]
	8	183	.410	.426	.362
	11	174	.545	.535	.432
	14	92	.517	.473	.297[3]
β-lipoprotein cholesterol[1]	5	111	.633	.670	.615
	8	180	.829	.786	.758
	11	173	.804	.795	.653
	14	92	.794	.826	.722
Pre-β-lipoprotein cholesterol[1]	5	111	.505	.234[4]	.439
	8	180	.433	.402	.433
	11	173	.480	.376	.440
	14	92	.585	.625	.516

[1]Fasting for all 4 examinations
[2]$p < 0.001$
[3]$p < 0.01$
[4]$p < 0.05$
All others $p < 0.0001$

nomenon that a large number of children are at risk for cardiovascular disease with values heretofore considered within normal limits. What number we identify with specific abnormalities then depends upon whatever criteria we arbitrarily select to define as abnormal. Generally, as in adults, the higher the level of the risk-factor, the greater the risk for disease. The higher the level, the more intense should be the effort toward further examination, monitoring, or treatment.

In contrast to studies of adults, we cannot equate risk-factor variable levels in children with end-organ or target-organ disease—morbidity or mortality. For instance, changes in the retina and kidney, alteration of creatinine clearance, and elevations of BUN do not occur or are not detectable in the early stages of hypertension. Therefore, we cannot define specific levels for the factors at risk, except for relative ranking (percentiles) in the population. Perhaps, from a practical standpoint we cannot screen all children, but we should try—since an overwhelming number are at risk for coronary artery disease and hypertension. Once identified, should we treat children that remain in the top 5 or 10%? We feel they should be treated. But such a task would overtax our professional resources. Therefore, public health measures and personal care through education may be the only realistic approaches for the total population at risk for these cardiovascular diseases.

WHAT RECOMMENDATIONS CAN WE MAKE TO PHYSICIANS?

We can now give guidelines to the practicing physician for monitoring and managing risk-factor variables detected early in life. They can be listed in simple terms of *who, what, when, where,* and *how*. But it must be emphasized that the guidelines we suggest must be modified as the knowledge of cardiovascular disease continues to increase.

Who? At present there is a controversy in pediatrics as to the extent of screening that should be undertaken in children. Some recommend screening only those children with a family history of cardiovascular disease, such as children with a parent who has had a myocardial infarction by age 50. We feel on the other hand, that *all* children should be examined for a complete risk-factor profile. From infant studies we begin to see predictability of lipid and lipoprotein levels at the age of six months. Indirect blood pressure is easy to measure beginning with

school-age children. Weight, height or length, and skinfold thickness
are easy to measure at all ages. The consistency of levels, ranking
within levels, and persistence of this ranking (tracking) is surprisingly
high, according to our observations over four consecutive annual examinations (see Table 26–3). Practical limits will determine the extent to which children are examined, but the effort to incorporate such
examinations into routine practice needs to be strongly encouraged.

What? The simplest observations include a family history; smoking
history; and measurements of height, weight, skinfold thickness,
serum lipids and lipoproteins, and blood pressure. The initial analysis
of serum lipoproteins can be done very simply and inexpensively by
combining the turbidity procedure (Berenson et al., 1972b; Srinivasan
et al., 1979a) which is an assay of β plus pre-β-lipoprotein cholesterol,
and a measure of serum total cholesterol. Together, these procedures
can exclude errors in interpreting relatively high serum total cholesterol in the presence of high α-lipoprotein levels.

Multiple observations of blood pressure and cholesterol levels must
be made to compensate for measurement and laboratory error. Three
or four visits are needed to approach representative blood pressure
levels, at least for a resting, basal value (Voors et al., 1979a). This is
particularly true when the initial measurement is high. The potential
error (95% confidence interval) of a single determination of serum
cholesterol or triglycerides in our laboratory has a range of 25–36
mg/dl.

When? We believe that measurements of blood pressure should begin
at least by school age and should become part of the general physical
examination of a child at various stages of growth. Serum lipids and
lipoproteins can be studied at any age for which it is practical to obtain blood samples.

Where? Wherever medicine is practiced. In our study population
many children are never seen by a physician. So that they will not be
denied the benefits of early risk factor detection, health clinics and
school health programs should incorporate these observations.

How? With all the intensity we can muster, since coronary artery disease and hypertension are epidemic in this country. Yet evidence ac-

cumulates that they are controllable. In this text we are referring to primary disease, so for each abnormality secondary causes need to be kept in mind and excluded when suspected.

In the attempt to prevent heart disease, we feel that practicing physicians should use more sophisticated modes of studying children for risk factor data. They, or preferably their nurses, should measure blood pressure in children regularly just as blood pressures are routinely obtained in adults. They should obtain analyses of serum lipoproteins or at least screen for hyper-β- or pre-β-lipoproteinemia by the turbidity method and serum total cholesterol, which will also indicate levels of α-lipoproteins. The tools are available, accessible, and easy to use.

We are beginning to appreciate that α-lipoproteins (HDL) may be a negative risk factor (Miller and Miller, 1975; Castelli et al., 1977b), so we can better assess both high and low risk. In the near future we will be able to study specific HDL fractions, and apoprotein chemistry will help us characterize more specific changes that occur as we attempt treatment by dietary modification and exercise.

WHAT ABOUT PREVENTION AND TREATMENT?

General preventive measures need to be practical. Weight control, regular exercise, reduced sodium intake, and acceptance of prudent diet are a minimum (Fig. 26–3) and should be recommended to our total population. More explicitly, individuals at high risk require treatment.

Again, the higher the level of the risk-factor variable, the greater the need for treatment and more intense management. Obviously, dietary changes to lower serum total cholesterol are not warranted if most of the cholesterol occurs as α-lipoproteins, and if β-lipoproteins are low. On the other hand, a high blood pressure level that persists over the 95th percentile and does not respond to weight control and reduction of dietary sodium requires graded drug therapy as outlined in the Task Force Report (Blumenthal et al., 1977).

Snacks have become dominant in children's diets. A stringent attack on diet may not be necessary when substitutes for the now "normal" diet are made available. Health education in the early school grades would be particularly helpful in the areas of personal habits, like smoking, as well as nutrition.

The problem is, how do we modify environmental factors, espe-

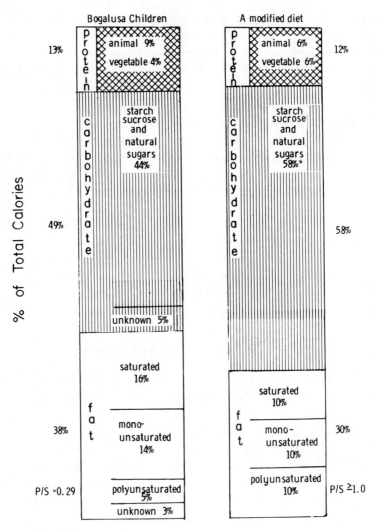

Figure 26–3. Composition of diets in Bogalusa children, age 10 years, and a suggested modification with a composition similar to the prudent diet. The desired changes are a reduction in total fat with increased P/S ratio and a reduction of refined sugars.

cially dietary factors? Should diets be specific for reducing dietary cholesterol, as suggested? Do we concentrate on exogenous cholesterol, or saturated fats or total fat, or refined sugars, or calories, or excessive intake of sodium chloride or all of these at once? Nutrition

studies of nonhuman primates suggest that all are important (Srinivasan et al., 1978b, 1979b, 1979c). We now have the advantage of being
able to monitor an individual's biochemical response to dietary
change, though how changes in a risk-factor variable will alter vascular disease remains uncertain. Epidemiologic observations suggest
that lowering the high-risk profile also lowers the potential for disease; experimental studies of nonhuman primates demonstrate this
anatomically.

Some dietary recommendations, i.e., reduction of saturated fat, exogenous cholesterol, sucrose, and sodium chloride, have been made
to the general public (American Heart Association, 1965, 1973, 1978;
United States Senate—Select Committee on Nutrition and Human
Needs, 1977). In making such recommendations, the hazards of dietary change should be kept in mind, but at present such caution by
physicians and laypersons is being used negatively to prevent
change in our current life style. Drastic changes are not being recommended, so that ill effects on growth and good nutritional status are
not apt to occur. Importantly, physical and biochemical changes can
be monitored.

Although lowering the total caloric intake may be difficult for most
children, it should be considered for the obese child. To date, the
most effective means in adults are group interaction methods (Stunkard, 1972). New techniques will have to be developed for children,
involving both family and school influences. A reduction of fat to
25–30% of total calories with a P/S ratio of 1:1 and a limitation of exogenous cholesterol to 200–300 mg for older children may be reasonable. Further reduction of fat (15%) to mimic diets of the Far East
might be considered. In our studies of nonhuman primates, sucrose in
high amounts enhances endogenous synthesis, and when coupled
with exogenous cholesterol, has a dramatic effect in elevating serum
total cholesterol (Srinivasan et al., 1978b, 1979b). In addition, we have
noted a potentiating effect of sucrose on salt-induced hypertension
(Srinivasan et al., 1979c).

Yudkin (1972) has indicated sucrose as a major culprit in cardiovascular disease, and he may be correct. So vegetables, fruits, legumes,
fish, chicken, lean beef, margarines with high P/S ratios, and selected
or prepared dairy products (skim milk, low-fat cheeses, yogurt), may
be the route to good health—and not the candy, hot dogs, hydrogenated fats, butter, whole milk, cake and desserts, ice cream, and
vegetables cooked with salted meats that our children are eating.

We have little data on exercise in children, but we know from dietary manipulations coupled with *dynamic exercise* in adults that we can change the serum lipoproteins, weight, and blood pressure to a profile more indicative of low risk.

What about the role of mental stress or *behavior?* Several clinical investigations are now obtaining meaningful data on the relationship between behavior and risk-factor variables, but the subject is broad and difficult to study. Our group is just beginning to explore this area.

And what about *cigarette smoking?* Clear, objective data from autopsy studies of young adults age 20–24 years demonstrate that raised lesions in coronary arteries are related to smoking (Strong and Richards, 1976). Clinically, the relation of smoking to myocardial infarction in young men and women without other risk-factor data is being seen. We have begun to study smoking behavior (Fig. 26–4) in third-grade children; but even younger children are smoking—children too young to answer our questionnaire. No additional comment seems necessary on the need to combat this habit.

Early evidence of *carbohydrate intolerance,* which is perhaps related to adult-onset diabetes or subclinical diabetes, has to be obtained. Overt diabetes mellitus and subclinical carbohydrate intolerance increase the risk for both atherosclerosis and hypertension. Currently, we know very little about the early onset of diabetes (at the subclinical phase), or about early abnormalities in metabolizing carbohydrates and their interrelation to *fat–cholesterol* metabolism in children; we are not sure of how to study these problems. Our leads are through family history, the occurrence of obesity, and the detection of hyper-pre-β-lipoproteinemia or mixed hyperlipoproteinemia by serum lipid analysis over time. Glucose tolerance tests and insulin determinations are done only on selected individuals. Not enough data have been collected from free-living children to know the role of carbohydrates in arteriosclerosis in the general public. The subject is of major importance.

FINALLY, WHAT IS OUR FUTURE ROLE?

Researchers are just beginning the effort to find out why risk-factor variables are high in some children and low in others. What are the early determinants of blood pressure levels or lipid values? Our data indicate that a person's general metabolic makeup, his overall genetic

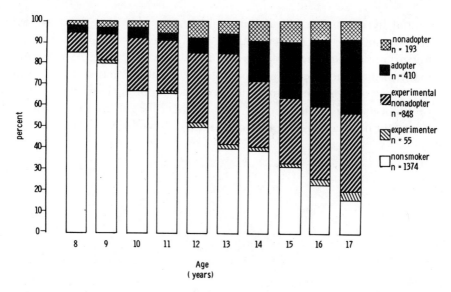

Figure 26–4. A questionnaire study of cigarette smoking behavior of children in Bogalusa, (unpublished data courtesy of Dr. Saundra Hunter). Experimenting begins in the second and third grade, age 7 and 8 years, and a progressive increase of smoking occurs as the children become older. Not shown, white boys begin earlier and have a high incidence of smoking by 14–15 years of age. White girls and black children increase to the level of white boys around 17 years. Some 30% are reported smoking at the young adult age. Nonsmoker —never smoked; experimenter—testing; experimental nonadopter—tested, but not smoking now; adopter—smoking regularly; nonadopter—smoked regularly at one time, but quit smoking.

milieu, probably plays the major role in the development of hyper-lipoproteinemia, hypertension, or cardiovascular disease. Just being primates, with lipid-laden fluid flowing through cardiovascular structures under pressure, exposes us to the risk of the two major cardiovascular diseases. Not only do clinical findings on risk factors show marked individual variability, but anatomic studies of blood vessels show wide variability of cardiovascular disease in our population (Berenson, 1961). Although all of the risk-factor observations we can make on individual children, including diet, seem to account for only a small part of this variability, we can change environmental conditions that account for that specific percentage of the variability.

How to prevent the development of coronary artery disease and essential hypertension is a major problem to tackle now for the next generation of adults (Berenson, 1978). We have accomplished much toward understanding the early natural history of arteriosclerosis, and many of these advances can be applied now at a practical level. If in any way we have helped to underscore the importance of this medical problem as beginning in early life and have begun to answer questions that need asking, then our efforts will have been rewarded.

Appendix. Percentile grids for selected risk-factor variables

Smoothed curves were developed for selected risk-factor variables for selected percentiles for children 2½–15 years of age. Curves for the 5th, 10th, 25th, 50th, 75th, 90th, and 95th percentiles are included. By drawing two lines connecting the child's age (also height or weight for blood pressure) along the abscissa and the value of the risk-factor variable along the ordinate, the proportion of children with lower values (percentile) can be determined. For example, for an 8-year-old boy with a height of 130 cm, some 75% of all 8-year-old boys would have a lower height (75th percentile). It is to be emphasized that these observations were obtained according to specific protocols as outlined in the various chapters in the text.

Percentile grids are given for the following risk-factor variables:

a. Height—Separate grids are given for boys and girls over the entire age range. The grids were developed for heights given in either centimeters or inches.

b. Weight—Separate grids are given for boys and girls over the entire age range. The grids were developed for weights given in either kilograms or pounds.

c. Triceps Skinfold Thickness—Separate grids are given for white boys, white girls, black boys, and black girls. Because the sample sizes tended to be small when separated by race and by sex, 95th percentiles are not included.

d. Blood-Pressure—Separate grids are given for both systolic and fourth-phase (diastolic) blood pressure. Because of instrumentation differences between school-age and preschool-age children, only data for school children (ages 5–15) are given. Grids developed are for blood pressure by age, by height, or by weight. Levels for preschool-age children are found in Chapter 15.

e. Serum Total Cholesterol—One grid, applicable for both races and both sexes over the entire age range, is given.

f. Serum Triglycerides—One grid, applicable for both races and both sexes for fasting children over the entire age range, is given.

g. Serum Lipoprotein Cholesterol—Separate grids for α-, β-, and pre-β-lipoprotein cholesterol are given. Each grid is applicable for fasting children of either sex or race for the entire age range.

The smoothing for each curve was achieved by determining the best fitting cubic equation to the actual raw percentile values. Because of this technique, certain exaggerations in the curves may have occurred, particularly for the 75th and 90th percentiles for triceps skinfold thickness and the 95th percentiles for diastolic blood pressure.

LIST OF GRIDS

Grid 1   Height by age (boys)
Grid 2   Height by age (girls)
Grid 3   Weight by age (boys)
Grid 4   Weight by age (girls)
Grid 5   Triceps skinfold thickness by age (white boys)
Grid 6   Triceps skinfold thickness by age (white girls)
Grid 7   Triceps skinfold thickness by age (black boys)
Grid 8   Triceps skinfold thickness by age (black girls)
Grid 9   Systolic blood pressure by age
Grid 10   Diastolic (fourth phase) blood pressure by age
Grid 11   Systolic blood pressure by height
Grid 12   Diastolic (fourth phase) blood pressure by height
Grid 13   Systolic blood pressure by weight
Grid 14   Diastolic (fourth phase) blood pressure by weight
Grid 15   Serum total cholesterol by age

Grid 1   Height by age (boys)

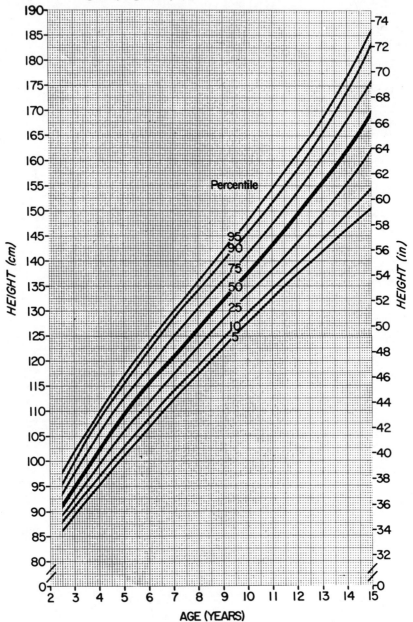

Grid 2   Height by age (girls)

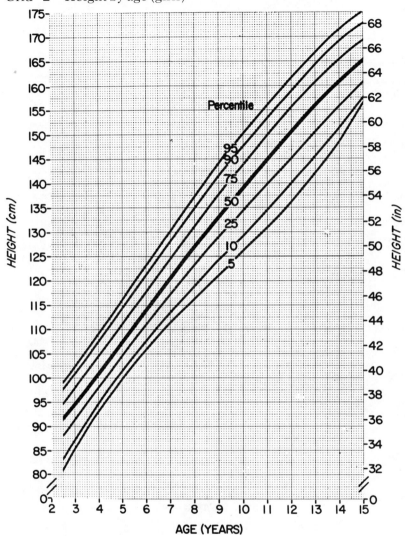

Grid 3   Weight by age (boys)

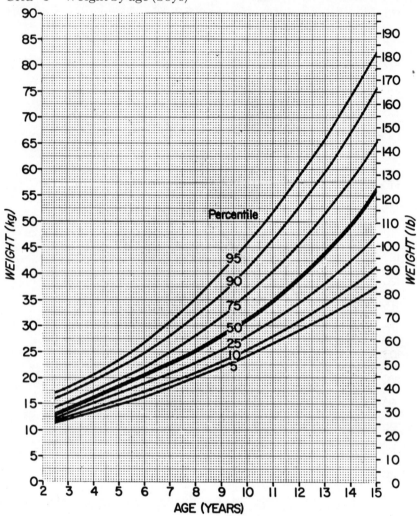

Grid 4 Weight by age (girls)

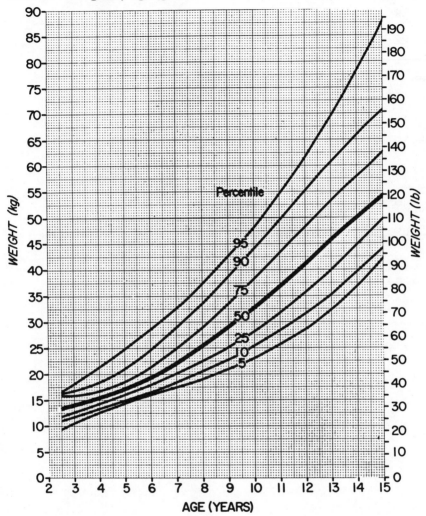

Grid 5   Triceps skinfold thickness by age (white boys)

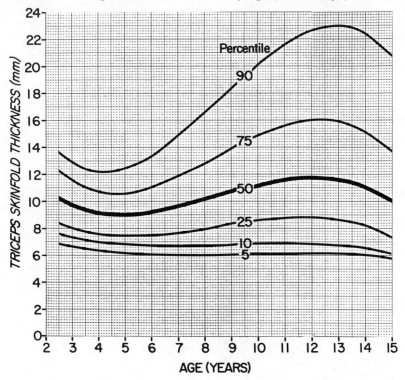

Grid 6 Triceps skinfold thickness by age (white girls)

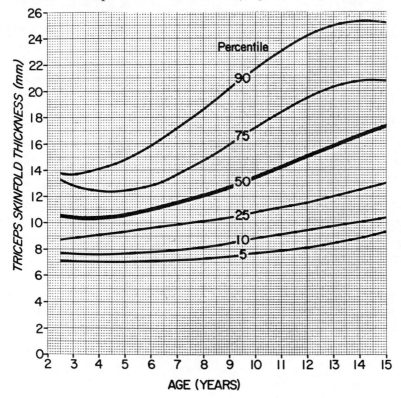

AGE (YEARS)

Grid 7   Triceps skinfold thickness by age (black boys)

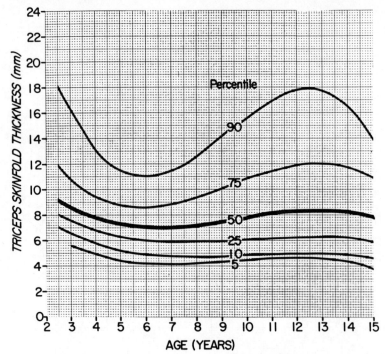

Grid 8   Triceps skinfold thickness by age (black girls)

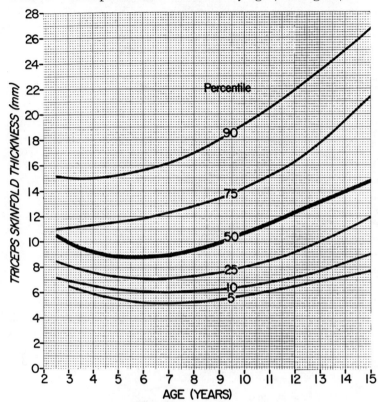

Grid 9   Systolic blood pressure by age

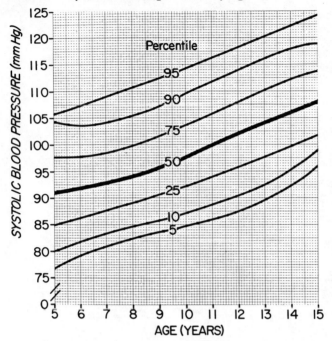

Grid 10   Diastolic (fourth phase) blood pressure by age

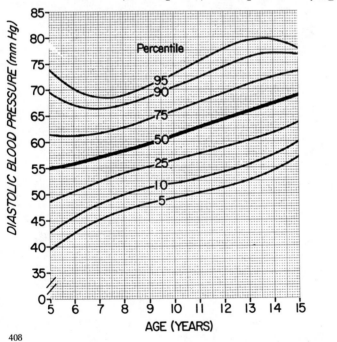

Grid 11 Systolic blood pressure by height

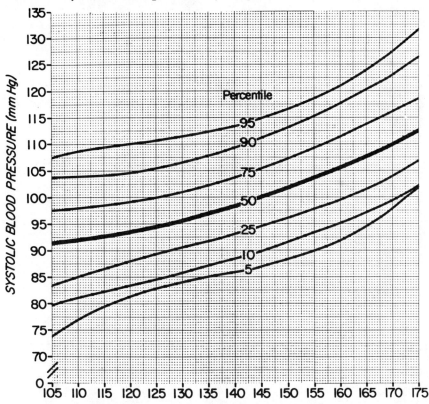

Grid 12 Diastolic (fourth phase) blood pressure by height

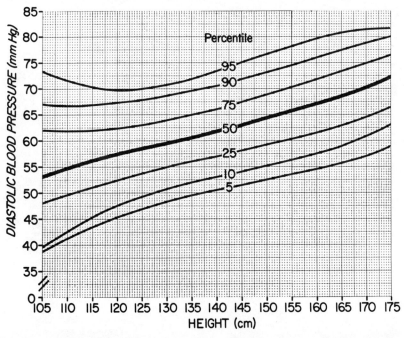

Grid 13 Systolic blood pressure by weight

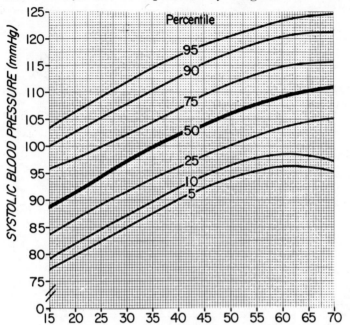

Grid 14 Diastolic (fourth phase) blood pressure by weight

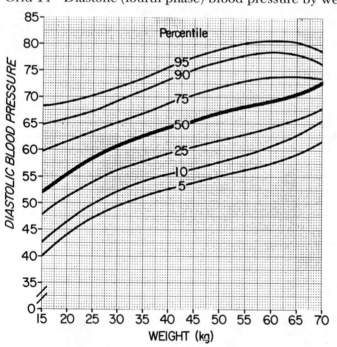

Grid 15 Serum total cholesterol by age

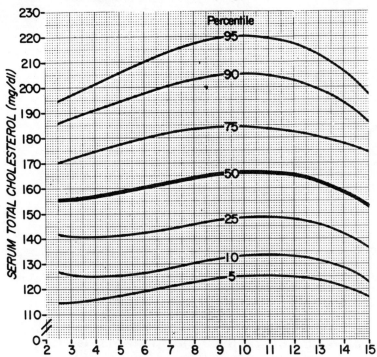

Grid 16 Serum triglycerides by age

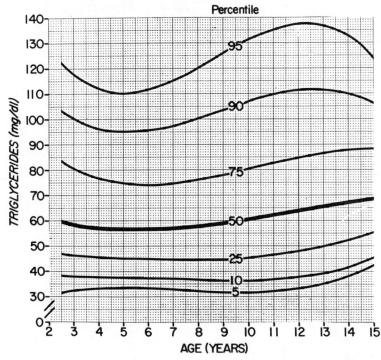

Grid 17   α-lipoprotein cholesterol by age

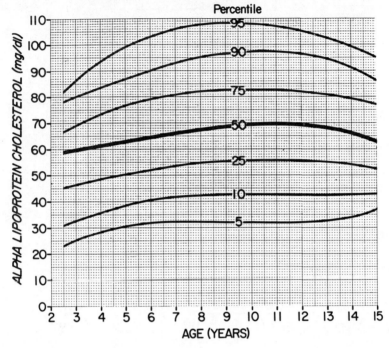

Grid 18   β-lipoprotein cholesterol by age

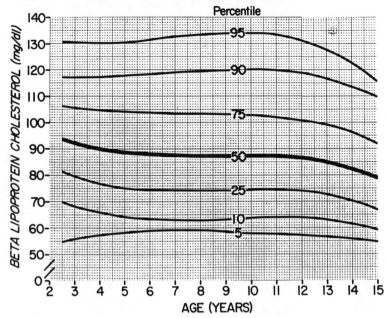

Grid 19   Pre-β-lipoprotein cholesterol by age

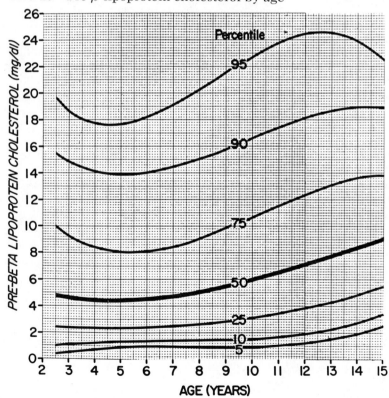

Bibliography

Abell, L. L., Levy, B. B., Brodie, B. B., and Kendall, F. E. 1952. A simplified method for the estimation of total cholesterol in serum. *J. Biol. Chem.* 195:357.

Abraham, S., National Center for Health Statistics, HANES (1971–1974), 1979. Personal communication.

Abraham, S., Collins, G., and Nordsieck, M. 1971. Relationship of childhood weight status to morbidity in adults. *HSMHA Health Reports (Public Health Reports)* 86:273.

Abraham, S., Lowenstein, F. W., and O'Connell, D. E. 1975. Preliminary findings of the first health and nutrition examination survey, United States, 1970–1972: Anthropometric and clinical findings. *DHEW Pub. No. (HRA) 75–1229*, Washington; U.S. Government Printing Office.

Alaupovic, P. 1971. Editorial: Apolipoproteins and lipoproteins. *Atherosclerosis* 13:141.

Alexander, J. K. 1963. Obesity and the circulation. *Mod. Concepts Cardiovasc. Dis.* 32:799.

Alexander, J. K., Dennis, E. W., Smith, W. G., Amad, K. H., Duncan, W. C., and Austin, R. C. 1962. Blood volume, cardiac output, and distribution of systemic blood flow in extreme obesity. *Cardiovasc. Res. Cent. Bull.* 1:39.

Alfin-Slater, R. 1969. Diet and heart disease. *J. Am. Diet. Assoc.* 54:486.

Allen, T. H., Peng, M. T., Chen, K. P., Huang, T. F., Chang, C., and Fang, H. S. 1956. Prediction of blood volume and adiposity in man from body weight and cube of height. *Metabolism* 5:328.

Allen-Williams, G. M. 1945. Pulse-rate and blood-pressure in infancy and early childhood. *Arch. Dis. Child.* 20:125.

American Academy of Pediatrics Committee on Nutrition. 1972. Childhood diet and coronary heart disease. *Pediatrics 49:*305.

American Heart Association. 1965. *Committee on Nutrition, Diet and Coronary Heart Disease.* New York: American Heart Association.

American Heart Association. 1968. The National Diet-Heart Study final report. *Circulation 37–38 (Suppl. 1):*1.

American Heart Association. 1970. Inter-Society Commission for Heart Disease Resources. Primary prevention of the arteriosclerotic disease. *Circulation 42:*1.

American Heart Association. 1972. Report of Inter-Society Commission for Heart Disease Resources. *Circulation 42:*31.

American Heart Association. 1973. *Committee on Nutrition, Diet and Coronary Heart Disease.* New York: American Heart Association.

American Heart Association. 1978. Diet modification in childhood. *Circulation 58(2):*381A.

Andersen, G. E., and Friis-Hansen, B. 1976. Neonatal hypertriglyceridemia. *Acta Paediatr. Scand.* 65:369.

Armitage, P., and Rose, G. A. 1966. The variability of measurements of casual blood pressure: I. A laboratory study. *Clin. Sci.* 30:325.

Armstrong, M. L. 1976. Regression of atherosclerosis. In *Atherosclerosis Reviews,* Vol. 1, R. Paoletti and A. M. Gotto, Jr. ed., p. 137. New York: Raven Press.

Arquembourg, P. C., Salvaggio, J. E., and Bickers, J. N. 1970. *Primer of Immunoelectrophoresis.* Basel, Switzerland: S. Karger.

Ashley, F. W., Jr., and Kannel, W. V. 1974. Relation of weight change to changes in atherogenic traits: The Framingham Study. *J. Chronic Dis.* 27:103.

Aygen, M. M., and Braunwald, E. 1962. Studies on Starling's Law of the Heart: VIII. Mechanical properties of human myocardium studied in vivo. *Circulation 26:*516.

Ayman, D., and Goldshine, A. D. 1940. Blood pressure determinations by patients with essential hypertension: 1. The difference between clinic and home readings before treatment. *Am. J. Med. Sci. 200:*465.

Bagshaw, R. J., Fronek, A., Peterson, L. H., and Zinsser, H. F. 1975. Dispersion of blood pressure and heart rate in essential hypertension. *IEEE Trans. Biomed. Eng. 22:*508.

Baker, H., Frank, O., Feingold, S., Christakis, G., and Ziffer, H. 1967. Vitamins, total cholesterol and triglycerides in 642 New York City school children. *Am. J. Clin. Nutr. 20:*850.

Barclay, M. 1972. Lipoprotein class distribution in normal and diseased states. In *Blood Lipids and Lipoproteins: Quantitation, composition, and metabolism,* G. J. Nelson, ed., p. 585. New York: Wiley-Interscience.

Barr, A. J., Goodnight, J. H., Sall, J. P., and Helwig, J. T. 1976. *A User's Guide to SAS 76.* Raleigh, N.C.: Sparis Press.

Bates, S. R., and Rothblat, G. H. 1974. Regulation of cellular sterol flux and synthesis by human serum lipoproteins. *Biochim. Biophys. Acta 360:*38.

Beaglehold, R., Salmond, C. E., and Prior, I. A. M. 1976. A family study of blood pressure in Polynesians. *Int. J. Epidemiol.* 4:217.

Beaumount, J. L., Carlson, L. A., Cooper, G. R., Fejfar, Z., Fredrickson, D. S., and Strasser, T. 1970. Classification of hyperlipidaemias and hyperlipoproteinemias. *WHO Bull.* 43:891.

Benn, R. T. 1971. Some mathematical properties of weight-for-height indices as measures of adiposity. *Br. J. Prev. Soc. Med.* 25:42.

Berenson, G. S. 1961. Studies of "ground substance" of vessel wall and alterations in disease. *J. Atherosclerosis Res.* 1:386.

Berenson, G. S. 1978. Children, the next generation of patients with myocardial infarction. In *Changes in the Medical Panorama*, G. Schettler, J. Drews, and H. Greten, eds., p. 75. Stuttgart: George Thieme.

Berenson, G. S., Radhakrishnamurthy, B., Dalferes, E. R., Jr. and Srinivasan, S. R. 1971a. Carbohydrate macromolecules and atherosclerosis. *Hum. Path.* 2:57.

Berenson, G. S., Srinivasan, S. R., Pargaonkar, P. S., Lindsey, S., Plavidal, F., Radhakrishnamurthy, B., Dalferes, E. R., Jr., Lopez-S., A., and Dugan, F. A. 1971b. The detection of individuals prone to coronary artery disease: A screening program conducted on medical students. *J. La. State Med. Soc.* 123:49.

Berenson, G. S., Srinivasan, S. R., Lopez-S., A., Radhakrishnamurthy, B., Pargaonkar, P. S., and Deupree, R. H. 1972a. Clinical appplication of an indirect method for quantitating serum lipoproteins. *Clin. Chim. Acta* 36:175.

Berenson, G. S., Srinivasan, S. R., Pargaonkar, P. S., Radhakrishnamurthy, B., and Dalferes, E. R., Jr. 1972b. A simplified primary screening procedure for detection of hyperlipidemias in healthy individuals. *Clin. Chem.* 18:1463.

Berenson, G. S., Radhakrishnamurthy, B., Srinivasan, S. R. and Dalferes, E. R., Jr. 1973. Pathogenesis of coronary artery disease, In *Nutrition and Metabolism in Medical Practice*, S. L. Halpern, A. L. Luhby, and G. S. Berenson, eds., p. 49. Mt. Kisco, New York: Futura.

Berenson, G. S., Radhakrishnamurthy, B., Srinivasan, S. R. and Dalferes, E. R., Jr. 1974a. Macromolecules in the arterial wall in relation to injury and repair—A survey. *Angiology* 25:649.

Berenson, G. S., Pargaonkar, P. S., Srinivasan, S. R., Dalferes, E. R., Jr., and Radhakrishnamurthy, B. 1974b. Studies of serum lipoprotein concentrations in children: A preliminary report. *Clin. Chim. Acta* 56:65.

Berenson, G. S., Srinivasan, S. R., and Frerichs, R. R. 1976. The not-so-hyper hyperlipoproteinemia and coronary artery disease. *Postgrad. Med.* 59:173.

Berenson, G. S., Foster, T. A., Frank, G. C., Frerichs, R. R., Srinivasan, S. R., Voors, A. W., and Webber, L. S. 1978a. Cardiovascular disease risk factor variables at the preschool age—The Bogalusa Heart Study. *Circulation* 57:603.

Berenson, G. S., Voors, A. W., Webber, L. S., and Frerichs, R. R. 1978b. Blood pressure in children and its interpretation. *Pediatrics 61:*333.

Berenson, G. S., Voors, A. W., Dalferes, E. R., Jr., Webber, L. S., and Shuler, S. E. 1979a. Creatinine clearance, electrolytes, and plasma renin activity related to the blood pressure of white and black children—The Bogalusa Heart Study. *J. Lab. Clin. Med. 93:*535.

Berenson, G. S., Srinivasan, S. R., Frerichs, R. R., and Webber, L. S. 1979b. Serum high density lipoprotein and its relationship to cardiovascular disease risk factor variables in children—The Bogalusa Heart Study. *Lipids 14:*91.

Berenson, G. S., Blonde, C. V., Farris, R. P., Foster, T. A., Frank, G. C., Srinivasan, S. R., Voors, A. W., and Webber, L. S. 1979c. Cardiovascular disease risk factor variables during the first year of life. *Am. J. Dis. Child. 10:*1049.

Berenson, G. S., Voors, A. W., Webber, L. S., Dalferes, E. R., Jr., and Harsha, D. W. 1979d. Racial differences of parameters associated with blood pressure levels in children—The Bogalusa Heart Study *Metabolism 12:*1218.

Berg, K. 1963. A new serum type system in man—the L_p system. *Acta Pathol. Microbiol. Scand. 59:*369.

Berg, K., Borresen, A. L., and Dahlen, G. 1976. Serum-high-density-lipoprotein and atherosclerotic heart disease. *Lancet 2:*499.

Bhandaru, R. R., Srinivasan, S. R., Pargaonkar, P. S., and Berenson, G. S. 1977. A simplified colorimetric micromethod for determination of serum cholesterol. *Lipids 12:*1078.

Bierman, E. L., and Porte, D., Jr. 1968. Carbohydrate intolerance and lipemia. *Ann. Intern. Med. 68:*926.

Bleiler, A., Yearick, E., Schnur, S., Singson, I. L., and Ohlson, M. A. 1963. Seasonal variation of cholesterol in serum of men and women. *Am. J. Clin. Nutr. 12:*12.

Blumenthal, S. 1973. Prevention of atherosclerosis. *Am. J. Cardiol. 31:*591.

Blumenthal, S., Jesse, M. J., Hennekens, C. H., Klein, B. E., Ferrer, P. L., and Gourley, J. E. 1975. Risk factors of coronary artery disease in children of affected families. *J. Pediatrics 87:*1187.

Blumenthal, S., Epps, R. P., Heavenrich, R., Lauer, R. M., Lieberman, E., Mirkin, B., Mitchell, S. C., Naito, V. B., O'Hare, D., Smith, W. McF., Tazari, R. C., and Upson, D. 1977. Report of the Task Force on Blood Pressure Control in Children. *Pediatrics 59:*797.

Bøe, J., Humerfelt, G., and Wedervang, F. 1957. The blood pressure in a population. *Acta Med. Scand. (Suppl. 321):*1.

Borst, J. G. G., and Borst, A.deG. 1963. Hypertension explained by Starling's theory of circulatory homoeostasis. *Lancet 1:*677.

Bortz, W. M. 1974. The pathogenesis of hypercholesterolemia. *Ann. Intern. Med. 80:*738.

Bosley, B. 1947. A practical approach to nutrition education for children. *J. Am. Diet. Assoc. 23:*304.

Boston City Hospital. Recording Sphygmomanometer Operator's Manual. Biomedical Engineering Division, Thorndike Memorial Laboratory, Boston (unpublished).

Breit, S. N., and O'Rourke, M. F. 1974. Comparison of direct and indirect arterial measurements in hospitalized patients. *Aust. N.Z. J. Med. 4:*485.

Brines, J. K., Gibson, J. G. II, and Kunkel, P. 1941. The blood volume in normal infants and children. *J. Pediatr. 18:*447.

Brook, C. G. D., and Lloyd, J. K., 1973. Adipose cell size and glucose tolerance in obese children and effects of diet. *Arch. Dis. Child. 48:*301.

Brooks, D. N. 1976. School screening for middle ear effusions. *Ann. Otol. Rhinol. Laryngol. 85 (Suppl. 25):*223.

Brozek, J., Chapman, C. B., and Keys, A. 1948. Drastic food restriction: Effect on cardiovascular dynamics in normotensive and hypertensive conditions. *J.A.M.A. 137:*1569.

Brunner, D., Altman, S., Posner, L., Bearman, J. E., Loebl, K., and Lewin, S. 1971. Heredity, environment, serum lipoproteins and serum uric acid. *J. Chronic Dis. 23:*763.

Brunner, H. R., Sealey, J. E., and Laragh, J. H. 1973. Renin subgroups in essential hypertension. *Circ. Res. 33 (Suppl. 1):*99.

Bryan, A. H., and Greenberg, B. C. 1952. Methodology in the study of physical measurements of school children: II. Sexual maturation—determination of immaturity points. *Hum. Biol. 24:*117.

Burch, G. E., and DePasquale, N. P. 1962. Primer of clinical measurement of blood pressure. St. Louis: C. V. Mosby.

Burke, S., Reed, R. B., Van Den Berg, A. S., and Stuart, H. C. 1959. Calorie and protein intakes in children between 1 and 18 years of age. *Pediatrics 24:*922.

Burstein, M., Scholnick, H. R., and Morfin, R. 1970. Rapid method for the isolation of lipoproteins from human serum by precipitation with polyanions. *J. Lipid Res. 11:*583.

Cagas, C. R., and Riley, H. D., Jr. 1970. Age of menarche in girls in a west-south-central community. *Am. J. Dis. Child. 120:*303.

Carlson, L. A. 1973. Clinical aspects of classification of primary hyperlipoproteinemias. *Adv. Exp. Med. Biol. 38:*89.

Carlson, L. A., and Bottiger, L. E. 1972. Ischemic heart disease in relation to fasting values of plasma triglycerides and cholesterol. *Lancet 1:*865.

Carlson, L. A., and Hardell, L. I. 1977. Sex differences in serum lipids and lipoproteins at birth. *Eur. J. Clin. Invest. 7:*133.

Carter, C. 1974. Genetic factors in coronary heart disease. *Acta Cardiol. (Suppl. XX):*27.

Castelli, W. P., Cooper, G. R., Doyle, J. T., Garcia-Palmieri, M., Gordon, T., Hames, C., Hulley, S. B., Kagan, A., Kuchmak, M., McGee, D., and Vicic, W. J. 1977a. Distribution of triglyceride and total LDL and HDL cholesterol in several populations: A cooperative lipoprotein phenotyping study. *J. Chronic Dis. 30:*147.

Castelli, W. P., Doyle, J. T., Gordon, T., Hames, C. G., Hjortland, M. C., Hulley, S. B., Kagan, A., and Zukel, W. J. 1977b. HDL cholesterol and other lipids in coronary heart-disease cooperative lipoprotein phenotyping study. *Circulation 55:767.*

Cawley, L. P. 1969. *Electrophoresis and Immunoelectrophoresis.* Boston: Little, Brown.

Chiang, B. N., Perlman, L. V., and Epstein, F. H. 1969. Overweight and hypertension: A review. *Circulation 39:403.*

Chiumello, G., Del Guercio, M. J., Carnelutti, M., and Bidone, G. 1969. Relationship between obesity, chemical diabetes and beta pancreatic function in children. *Diabetes 18:238.*

Christian, J. C., Cheung, S. W., Kang, K., Harmath, F. P., Huntzinger, D. J., and Powell, R. C. 1976. Variance of plasma free and esterified cholesterol in adult twins. *Am. J. Hum. Genet. 28:174.*

Christou, G. C. 1973. *Migration in Louisiana.* New Orleans: University of New Orleans, College of Business Administration, Division of Business and Economic Research, Research Study No. 17.

Clark, E. G., Schweitzer, M. D., Glock, C. Y., and Vought, P. L. 1956. Studies in hypertension: III. Analysis of individual blood pressure changes. *J. Chronic Dis. 4:477.*

Clarke, R. P., Merrow, S. B., Morse, E. H., and Keyser, D. E. 1970. Interrelationships between plasma lipids, physical measurements, and the body fatness of adolescents in Burlington, Vermont. *Am. J. Clin. Nutr. 23:754.*

The Clinical Measurement of Blood Pressure. 1969. Copiague, N.Y.: W. A. Baum.

Comstock, G. W. 1957. An epidemiologic study of blood pressure levels in a biracial community in the southern United States. *Am. J. Hyg. 65:271.*

Connor, W. E. 1970. The effects of dietary lipid and sterols on the sterol balance. In *Atherosclerosis,* R. J. Jones, ed., p. 253. New York: Springer-Verlag.

Connor, W. E., Cerqueira, M. T., Connor, R. W., Wallace, R. B., Malinow, M. R., and Casdorph, H. R. 1978. The plasma lipids, lipoproteins, and diet of the Tarahumara Indians of Mexico. *Am. J. Clin. Nutr. 31:1131.*

Connor, W. E., and Connor, S. L. 1972. The key role of nutritional factors in the prevention of coronary heart disease. *Prev. Med. 1:49.*

Cornfield, J. 1962. Joint dependence of risk of coronary heart disease on serum cholesterol and systolic blood pressure: A discriminant function analysis. *Fed. Proc. 21:58.*

Cornfield, J., and Mantel, N. 1950. Some new aspects of the application of maximum likelihood to the calculation of the dosage response curve. *J. Am. Stat. Assoc. 45:181.*

Corns, R. H. 1976. Maintenance of blood pressure equipment. *Am. J. Nurs. 76:776.*

Court, J. M., and Dunlop, M. 1975. Plasma lipid values and lipoprotein patterns during adolescence in boys. *J. Pediatrics 86:453.*

Court, J. M., Hill, G. J., Dunlop, M., and Boulton, T. J. C. 1974. Hypertension and childhood obesity. *Aust. Paediatr. J. 10:296.*

Cresanta, J. L., Srinivasan, S. R., Webber, L. S., and Berenson, G. S. 1979. Changes of serum lipoprotein cholesterol in children with age and maturation. South. Soc. of Clin. Invest. *Clin. Res. 26:*789A.

Cress, H. R., Shahet, R. M., Laffin, R., and Karpowicz, K. 1977. Cord blood hyperlipoproteinemia and perinatal stress. *Pediatr. Res. 11:*19.

Darmady, J. M., Fosbrooke, A. S., and Lloyd, J. K. 1972. Prospective study of serum cholesterol levels during first year of life. *Br. Med. J. 2:*685.

deLalla, O. F., and Gofman, J. W. 1954. Ultracentrifugal analysis of serum lipoproteins. *Methods Biochem. Anal. 1:*459.

Deschamps, I., Giron, B. J., and Lestradet, H. 1977. Blood glucose, insulin, and free fatty acid levels during oral glucose tolerance tests in 158 obese children. *Diabetes 26:*89.

De Swiet, M., Fancourt, R., and Peto, J. 1975. Systolic blood pressure variation during the first 6 days of life. *Clin. Sci. Mol. Med. 49:*557.

Deutscher, S., Epstein, F. H., and Kjelsberg, M. O. 1966. Familial aggregation of factors associated with coronary heart disease. *Circulation 33:*911.

de Waard, F. 1975. Breast cancer incidence and nutritional status with particular reference to body weight and height. *Cancer Res. 35:*3351.

Diehl, H. S., and Lees, H. D. 1929. The variability of blood pressure: II. A study of systolic pressure at five minute intervals. *Arch. Intern. Med. 44:*229.

Dixon, W. J., and Massey, F. J. 1969. *Introduction to Statistical Analysis.* New York: McGraw-Hill.

Dodge, W. F., West, E. F., Smith, E. H., and Bunce, H. 1976. Proteinuria and hematuria in schoolchildren: Epidemiology and early natural history. *J. Pediatr. 88:*327.

Doyle, J. T., Kinch, S. H., and Brown, D. F. 1965. Seasonal variation in serum cholesterol concentration. *J. Chronic Dis. 18:*657.

Drash, A. 1973. Relationship between diabetes mellitus and obesity in the child. *Metabolism 22:*337

Drash, A. 1975. Diabetes mellitus. In *Nelson Textbook of Pediatrics,* 10th ed., V. C. Vaughan and R. J. McKay, eds., p. 1259. Philadelphia: Saunders.

Dustan, H. P. 1976. Evaluation and therapy of hypertension—1976. *Mod. Concepts Cardiovasc. Dis. 45:*97.

Dyer, A. R., Stamler, J., Berkson, D. M., and Lindberg, H. 1975. Relationship of relative weight and body mass index to the 14-year mortality in the Chicago People's Gas Company Study. *J. Chronic Dis. 28:*109.

Dyerberg, J., and Hjorne, N. 1973. Plasma lipid and lipoprotein levels in childhood and adolescence. *Scand. J. Clin. Lab. Invest. 31:*473.

Eisenberg, S., and Levy, R. I. 1975. Lipoprotein metabolism. *Adv. Lipid Res. 13:*1.

Ellefson, R. D., Elveback, L. R., Hodgson, P. A., and Weidman, W. H. 1978. Cholesterol and triglycerides in serum lipoproteins of young persons in Rochester, Minnesota. *Mayo Clin. Proc. 53:*307.

Emmons, L., and Hayes, M. 1973. Accuracy of 24-hr. recalls of young children. *J. Am. Diet. Assoc. 62:*409.

Enos, W. F., Holmes, R. H., and Beyer, J. 1953. Coronary disease among United States soldiers killed in action in Korea: Preliminary report. *J.A.M.A. 152:*1090.

Epstein, F. H. 1976. Genetics of ischaemic heart disease. *Postgrad. Med. J. 52:*477.

Epstein, F. H., Francis, T., Hayner, N. S., Johnson, B. C., Kjelsberg, M.O., Napier, J. A., Ostrander, L. D., Payne, M. W., and Dodge, H. J. 1965. Prevalance of chronic diseases and distribution of selected physiologic variables in a total community—Tecumseh, Michigan. *Am. J. Epidemiol. 81:*307.

Ertel, P. Y., Lawrence, M., Brown, R. K., and Stern, A. M. 1966. Stethoscope acoustics: 2. Transmission and filtration patterns. *Circulation 34:*899.

Faber, H. K., and James, C. A. 1921. The range and distribution of blood pressures in normal children. *Am. J. Dis. Child. 22:*7.

Fabry, P., Hejda, S., Cerny, K., Osancova, K., and Pechar, J. 1966. Effect of meal frequency in school children. Changes in the weight-height proportion and skinfold thickness. *Am. J. Clin. Nutr. 18:*358.

Falconer, D. S. 1965. The inheritance of liability to certain diseases, estimated from the incidence among relatives. *Ann. Hum. Genet. 29:*51.

Fallat, R. W., Tsang, R. C., and Glueck, C. J. 1974. Hypercholesterolemia and hypertriglyceridemia in children. *Prev. Med. 3:*390.

Feinleib, M., Garrison, R., Borhani, N., Rosenman, R., and Christian, J. 1975. Studies of hypertension in twins. In *Epidemiology and the Control of Hypertension*, O. Paul, ed., p. 3. New York: Stratton.

Feldman, J. G., Ibrahim, M. A., and Sultz, H. 1973. Differential filial aggregation of coronary risk factors. *Hum. Biol. 45:*541.

Fernandez, H., and Robinson, R. 1971, The automatic device for recording blood pressure. *Aerosp. Med. 42:*209.

Fishberg, A. M. 1954. Essential hypertension: 3. Clinical picture. In *Hypertension and Nephritis*. p. 757. Philadelphia: Lea & Febiger.

Fisher, R. A. 1954. *Statistical Methods for Research Workers*, 12th ed. New York: Hafner.

Fletcher, M. J. 1972. Standardization of triglyceride methodology. *Ann. Clin. Lab. Sci. 2:*389.

Florey, C. duV., Uppal, S., and Clavy, C. 1976a. Relation between blood pressure, weight, and plasma sugar and serum insulin levels in school children aged 9–12 years in Westland, Holland. *Br. Med. J. 1:*1368.

Florey, C. duV., Lowy, C., and Uppal, S. 1976b. Serum insulin levels in school children aged 9–12 in Westland, Holland. *Diabetologia 12:*313.

Fogarty, T. J., Nolan, S. P., and Morrow, A. G. 1967. Effects of normovolemic polycythemia and anemia on cardiac performance and peripheral vascular resistance. *Surg. Forum 18:*162.

Fomon, S. J. 1971. A pediatrician looks at early nutrition. *Bull. N.Y. Acad. Med. 47:*569.

Food and Nutrition Board Recommended Dietary Allowances, 8th rev. ed. 1974. Washington: National Academy of Science.

Ford, C. H., McGandy, R. B., and Stare, F. J. 1972. An institutional approach to the dietary regulation of blood cholesterol in adolescent males. *Prev. Med. 1:*426.

Foster, T. A., Voors, A. W., Webber, L. S., Frerichs, R. R., and Berenson, G. S. 1977. Anthropometric and maturation measurements of children, ages 5–14 years, in a biracial community—The Bogalusa Heart Study. *Am. J. Clin. Nutr. 30:*582.

Frank, G. C., Berenson, G. S., Schilling, P. E., and Moore, M. C. 1977a. Adapting the 24-hour recall for epidemiologic studies of school children. *J. Am. Diet. Assoc. 71:*26.

Frank, G. C., Voors, A. W., Schilling, P. E., and Berenson, G. S. 1977b. Dietary studies of rural school children in a cardiovascular survey. *J. Am. Diet. Assoc. 71:*31.

Frank, G. C., Berenson, G. S., and Webber, L. S. 1978. Dietary studies and the relationship of diet to cardiovascular disease risk factor variables in ten-year-old children—The Bogalusa Heart Study. *Am. J. Clin. Nutr. 31:*328.

Frank, G. C., Farris, R. P., Webber, L. S., Srinivasan, S. R., and Berenson, G. S. 1979a. The relationship of infant feeding patterns to coronary risk factor variables in the first year of life. *Cardiovascular Disease Epidemiology Newsletter 26:*56.

Frank, G. C., Farris, R. P., Major, C. R., Webber, L. S. and Berenson, G. S. 1979b. Infant feeding patterns and their relationship to cardiovascular risk factor variables in the first year of life. Submitted.

Fraser, G. R., Volkers, W. S., Bernini, L. F., DeGreve, W. B., Van Loghem, E., Kahn, P. M., Nijenhuis, L. E., Vehkamp, J. J., Vogel, G. P., and Went, L. N. 1974. A search for associations between genetic polymorphic systems and physical, biochemical and haematological variables. *Hum. Hered. 24:*424.

Fredrickson, D. S., and Breslow, J. L. 1973. Primary hyperlipoproteinemia in infants. *Ann. Rev. Med. 24:*315.

Fredrickson, D. S., and Levy, R. I. 1972. Familial hyperlipoproteinemias. In *The Metabolic Basis of Inherited Disease,* J. B. Stanbury, J. B. Wyngaarden, and D. S. Fredrickson, eds., p. 545. New York: McGraw-Hill.

Fredrickson, D. S., Levy, R. I., and Lees, R. S. 1967. Fat transport in lipoproteins—An integrated approach to mechanisms and disorders. *N. Engl. J. Med. 276:*148.

Frerichs, R. R., Srinivasan, S. R., Webber, L. S., and Berenson, G. S. 1976. Serum cholesterol and triglyceride levels in 3,446 children from a biracial community—The Bogalusa Heart Study. *Circulation 54:*302.

Frerichs, R. R., Webber, L. S., Srinivasan, S. R., and Berenson, G. S. 1977. Hemoglobin levels in children from a biracial Southern community. *Am. J. Public Health 67:*841.

Frerichs, R. R., Srinivasan, S. R., Webber, L. S., Rieth, M. C., and Berenson, G. S. 1978a. Serum lipids and lipoproteins at birth in a biracial community. *Pediatr. Res. 12:*858.

Frerichs, R. R., Webber, L. S., Srinivasan, S. R., and Berenson, G. S. 1978b. Relation of serum lipids and lipoproteins to obesity and sexual maturation in white and black children. *Am. J. Epidemiol. 108:*486.

Frerichs, R. R., Webber, L. S., Voors, A. W., Srinivasan, S. R., and Berenson, G. S. 1979. Cardiovascular disease risk factor variables in children at two successive years—The Bogalusa Heart Study. *J. Chronic Dis. 32:*251.

Friedewald, W. T., Levy, R. I., and Fredrickson, D. S. 1972. Estimation of the concentration of low-density lipoprotein cholesterol in plasma, without use of the preparative ultracentrifuge. *Clin. Chem. 18:*499.

Friedman, G., and Goldberg, S. J. 1972. Comparison of serum cholesterol at one year of infants initially fed high and no cholesterol milk formula. *Circulation 46(Suppl. 11):*85.

Friedman, G., and Goldberg, S. J. 1973. Normal serum cholesterol values, percentile ranking in a middle-class pediatric population. *J.A.M.A. 225:*610.

Frisch, R. E. 1974. A method of predicting age of menarche from height and weight at ages 9 through 13 years. *Pediatrics 53:*587.

Frohlich, E. D., Kozul, V. J., Tarazi, R. C., and Dustan, H. P. 1970. Physiological comparison of labile and essential hypertension. *Circ. Res. 27 (Suppl. 1):*55.

Fujita, Y., Gotto, A. M., and Unger, R. H. 1975. Basal and postprotein insulin and glucagon levels during high and low carbohydrate intake and their relationships to plasma triglycerides. *Diabetes 24:*552.

Furman, R. H., Alaupovic, P., and Howard, R. P. 1967. Effects of androgens and estrogens on serum lipids and the composition and concentration of serum lipoproteins in normolipemic and hyperlipidemic states. *Progr. Biochem. Pharmacol. 2:*215.

Galbraith, W., Connor, W., and Stone, D. 1966. Weight loss and serum lipid changes in obese subjects given low calorie diets of varied cholesterol content. *Ann. Intern. Med. 64:*268.

Gardner, M. J., and Heady, J. A. 1973. Some effects of within-person variability in epidemiological studies. *J. Chronic Dis. 26:*781.

Garn, S. M. 1971. *Human Races*, 3rd ed. Springfield, Ill.: Charles C. Thomas.

Garn, S. M., and Clark, D. C. 1976. Trends in fatness and the origins of obesity. *Pediatrics 57:*443.

Garn, S. M., and Haskell, J. A. 1960. Fat thickness and developmental status in childhood and adolescence. *Am. J. Dis. Child. 99:*746.

Geddes, L. A. 1970. *The Direct and Indirect Measurement of Blood Pressure.* Chicago: Year Book Medical Publishers.

Genest, J. 1974. Basic mechanisms in benign essential hypertension. *Hosp. Pract. 9:*97.

Gerson, L. W., and Fodor, V. G. 1975. Family aggregation of high blood pressure groups in two Newfoundland communities. *Can. J. Public Health 66:*294.

Gertler, M. M., and White, P. D. 1954. *Coronary Heart Disease in Young*

Adults: A Multidisciplinary Study. Cambridge, Mass.: Harvard University Press.

Gilbert, A., Lewis, A., and Day, R. W. 1967. Project Head Start: An evaluation of the medical components in California. *Calif. Med. 106:*382.

Gleibermann, L. 1973. Blood pressure and dietary salt in human populations. *Ecol. Food. Nutr. 2:*143.

Glock, C. Y., Vought, R. L., Clark, E. G., and Schweitzer, M. D. 1956. Studies in hypertension: II. Variability of daily blood pressure measurements in the same individuals over a three-week period. *J. Chronic Dis. 4:*469.

Glomset, J. A., and Norum, K. R. 1973. The metabolic role of lecithin: cholesterol acyltransferase: Perspectives from pathology. *Adv. Lipid Res. 11:*1.

Glueck, C. J., Heckman, F., Schoenfeld, M., Steiner, P., and Pearce, W. 1971. Neonatal familial Type 11 hyperlipoproteinemia: Cord blood cholesterol in 1,800 births. *Metabolism 20:*597.

Glueck, C. J., and Tsang, R. C. 1972. Pediatric familial type II hyperlipoproteinemia: Effects of diet on plasma cholesterol in the first year of life. *Am. J. Clin. Nutr. 25:*224.

Glueck, C. J., Tsang, R. C., Fallat, R., and Balistieri, W. 1972. Plasma and dietary cholesterol in infancy: Effects of early low or moderate dietary cholesterol intake on subsequent response to increased dietary cholesterol. *Metabolism 21:*1181.

Glueck, C. J., Steiner, P., and Leuba, V. 1973. Cord-blood low-density lipoprotein cholesterol: Estimation versus measurement with the preparative ultracentrifuge. *J. Lab. Clin. Med. 82:*467.

Glueck, C. J., Fallat, R. W., Tsang, R., and Buncher, C. R. 1974. Hyperlipidemia in progeny of parents with myocardial infarction before age 50. *Am. J. Dis. Child. 127:*70.

Glueck, C. J., Fallat, R. W., Millett, F., Gartside, P., Elston, R. C., and Go, R. C. P. 1975. Familial hyperalphalipoproteinemia: Studies in eighteen kindreds. *Metabolism 24:*1243.

Glueck, C. J., Gartside, P. S., Tsang, R. C., Mellies, M., and Steiner, P. M. 1977. Black-white similarities in cord blood lipids and lipoproteins: A preliminary report. *Metabolism 26:*347.

Godfrey, R. C., Stenhouse, N. S., Cullen, K. J., and Blackman, V. 1972. Cholesterol and the child: Studies of the cholesterol levels of Busselton school children and their parents. *Aust. Paediatr. J. 8:*72.

Gofman, J. W., DeLalla, O., Glazier, F., Freeman, N. K., Lindgren, F. T., Nichols, A. V., Strisower, B., and Tamplin, A. R. 1954. The serum lipoprotein transport system in health, metabolic disorders, atherosclerosis and coronary heart disease. *Plasma 2:*413.

Golden, D. P., Wolthuis, R. A., Hoffler, G. W., and Cowen, R. J. 1974. Development of a Korotkov sound processor for automatic identification of auscultatory events: 1. Specification of preprocessing bandpass filters. *IEEE Trans. Biomed. Eng. 21:*114.

Goldring, W., and Chasis, H. 1944. Clinical aspects of hypertensive disease. In *Hypertension and Hypertensive Disease*, W. Goldring and H. Chasis, eds., p. 14. New York: The Commonwealth Fund.

Goldstein, J. L., Hazzard, W. R., Schrott, H. G., Bierman, E. L., and Motulsky, A. G. 1973a. Hyperlipidemia in coronary heart disease. I. Lipid levels in 500 survivors of myocardial infarction. *J. Clin. Invest. 52:*1533.

Goldstein, J. L., Schrott, H. G., Hazzard, W. R., Bierman, E. L., and Motulsky, A. G. 1973b. Hyperlipidemia in coronary disease: II. Genetic analysis of lipid levels in 176 families and delineation of a new inherited disorder, combined hyperlipidemia. *J. Clin. Invest. 52:*1544.

Goldstein, J. L., Albers, J. J., Schrott, H. G., Hazzard, W. R., Bierman, E. L., and Motulsky, A. G. 1974. Plasma lipid levels and coronary heart disease in adult relatives of newborns with normal and elevated cord blood lipids. *Am. J. Hum. Genet. 26:*727.

Goldstein, J. L., and Brown, M. S. 1974. Binding and degradation of low density lipoproteins by cultured human fibroblasts: Comparison of cells from a normal subject and from a patient with homozygous familial hypercholesterolemia. *J. Biol. Chem. 249:*5153.

Gordon, T. 1964. Blood pressure of adults, by age and sex—United States, 1960–1962. *Vital Health Stat.*, PHS Pub. No. 1000, series 11, no. 4. Public Health Service. Washington: U.S. Government Printing Office.

Gordon, T. 1973. Blood pressure of adults by race and area—United States, 1960–1962. *Vital Health Stat.*, PHS Pub. No. 1000, series 11, no. 5. Public Health Service. Washington: U.S. Government Printing Office.

Gordon, T., and Devine, B. 1966. Hypertension and hypertensive heart disease in adults. *Vital Health Stats.*, PHS Pub. No. 1000, series 11, no. 13. Public Health Service. Washington: U.S. Government Printing Office.

Gordon, T., Castelli, W. P., Hjortland, M. C., Kannel, W. B., and Dawber, T. R. 1977. High density lipoprotein as a protective factor against coronary heart disease—The Framingham Study. *Am. J. Med. 62:*70.

Graham, A. W., Hines, E. A., and Gage, R. P. 1945. Blood pressures in children between the ages of five and sixteen years. *Am. J. Dis. Child. 69:*203.

Grant, W. W., Fearnow, R. G., Hebertson, L. M., and Henderson, A. L. 1973. Health screening in school age children. *Am. J. Dis. Child. 125:*520.

Greten, H., ed. 1976. *Lipoprotein Metabolism.* New York: Springer-Verlag.

Greten, H., Wengeler, H., and Wagner, H. 1973. Early diagnosis of familial Type II hyperlipoproteinemia. *Nutr. Metabol. 15:*128.

Grove, R. D., and Hetzel, A. M. 1968. Vital statistics rates in the United States, 1940–1960. Washington, D.C.: National Center for Health Statistics.

Guyton, A. C. 1977. An overall analysis of cardiovascular regulation. Fifteenth Annual Baxter-Travenol Lecture. *Anesth. Analg. 56:*761.

Guyton, A. C., Jones, C. E., and Coleman, T. G. 1973. *Circulatory Physiology: Cardiac Output and Its Regulation.* Philadelphia: Saunders.

Guyton, A. C., Cowley, A. W., Jr. Coleman, T. G., DeClue, J. W., Norman,

R. A., and Manning, D. A. 1974. Hypertension: A disease of abnormal circulatory control. *Chest* 65:328.

Hald, A. 1952. Statistical theory with engineering applications. New York: Wiley.

Hames, C. G., and Greenberg, B. G. 1961. A comparative study of serum cholesterol levels in school children and their possible relation to atherogenesis. *Am. J. Public Health* 51:374.

Hamilton, M., Pickering, G. W., Fraser-Roberts, J. A., and Sowry, G. S. C. 1954. The aetiology of essential hypertension: 1. The arterial pressure in the general population. *Clin. Sci.* 13:11.

Hankins, G. J., Eccles, T. J., Jr., Judlin, B. C., and Moore, M. C. 1965. Data processing of dietary survey data—old and new: 1. A computer system for processing dietary data. *J. Am. Diet. Assoc.* 46:387.

Hansen, R. L., and Stickler, G. B. 1966. The 'nonhypertension' or 'small-cuff' syndrome. *Clin. Pediatr.* 5:579.

Harlan, W. R., Osborne, R. K., and Graybiel, A. 1964. Prognostic value of the cold pressor test and the basal blood pressure. *Am. J. Cardiol.* 13:683.

Harlan, W. R., Jr., Winesett, P. S., and Wasserman, A. J. 1967. Tissue lipoprotein lipase in normal individuals and in individuals with exogenous hypertriglyceridemia and the relationship of this enzyme to assimilation of fat. *J. Clin. Invest.* 46:239.

Harlan, W. R., Oberman, A., Mitchel, R. E., and Graybiel, A. 1973. A 30-year study of blood pressure in a white male cohort. In *Hypertension: Mechanisms and Management*, G. Onesti, K. E. Kim, and J. H. Moyer, eds., p. 85. New York: Grune & Stratton.

Hartog, C. D., Buzina, K., Fidanza, F., Keys, A., and Roine, P. 1968. *Dietary Studies and Epidemiology of Heart Diseases*. The Netherlands: The Hague.

Hatano, S. 1979. Personal communication.

Hatch, F. T., and Lees, R. S. 1968. Practical methods for plasma lipoprotein analysis. *Adv. Lipid Res.* 6:1.

Hatch, F. T., Lindgren, F. T., Adamson, G. L., Jenson, L. C., Wong, A. W., and Levy, R. I. 1973. Quantitative agarose gel electrophoresis of plasma lipoproteins: A simple technique and two methods for standardization. *J. Lab. Clin. Med.* 81:946.

Hawksley/Gelman. Hawksley Random Zero Sphygmomanometer. Sussex, England. Unpublished.

Hayes, C. G., Tyroler, H. A., and Cassel, J. C. 1971. Family aggregation of blood pressure in Evans County, Georgia. *Arch. Intern. Med.* 128:965.

Hennekens, C. H., Jesse, M. J., Klein, B. E., Gourley, J. E., and Blumenthal, S. 1976. Cholesterol among children of men with myocardial infarction. *Pediatrics* 58:211.

Heptinstall, R. H. 1976. Relation of hypertension to changes in the arteries. *Prog. Cardiovasc. Dis.* 17:25.

Herrick, J. B. 1912. Clinical features of sudden obstruction of the coronary arteries. *J.A.M.A.* 59:2015.

Heyden, S., Bartel, A. G., Hames, C. G., and McDonough, J. R. 1969. Elevated blood pressure levels in adolescents, Evans County, Georgia. *J.A.M.A.* *209:*1683.

Hickie, J. B., Sutton, J., Russo, P., Ruys, J., and Kraegen, E. W. 1974. Serum cholesterol and serum triglyceride levels in Australian adolescent males. *Med. J. Aust. 1:*825.

Hochberg, H. M. and Saltzman, M. B. 1971. Accuracy of an ultrasound blood pressure instrument in neonates, infants, and children. *Curr. Ther. Res. 13:*482.

Hodges, R. E. and Krehl, W. A. 1965. Nutritional status of teen-agers in Iowa. *Am. J. Clin. Nutr. 17:*200.

Hoffman-LaRoche, Inc. Arteriosonde Ultrasonic Indirect Blood Pressure Monitor. Cranberry, N.J., Roche Medical Electronics Division. Unpublished.

Holland, W. W. and Humerfelt, S. 1964. Measurement of blood pressure: Comparison of intra-arterial and cuff values. *Br. Med. J. 2:*1241.

Holman, R. L., McGill, H. C., Strong, J. P., and Geer, J. C. 1958. The natural history of atherosclerosis: The early aortic lesions as seen in New Orleans in the middle of the 20th century. *Am. J. Pathol. 34:*209.

Hunt, E. E., Cocke, G., and Gallagher, J. R. 1958. Somatotype and sexual maturation in boys: A method of developmental analysis. *Hum. Biol. 30:*73.

Hunter, S. M., Frerichs, R. R., Webber, L. S., and Berenson, G. S. 1979. Social status and cardiovascular disease risk factor variables in children—The Bogalusa Heart Study. *J. Chronic Dis., 32:*441.

Irvine, R. O. H. 1967. The influence of arm girth and cuff size on the measurement of blood pressure. *N. Z. Med. J. 67:*279.

Irwin, J. O., and Cheeseman, E. A. 1939. On an approximate method of determining the mean effective dose and its error, in the case of quantal response. *J. Hyg. (Camb.) 39:*574.

Jensen, J., and Blankenhorn, D. H. 1972. The inheritance of familial hypercholesterolemia. *Am. J. Med. 52:*499.

Johnson, A. L., Cornoni, J. C., Cassel, J. C., Tyroler, H. A., Heyden, S., and Hames, C. G. 1975. Influence of race, sex and weight on blood pressure behavior in young adults. *Am. J. Cardiol. 35:*523.

Johnson, B. C., Epstein, F. H., and Kjelsberg, M. O. 1965. Distributions and familial studies of blood pressure and serum cholesterol levels in a total community—Tecumseh, Michigan. *J. Chronic Dis. 18:*147.

Johnson, B. C., Karunas, T. M., and Epstein, F. H. 1973. Longitudinal change in blood pressure in individuals, families, and social groups. *Clin. Sci. Mol. Med. 45 (Suppl. 1):*35s.

Johnson, M. L., Burke, B. S., and Mayer, J. 1956. Relative importance of inactivity and overeating in the energy balance of obese high school girls. *Am. J. Clin. Nutr. 4:*37.

Johnston, F. D., and Kline, E. M. 1940. An acoustical study of the stethoscope. *Arch. Intern. Med. 65:*328.

Johnston, F. E., Hamill, P. V. V., and Lemeshow, S. 1974. Skinfold thickness of youths 12–17 years—United States. *Vital Health Stat.*, DHEW Pub. No. (HRA) 74-1614, series 11, no. 132. Public Health Service. Washington: U.S. Government Printing Office.

Johnston, F. E., and Beller, A. 1976. Anthropometric evaluation of the body composition of black, white, and Puerto Rican newborns. *Am. J. Clin. Nutr.* 29:61.

Johnston, J. A. 1957. Protein requirements of adolescents. *Ann. N.Y. Acad. Sci.* 69:881.

Joossens, J. V., Willems, J., Claessens, J., Claes, J., and Lissens, W. 1970. Sodium and hypertension. In *Nutrition and Cardiovascular Diseases*, F. Fidanza, A. Keys, G. Ricci, and J. C. Somogy, eds., p. 91. Rome: Morgagni Edizione Scientifiche.

Kagan, A., Gordon, T., Kannel, W. B., and Dawber, T. R. 1959. Blood pressure and its relation to coronary heart disease in the Framingham study. *Hypertension* 7:53.

Kannel, W. B. 1972. *Handbook of Coronary Risk Probability*. New York: American Heart Association.

Kannel, W. B. 1974. Role of blood pressure in cardiovascular morbidity and mortality. *Prog. Cardiovasc. Dis.* 17:5.

Kannel, W. B., and Dawber, T. R. 1972. Atherosclerosis as a pediatric problem. *J. Pediatr.* 80:544.

Kannel, W. B., and Gordon, T., eds. 1970. The Framingham Study: An epidemiological investigation of cardiovascular disease. Section 24 of *The Framingham Diet Study: Diet and the Regulation of Serum Cholesterol*. USD HEW NIH. Washington: U.S. Government Printing Office.

Kannel, W. B., Brand, N., Skinner, J. J., Jr., Dawber, T. R., and McNamara, P. M. 1967a. The relationship of adiposity to blood pressure and development of hypertension—The Framingham Study. *Ann. Intern. Med.* 67:48.

Kannel, W. B., LeBauer, E. J., Dawber, T. R., and McNamara, P. M. 1967b. Relation of body weight to the development of coronary heart disease—The Framingham Study. *Circulation* 35:734.

Kannel, W. B., Castelli, W. P., Gordon, T., and McNamara, P. M. 1971a. Serum cholesterol, lipoproteins, and the risk for coronary heart disease—The Framingham Study. *Ann. Intern. Med.* 74:1.

Kannel, W. B., Garcia, M. J., McNamara, P. M., and Pearson, G. 1971b. Serum lipid precursors of coronary heart disease. *Hum. Pathol.* 2:129.

Karvonen, M. J., Telivuo, L. J., and Jaervinen, E. J. K. 1964. Sphygmomanometer cuff size and the accuracy of indirect measurement of blood pressure. *Am. J. Cardiol.* 13:688.

Keys, A. 1975. Coronary heart disease—the global picture. *Atherosclerosis* 22:149.

Keys, A., Mickelsen, O., Miller, E., Hayes, E. R., and Todd, R. L. 1950. The concentration of cholesterol in the blood serum of normal man and its relation to age. *J. Clin. Invest.* 29:1347.

Keys, A., Anderson, J. L., Mickelson, O., Adelson, S. F., and Fidanza, F. 1956. Diet and serum cholesterol in man: Lack of effect of dietary cholesterol. *J. Nutr.* 59:39.

Keys, A., Aravanis, C., Blackburn, H., Van Buchem, F. S. P., Buzina, R., Djordjevic, B. S., Fidanza, F., Karvonen, M. J., Menotti, A., Puddu, V., and Taylor, H. L. 1972. Coronary heart disease: Overweight and obesity as risk factors. *Ann. Intern. Med.* 77:15.

King, G. E. 1967. Errors in clinical measurement of blood pressure in obesity. *Clin. Sci.* 32:223.

Kirk, T. R., Rice, R. G., and Allen, P. M. 1976. EPSDT—One quarter million screenings in Michigan. *Am.'J. Public Health* 66:482.

Kirkendall, W. M., Burton, A. C., Epstein, F. H., and Freis, E. D. 1967. Recommendations for human blood pressure determination by sphygmomanometers. *Circulation* 36:980.

Kitterman, J. A., Phibbs, R. H., and Tooley, W. H. 1969. Aortic blood pressure in normal newborn infants during the first 12 hours of life. *Pediatrics* 44:959.

Klein, B. E. K., Cornoni, J. C., Jones, F., and Boyle, E., Jr. 1973. Overweight indices as correlates of coronary heart disease and blood pressure. *Hum. Biol.* 45:329.

Kohn, R. M., Ibrahim, M. A., Winkelstein, W., Jr., Pinsky, W., Borden, H., and Binette, P. J. 1969. Identifying coronary prone families by screening of school populations. *Israel J. Med. Sci.* 5:683.

Koran, L. M. 1975. The reliability of clinical methods, data and judgements. *N. Engl. J. Med.* 293:642.

Kornerup, V. 1950. Concentrations of cholesterol, total fat and phospholipid in serum of normal man. *Arch. Intern. Med.* 85:398.

Kromhout, D., van der Haar, F., Hautvast, J.G.A.J. 1977. Coronary heart disease risk factors in Dutch schoolchildren—results of a pilot-study. *Prev. Med.* 6:500.

Kwiterovich, P. O., Jr. 1974. Neonatal screening for hyperlipidemia. *Pediatrics* 53:455.

Kwiterovich, P. O., Jr., Levy, R. I., and Fredrickson, D. S. 1973. Neonatal diagnosis of familial Type II hyperlipoproteinemia. *Lancet* 1:118.

Kwiterovich, P. O., Jr., Fredrickson, D. S., and Levy, R. I. 1974. Familial hypercholesterolemia (one form of familial type II hyperlipoproteinemia): A study of its biochemical, genetic and clinical presentation in childhood. *J. Clin. Invest.* 53:1237.

Labarthe, D. R., Hawkins, C. M., and Remington, R. D. 1973. Evaluation of performance of selected devices for measuring blood pressure. *Am. J. Cardiol.* 32:546.

Langford, H. G., Watson, R. L., and Douglas, B. H. 1968. Factors affecting blood pressure in population groups. *Trans. Assoc. Am. Physicians* 81:135.

Laragh, J. H. 1973. Vasoconstriction-volume analysis for understanding and treating hypertension: The use of renin and aldosterone profile. *Am. J. Med.* 55:261.

Larsen, R., Glueck, C. J., and Tsang, R. 1974. Special diet for familial Type II hyperlipoproteinemia. *Am. J. Dis. Child. 128:*67.

Laska-Mierzejewska, T. 1970. Morphological and developmental difference between Negro and white Cuban youths. *Hum. Biol. 42:*581.

Lauer, R. M., Connor, W. E., Leaverton, P. E., Reiter, M. A., and Clarke, W. R. 1975. Coronary heart disease risk factors in school children—The Muscatine Study, *J. Pediatr. 86:*697.

Lee, V. A. 1967. Individual trends in the total serum cholesterol of children and adolescents over a ten-year period. *Am. J. Clin. Nutr. 20:*5.

Lee, Y. H., Rosner, B., Gould, J. B., Lowe, E. W., and Kass, E. H. 1976. Familial aggregation of blood pressures of newborn infants and their mothers. *Pediatrics 58:*722.

Levine, R. J., and Cohen, E. D. 1974. Editorial: The Hawthorne Effect. *Clin. Res. 22:*111.

Levy, P. S., Hamill, P. V. V., Heald, F., and Rowland, M. 1976. Total serum cholesterol values of youths 12–17 years. *Vital Health Stat.*, series 11, no. 156. DHEW Pub. No. (HRA) 76-1638. Public Health Service. Washington: U.S. Government Printing Office.

Levy, R. I. 1978. Progress toward prevention of cardiovascular disease—a thirty year retrospective. *Mod. Concepts Cardiovasc. Dis. 47:*103.

Levy, R. I., and Rifkind, B. M. 1973. Diagnosis and management of hyperlipoproteinemia in infants and children. *Am. J. Cardiol. 31:*547.

Levy, R. L., White, P. D., Stroud, W. D., and Hillman C. C. 1946. Overweight: Its prognostic significance in relation to hypertension and cardiovascular-renal disease. *J.A.M.A. 131:*951.

Lie, J. T. 1978. Recognizing coronary heart disease—Selected historical vignettes from the period of William Harvey (1578–1657) to Adam Hammer (1818–1878). *Mayo Clin. Proc. 53:*811.

Lindgren, F. T., Jensen, L. C., and Hatch, F. T. 1972. The isolation and quantitative analysis of serum lipoproteins. In *Blood Lipids and Lipoproteins: Quantitation, Composition, and Metabolism*, G. J. Nelson, ed., p. 181. New York: Wiley-Interscience.

Lipid Research Clinics Program. 1974. *Manual of Laboratory Operations. Vol 1: Lipid and Lipoproteins Analysis.* DHEW Pub. No. (NIH) 75-628. Washington: U.S. Government Printing Office.

Loggie, J. M. H. 1971. Systemic hypertension in children and adolescents. *Pediatr. Clin. North Am. 18:*1273.

Loggie, J. M. H. 1975. Hypertension in children and adolescents. *Hospital Practice 10 (6):*81.

Londe, S. 1968. Blood pressure standards for normal children as determined under office conditions. *Clin. Pediatr. 7:*400.

Londe, S., and Goldring, D. 1972. Hypertension in children. *Am. Heart J. 84:*1.

Londe, S., and Goldring, D. 1976. High blood pressure in children: Problems and guidelines for evaluation and treatment. *Am. J. Cardiol. 37:*650.

Londe, S., Bourgoignie, J. J., Robson, A. M., and Goldring, D. 1971. Hypertension in apparently normal children. *J. Pediatr.* 78:569.

Lopez-S. A., Srinivasan, S. R., Dugan, F. A., Radhakrishnamurthy, B., and Berenson, G. S. 1971. Detection of subtle abnormalities of serum β- and pre-β-lipoproteins in "normal" individuals by turbidimetric and electrophoretic methods. *Clin. Chim. Acta 31:*123.

Lovell, R. H. H. 1967. Race and blood pressure, with special reference to Oceania. In *The Epidemiology of Hypertension,* J. Stamler, R. Stamler, and T. N. Pullman, eds., p. 122. New York: Grune and Stratton.

Luft, F. C., Grim, C. E., Higgins, J. T., and Weinberger, M. H. 1977. Differences in response to sodium administration in normotensive white and black subjects. *J. Lab. Clin. Med.* 90:555.

Lups, S., and Francke, C. 1947. On the changes in blood pressure during the period of starvation (September 1944 to May 1945) and after the liberation (May 1945 to September 1945) in Utrecht, Holland. *Acta Med. Scand. 126:*449.

McDonough, J. R., Garrison, G. E., and Hames, C. G. 1964. Blood pressure and hypertensive disease among negroes and whites: A study in Evans County, Georgia. *Ann. Intern. Med. 61:*208.

McDonough, J. R., Hames, C. G., Garrison, G. E., Stulb, S. C., Lichtman, M. A., and Hefelfinger, D. C. 1965. The relationship of hematocrit to cardiovascular states of health in the negro and white population of Evans County, Georgia. *J. Chronic Dis. 18:*243.

McGandy, R. B. 1971. Adolescence and the onset of atherosclerosis. *Bull. N.Y. Acad. Med. 47:*590.

McGill, H. C., ed. 1968. *The Geographic Pathology of Atherosclerosis.* Baltimore: Williams and Wilkins.

McGill, H. C., Jr., Geer, J. C., and Strong, J. P. 1963. Natural history of human atherosclerotic lesions. In *Atherosclerosis and Its Origin,* M. Sandler and G. H. Bourne, eds., p. 39. New York: Academic Press.

McMahan, C. A. 1967. *Rudiments of Biometry.* Ann Arbor, Michigan: Edwards Brothers.

McMahan, C. A. 1970. *Retriever Theory.* Ann Arbor, Mich.: Edwards Brothers.

McMahan, C. A., and Strong, J. P. 1965. Factorial experiments for pilot studies of serum cholesterol in baboons. In *The baboon in medical research: Proceedings of the first international symposium on the baboon and its use as an experimental animal,* p. 485. Austin: University of Texas Press.

McMillan, G. C. 1973. Development of arteriosclerosis. *Am. J. Cardiol. 31:*542.

McNamara, J. J., Molot, M. A., and Stremple, J. F. 1971. Coronary artery disease in combat casualties in Viet Nam. *J.A.M.A. 216:*1185.

Mann, G., Teel, K., Hayes, O., McNally, A., and Bruno, D. 1955. Exercise in the disposition of dietary calories-regulation of serum lipoprotein and cholesterol levels in human subjects. *N. Engl. J. Med. 253:*349.

Martin, M. M. and Martin, L. A. 1973. Obesity, hyperinsulinism and diabetes mellitus in childhood. *J. Pediatrics 82:*192.

Mathewson, F. A. L., Corne, R. A., Nelson, N. A., and Hill, N. L. 1972. Blood pressure characteristics of a select group of North American males, followed for 20 years. *Can. Med. Assoc. J. 106:*549.

Maurer, A. H. and Noordergraaf, A. 1976. Korotkoff sound filtering for automated three-phase measurement of blood pressure. *Am. Heart J. 91:*584.

Maxwell, A. E. 1961. *Analysing Qualitative Data.* London: Methuen.

Meredith, A., Matthews, A., Zickefoose, M., Weagley, E., Wayave, M., and Brown, E. G. 1951. How well do school children recall what they have eaten? *J. Am. Diet Assoc. 27:*749.

Miall, W. E., and Chinn, S. 1973. Blood pressure and aging: Results of a 15–17 year follow-up study in South Wales. *Clin. Sci. Mol. Med. 45 Suppl. 1:*23s.

Miall, W. E., and Lovell, H. G. 1967. Relation between change of blood pressure and age. *Br. Med. J. 2:*660.

Miall, W. E., Heneage, P., Khosla, T., Lovell, H. G., and Moore, F. 1967. Factors influencing the degree of resemblance in arterial pressure of close relatives. *Clin. Sci. 33:*271.

Miall, W. E., Bell, R. A., and Lovell, H. G. 1968. Relation between change in blood pressure and weight. *Br. J. Prev. Soc. Med. 22:*73.

Miettinen, T. A. 1971. Cholesterol production in obesity. *Circulation 44:*842.

Miller, G. J., and Miller, N. E. 1975. Plasma-high-density-lipoprotein concentration and development of ischaemic heart-disease. *Lancet 1:*16.

Mitchell, S. C., and Jesse, M. J. 1973. Risk factors of coronary heart disease: their genesis and pediatric implications. *Am. J. Cardiol. 31:*588.

Modanlou, H., Yeh, S-Y., Siassa, B., and Hon, E. H. 1974. Direct monitoring of arterial blood pressure in depressed and normal newborn infants during the first hour of life. *J. Pediatr. 85:*553.

Montoye, H. J., Epstein, F. J., and Kjelsberg, M. D. 1966. Relationship between serum cholesterol and body fatness: An epidemiologic study. *Am. J. Clin. Nutr. 18:*397.

Moore, M. C., Judlin, B. C., and Kennemur, P.McA. 1967. Using graduated food models in taking dietary histories. *J. Am. Diet. Assoc. 51:*447.

Moore, M. C., Goodloe, M. H., and Schilling, P. E. 1974. *Extended Table of Nutrient Values (ETNV).* Atlanta: International Dietary Information Foundation. (Data tapes at Louisiana State University Computer Center)

Morrison, J. A., deGroot, I., Edwards, B. K., Kelly, K. A., Mellies, M. J., Khoury, P., and Glueck, C. J. 1978. Lipids and lipoproteins in 927 school children, ages 6 to 17 years. *Pediatrics 62:*990.

Morse, M., Cassels, D. E., and Schlutz, F. W. 1947. Blood volumes of normal children. *Am. J. Physiol. 151:*448.

Moss, A. J. 1962. Blood pressure in children with diabetes mellitus. *Pediatrics 30:*932.

Moss, A. J., and Adams, F. H. 1962. *Problems of Blood Pressure in Childhood.* Springfield, Ill.: C. C. Thomas

Moss, A. J., and Adams, F. H. 1965. Auscultatory and intra-arterial pressure: A comparison in children with special reference to cuff width. *J. Pediatr.* 66:1094.

Motulsky, A. G. 1976. Genetic basis of hyperlipoproteinemia. Task force on genetic factors in atherosclerotic disease, *DHEW Pub. No. (NIH) 76-922.* Washington: U.S. Government Printing Office.

Moyer, J. H., Heider, C., Pevey, K., and Ford, R. V. 1958. The vascular status of a heterogeneous group of patients with hypertension, with particular emphasis on renal function. *Am. J. Med. 24:*164.

Nance, W. E., Krieger, H., Azevedo, E., and Mi, M. P. 1965. Human blood pressure and the ABO blood group system: An apparent association. *Hum. Biol. 37:*238.

Nankin, H. R., Sperling, M., Kenny, F. M., Drash, A. L., and Troen, P. 1974. Correlation between sexual maturation and serum gonadotropins: Comparison of black and white youngsters. *Am. J. Med. Sci. 268:*139.

National Center for Health Statistics. 1970. Height and weight of children, United States. *Vital Health Stat.*, series 11, no. 104, PHS Pub. No. 1000, Public Health Service. Washington: U.S. Government Printing Office.

National Center for Health Statistics. 1972. Skinfold thickness of children 6–11 years, United States. *Vital Health Stat.*, series 11, no. 120. DHEW Pub. No. (HSM) 73–1602, Public Health Service. Washington: U.S. Government Printing Office.

National Center for Health Statistics. 1973a. Age at menarche, United States. *Vital Health Stat.*, series 11, no. 133. DHEW Pub. No. (HRA) 74–1615, Public Health Service. Washington: U.S. Government Printing Office.

National Center for Health Statistics. 1973b. Examination and health history findings among children and youths, 6–17 years. *Vital Health Stat.*, series 11, no. 129. DHEW Pub. No. (HRA) 74–1611, Public Health Service. Washington: U.S. Government Printing Office.

National Center for Health Statistics. 1973c. Height and weight of youths 12–17 years, United States. *Vital Health Stat.*, series 11, no. 124, DHEW Pub. No. (HSM) 73–1606, Public Health Service. Washington: U.S. Government Printing Office.

National Center for Health Statistics. 1974. Skinfold thickness of youths 12–17 years, United States. *Vital Health Stat.*, series 11, no. 132. DHEW Pub. No. (HRA) 74–1614, Public Health Service. Washington: U.S. Government Printing Office.

National Center for Health Statistics. 1977. Total serum cholesterol levels of children 4–17 years of age, United States (1971–74) Advance data from *Vital Health Stat.*, series 8, no. 8, Public Health Service. Washington: U.S. Government Printing Office.

National Diet Heart Study Research Group. 1968. The national diet-heart study, final report. *Circulation 37 (I):*1.

National Heart, Lung, and Blood Institute. 1978. *Cardiovascular Profile of 15,000 Children of School Age in Three Communities, 1971–1975.* DHEW Pub. No. (NIH) 78–1472. Washington: U.S. Government Printing Office.

National Institutes of Health. 1971. Arteriosclerosis—A report by the National Heart and Lung Institute Task Force on Arteriosclerosis. vol. 1, DHEW Pub. No. (NIH) 72–137, vol II:72–219. Washington: U.S. Government Printing Office.

Nestel, P. J., Schreibman, P. H., and Ahrens, E. H., Jr. 1973. Cholesterol metabolism in human obesity. *J. Clin. Invest. 52:*2389.

New, M. I., Baum, C. J., and Levine, L. S. 1977. Nomograms relating aldosterone excretion to urinary sodium and potassium in the pediatric population: their application to the study of childhood hypertension. *Am. J. Cardiol. 37:*658.

Newman, R. W. 1956. Skinfold measurements in young American males. *Hum. Biol. 28:*154.

Newman, R., W., and Munro, E. H. 1955. The relation of climate and body size in U.S. males *Am. J. Phys. Anthropol. 13:*1.

Nichols, A. V. 1967. Human serum lipoproteins and their interrelationships. *Adv. Biol. Med. Phys. 11:*109.

Nichols, A. V. 1969. Functions and interrelationships of different classes of plasma lipoproteins. *Proc. Natl. Acad. Sci. U.S. 64:*1128.

Nichols, A. V., Ravenscroft, C., Lamphiear, D.-E., and Ostrander, L. D., Jr. 1976. Independence of serum lipid levels and dietary habits: The Tecumseh Study. *J.A.M.A. 236:*1948.

Nielson, P. E., and Janniche, H. 1974. The accuracy of auscultatory measurement of arm blood pressure in very obese subjects. *Acta Med. Scand. 195:*403.

Noble, R. P. 1968. Electrophoretic separation of plasma lipoproteins in agarose gel. *J. Lipid Res. 9:*693.

Nuessle, W. F. 1956. The importance of a tight blood pressure cuff. *Am. Heart J. 52:*905.

Oberman, A., Lane, N. E., Harlan, W. R., Graybiel, A., and Mitchell, R. E. 1967. Trends in systolic blood pressure in the thousand aviator cohort over a twenty-four-year period. *Circulation 36:*812.

Oldham, P. D. 1968. *Measurement in Medicine, the Interpretation of Numerical Data,* p. 148. Philadelphia: Lippincott.

Olefsky, J. M., Farquhar, J. W., and Reaven, G. M. 1974. Reappraisal of the role of insulin in hypertriglyceridemia. *Am. J. Med. 57:*551.

Oliver, W. J., Cohen, E. L., and Neel, J. V. 1975. Blood pressure, sodium intake, and sodium related hormones in the Yanomamo Indians, a "no-salt" culture. *Circulation 52:*146.

O'Neal, R. M., Johnson, O. C., and Schaefer, A. E. 1970. Guidelines for classification and interpretation of group blood and urine data collected as part of the National Nutrition Survey. *Pediatr. Res. 4:*102.

Ose, L. 1975. LDL and total cholesterol in cord-blood screening for familial hypercholesterolemia. *Lancet 2:*615.

Ostle, B. 1963. *Statistics in Research,* 2nd ed. Ames, Iowa: Iowa State University Press.

Owen, G. M., and Lubin, A. H. 1973. Anthropometric differences between black and white preschool children. *Am. J. Dis. Child. 126:*168.

Owen, G. M., Kram, K. M., Garry, P. J., Lowe, J. E., and Lubin, A. H. 1974. A study of nutritional status of preschool children in the United States, 1968–1970. *Pediatrics 53:*597.

Paffenbarger, R. S., Jr., Thorne, M. C., and Wing, A. L. 1968. Chronic disease in former college students. VIII. Characteristics in youth predisposing to hypertension in later years. *Am. J. Epidemiol. 88:*25.

Page, I. H., and Dustan, H. P. 1962. Persistence of normal blood pressure after discontinuing treatment in hypertensive patients. *Circulation 25:*433.

Perry, H. M., and Schroeder, H. A. 1955. Evidence for reversal of the hypertensive process when blood pressure is controlled by drugs. *Circulation 12:*759.

Physiometrics, Inc. 1971. Instruction Manual for Automated Blood Pressure Recorder Model USM-105. Malibu, Calif.: Unpublished.

Pickering, G. 1968. *High Blood Pressure*, p. 38. London: J. & A. Churchill.

Pillsbury, D. M., Shelley, W. B., and Kligman, A. M. 1956. In *Dermatology*, p. 807. Philadelphia: W. B. Saunders.

Pincherle, G. 1971. Factors affecting the mean serum cholesterol. *J. Chronic. Dis. 24:*289.

Puska, P., Virtamo, J., Tuomilehto, J., Maki, J., and Neittaaumaki, L. 1978. Cardiovascular risk factor changes in a three-year follow-up of a cohort in connection with a community programme (the North Karelia Project). *Acta Med. Scand. 204(5):* 381.

Pykalisto, O. J., Brunzell, J. D., and Bierman, E. L. 1975. Decreased adipose tissue lipoprotein lipase activity in hypothyroid subjects. *Clin. Res. 23:*113A.

Rafstedt, S. 1955. Studies on serum lipids and lipoproteins in infancy and childhood. *Acta Pediatr. (Uppsala) 44 (Suppl. 102):*1.

Raftery, E. G., and Ward, A. P. 1968. The indirect method of recording blood pressure. *Cardiovasc. Res. 2:*210.

Ragan, C., and Bordley, J. 1941. The accuracy of clinical measurements of arterial blood pressure. *Bull. Johns Hopkins Hosp. 69:*504.

Rao, D. C., MacLean, C. J., Morton, N. E., and Yee, S. 1975. Analysis of family resemblance. V. Height and weight in northeastern Brazil. *Am. J. Hum. Genet. 27:*509.

Räsänen, L., Wilska, M., Kantero, R-L., Näntö, V., Ahlström, A., and Hallman, N. 1978. Nutrition survey of Finnish rural children. IV. Serum cholesterol values in relation to dietary variables. *Am. J. Clin. Nutr. 31:*1050.

Rauh, J. L., and Schumsky, D. A. 1968. An evaluation of triceps skinfold measures from urban school children. *Hum. Biol. 40:*363.

Ravin, A. The clinical significance of the sounds of Korotkoff. University of Colorado School of Medicine. An audio-cassette program previously distributed by Merck, Sharp and Dohme.

Reiss, A. J., Jr., Duncan, O. D., Hatt, P., and North, C. C. 1961. *Occupations and Social Status.* Glencoe, Ill: The Free Press of Glencoe.

Reynolds, E. L. 1946. Sexual maturation and the growth of fat, muscle and bone in girls. *Child. Dev. 17:*121.

Rhoads, G. G., Gulbrandsen, C. L., and Kagan, A. 1976. Serum lipoproteins and coronary heart disease in a population study of Hawaii Japanese men. *N. Engl. J. Med. 294:*293.

Richardson, B. D., and Walker, A. R. P. 1975. Prevalences of leg and chest abnormalities in four South African school child populations with special reference to Vitamin D status *Postgrad. Med. J. 51:*22.

Rifkind, B. B., Gale, M., and Lawson, D. 1968. Serum cholesterol and triglyceride levels and adiposity. *Cardiovasc. Res. 2:*143.

Roberts, J., and Maurer, K. 1976. Blood pressure of persons 6–74 years of age in the United States. Advance data from *Vital Health Stat.*, series 1, no. 1. Public Health Service. Washington: U.S. Government Printing Office.

Roberts, L. N., Smiley, J. R., and Manning, G. W. 1958. A comparison of direct and indirect blood pressure determinations. *Circulation 8:*232.

Robinow, M., Hamilton, W. F., Woodbury, R. A., and Volpitto, P. P. 1939. Accuracy of clinical determinations of blood pressure in children, with values under normal and abnormal conditions. *Am. J. Dis. Child. 58:*102.

Robinson, S. C., and Brucer, M. 1939. Range of normal blood pressure: A statistical and clinical study of 11,383 persons. *Arch. Intern. Med. 64:*409.

Roche, A. F., and McKigney, J. I. 1976. Physical growth of ethnic groups comprising the U.S. population. *Am. J. Dis. Child. 130:*62.

Rose, G. A., and Blackburn, H. 1968. Cardiovascular survey methods, Monograph Series No. 56. Geneva: World Health Organization.

Rosenman, R. H., Brand, R. J., Jenkins, C. D., Friedman, M., Straus, R., and Wurm, M. 1975. Coronary heart disease in the western collaborative group study—final follow-up experience of 8½ years. *J.A.M.A. 233:*872.

Russell, S. J. M. 1949. Blood volume studies in healthy children. *Arch. Dis. Child. 24:*88.

Sackett, D. L. 1975. Studies of blood pressure in spouses. In *Epidemiology and the Control of Hypertension*, O. Paul, ed., p. 21. New York: Stratton Intercontinental.

Salhanick, H. A., Kipnis, D. M., and Wiele, R. L. 1969. *Metabolic Effects of Gonadal Hormones and Contraceptive Steroids.* New York: Plenum Press.

Savage, P. J., Hamman, R. F., Bartha, G., Dippe, S. E., Miller, M., and Bennet, P. H. 1976. Serum cholesterol levels in American (Pima) Indian children and adolescents. *Pediatrics 58:*274.

Scanu, A. M., Edelstein, C., and Kiem, P. 1975. Serum lipoproteins. In *The Plasma Proteins: Structure, Function and Genetic Control*, F. W. Putnam, ed., Vol. 1, p. 318. New York: Academic Press.

Schubert, W. K. 1973. Fat nutrition and diet in childhood. *Am. J. Cardiol.* 31:581.

Schwalb, H., and Schimert, G. 1970. Das Herz bei Fettsucht. *Med. Klin.* 65:1908.

Schwartz, M. K., and Hill, P. 1972. Problems in the interpretation of serum cholesterol values. *Prev. Med. 1:*167.

Scrimshaw, N. S., Balsam, A., and Arroyave, G. 1957. Serum cholesterol levels in school children from three socio-economic groups. *Am. J. Clin. Nutr.* 5:629.

Selby, S. M., ed. 1970. *Standard Mathematical Tables,* 18th ed. Cleveland, Ohio: The Chemical Rubber Company.

Shock, N. W. 1944. Basal blood pressure and pulse rate in adolescents. *Am. J. Dis. Child. 68:*16.

Shorey, R. A. L., Sewell, B., and O'Brien, M. 1976. Efficacy of diet and excercise in the reduction of serum cholesterol and triglyceride in free-living adult males. *Am. J. Clin. Nutr. 29:*512.

Siegel, S. 1956. *Nonparametric Statistics for the Behavioral Sciences.* New York: McGraw-Hill.

Simpson, J. A., Jamieson, G., Dickhaus, D. W., and Grover, R. F. 1965. Effect of size of cuff bladder on accuracy of measurement of indirect blood pressure. *Am. Heart J. 70:*208.

Singh, S. P., and Page, L. B. 1967. Hypertension in early life. *Am. J. Med. Sci.* 253:255.

Smirk, F. H. 1957. *High Arterial Pressure,* p. 365. Springfield, Ill.: C. C. Thomas.

Smith, W. M. 1978. Mild essential hypertension: benefit of treatment: discussion. *Ann. N. Y. Acad. Sci. 304:*74.

Snedecor, G. W., and Cochran, W. G. 1967. *Statistical Methods,* 6th ed. Ames, Iowa: Iowa State University Press.

Sneiderman, C., Heyden, S., Heiss, G., Tyroler, H., and Hames, C. 1976. Predictors of blood pressure over a 16-year follow-up of 163 youths. *Circulation 54, (suppl. 2):*II–24.

Society of Actuaries. 1959. Build and blood pressure study. Chicago.

Sokal, R. R., and Rohlf, F. J. 1969. *Biometry.* San Francisco: W. H. Freeman.

Spellacy, W. N., Ashbacker, L. V., Harris, G. K., and Buhi, W. C. 1974. Total cholesterol content in maternal and umbilical vessels in term pregnancies. *Obstet. Gynecol. 44:*661.

Srinivasan, S. R., Lopez-S, A., Radhakrishnamurthy, B., and Berenson, G. S. 1970a. A simplified technique for semi-quantitative, clinical estimation of serum β- and pre-β-lipoproteins. *Angiologica 7:*344.

Srinivasan, S. R., Lopez-S, A., Radhakrishnamurthy, B., and Berenson, G. S. 1970b. Complexing of serum pre-β- and β-lipoproteins and acid mucopolysaccharides. *Atherosclerosis 12:*321.

Srinivasan, S. R., Frerichs, R. R., and Berenson, G. S. 1975a. Serum lipid and lipoprotein profile in school children from a rural community. *Clin. Chim. Acta 60:*293.

Srinivasan, S. R., Radhakrishnamurthy, B., and Berenson, G. S., 1975b. Studies on the interaction of heparin with serum lipoproteins in the presence of Ca^{++}, Mg^{++}, and Mn^{++}. *Arch. Biochem. Biophys. 170:*334.

Srinivasan, S. R., Frerichs, R. R., Webber, L. S., and Berenson, G. S. 1976a. Serum lipoprotein profile in children from a biracial community—The Bogalusa Heart Study. *Circulation 54:*309.

Srinivasan, S. R., Smith, C. C., Radhakrishnamurthy, B., Wolf, R. H., and Berenson, G. S. 1976b. Phylogenetic variability of serum lipids and lipoproteins in nonhuman primates fed diets with different contents of dietary cholesterol. *Adv. Exp. Med. Biol. 67:*65.

Srinivasan, S. R., Ellefson, R. D., Whitaker, C. F., and Berenson, G. S. 1978a. Lipoprotein cholesterol in the serum of children, as determined independently by two different methods. *Clin. Chem. 24:*157.

Srinivasan, S. R., Radhakrishnamurthy, B., Webber, L. S., Dalferes, E. R., Jr., Kokatnur, M. G., and Berenson, G. S. 1978b. Synergistic effects of dietary carbohydrate and cholesterol on serum lipids and lipoproteins in squirrel and spider monkeys. *Am. J. Clin. Nutr. 31:*603.

Srinivasan, S. R., Foster, T. A., and Berenson, G. S. 1979a. Efficacy of a simplified primary screening procedure for detection of hyperlipoproteinemias in a pediatric population. *Clin. Chem. 25:*242.

Srinivasan, S. R., Clevidence, B. A., Pargaonkar, P. S., Radhakrishnamurthy, B., and Berenson, G. S. 1979b. Varied effects of dietary sucrose and cholesterol on serum lipids, lipoproteins and apolipoproteins in rhesus monkeys. *Atherosclerosis. 33:*301.

Srinivasan, S. R., Berenson, G. S., Radhakrishnamurthy, B., Dalferes, E. R., Jr., Underwood, D., and Foster, T. A. 1979c. Effects of dietary sodium and sucrose on the induction of hypertension in spider monkeys. *Am. J. Clin. Nutr.* (published March 1980).

Stamler, J. 1967. Discussion of paper by H. L. Taylor: Body composition and elevated blood pressure. In *The Epidemiology of Hypertension,* J. Stamler, R. Stamler, and T. N. Pullman, eds., p. 101. New York: Grune & Stratton.

Stamler, J. 1973. Epidemiology of coronary heart disease. *Med. Clin. North Am. 57:*5.

Stamler, J., Forman, S., and Krol, W. F. 1978. Natural history of myocardial infarction in the coronary drug project: Long-term prognostic importance of serum lipid levels. *Am. J. Cardiol. 42:*489.

Stanhope, J. M., and Sampson, V. M. 1977. High-density-lipoprotein cholesterol and other serum lipids in a New Zealand biracial adolescent sample. The Wairoa College Survey. *Lancet 1:*968.

Starr, P. 1971. Hypercholesterolemia in school children: A preliminary report. *Am. J. Clin. Pathol. 56:*515.

Steele, J. M. 1942. Comparison of simultaneous indirect (auscultatory) and direct (intra-arterial) measurements of arterial pressure in man. *J. Mt. Sinai Hosp. 8:*1042.

Steinberg, D. 1969. Opening remarks. *Drugs Affecting Lipid Metabolism.* In *Adv. Exp. Med. Biol. 4:*1.

Steinfeld, L., Alexander, H., and Cohen, M. L. 1974. Updating sphygmomanometry. *Am. J. Cardiol. 33:*107.

Stine, O. C., Hepner, R., and Greenstreet, R. 1975. Correlation of blood pressure with skinfold thickness and protein levels. *Am. J. Dis. Child. 129:*905.

Stocks, P. 1924. Blood pressure in early life. *Draper's Company Research Memoirs: Studies in National Deterioration. II.* Cambridge, Engl.: Cambridge University Press, As quoted by Hamilton *et al.,* 1954.

Stone, M. C., Thorp, J. M., Mills, G. L., and Dick, T. B. S. 1970. Comparison of membrane filtration and nephelometry with analytical ultracentrifugation for the quantitative analysis of low density lipoprotein fractions. *Clin. Chim. Acta 30:*809.

Strong, J. P., and Eggen, D. A. 1969. Risk factors and atherosclerotic lesions, In *Atherosclerosis: Proceedings of the Second International Symposium,* R. J. C. Jones, ed., p. 355. New York: Springer-Verlag.

Strong, J. P., and McGill, H. C., Jr. 1969. The pediatric aspects of atherosclerosis. *J. Atheroscler. Res. 9:*251.

Strong, J. P., and Richards, M. L. 1976. Cigarette smoking and atherosclerosis in autopsied men. *Atherosclerosis 23:*451.

Strong, J. P., Eggen, D. A., Oalmann, M. C., Richards, M. L., and Tracy, R. E. 1972. Pathology and epidemiology of atherosclerosis. *J. Am. Diet. Assoc. 62:*262.

Stunkard, A. 1972. New therapies for eating disorders: behavior modification of obesity and anorexia nervosa. *Arch. Gen. Psychiatry 26:*391.

Sundelin, C., and Vuille, J.-C. 1975. Health screening of four-year-olds in a Swedish county. 1. Organization, methods and participation. *Acta Pediatr. Scand. 64:*795.

Tamir, I., Bojanower, Y., Levtow, O., Heldenberg, D., Dickerman, Z., and Werbin B. 1972. Serum lipids and lipoproteins in children from families with early coronary heart disease. *Arch. Dis. Child. 47:*808.

Tanner, J. M. 1962. *Growth at Adolescence,* 2nd ed. Oxford: Blackwell Scientific Publications.

Tanner, J. M., and Whitehouse, R. H. 1975. Revised standards for triceps and subscapular skinfolds in British children. *Arch. Dis. Child. 50:*14.

Tejada, C., Strong, J. P., Montenegro, M. R., Restrepo, C., and Solberg, L. A. 1968. Distribution of coronary and aortic atherosclerosis by geographic location, race, and sex. *Lab. Invest. 18:*509.

Thomas, C. B., Holljes, H. W. D., and Eisenberg, F. F. 1961. Observations on seasonal variations in total serum cholesterol level among healthy young prisoners. *Ann. Intern. Med. 54:*413.

Tracy, R. E. 1970. Correlation of lengthy hospital records of blood pressure with nephrosclerosis. *Am. J. Epidemiol. 91:*32.

Tsang, R. C., Fallat, R. W., and Glueck, C. J. 1974a. Cholesterol at birth and age 1. Comparison and normal and hypercholesterolemic neonates. *Pediatrics 53:*458.

Tsang, R., Glueck, C. J., Evans, G., and Steiner, P. M. 1974b. Cord blood hypertriglyceridemia. *Am. J. Dis. Child. 127:*78.

Tsang, R. C., Glueck, C. J., Fallat, R. W., and Mellies, M. 1975. Neonatal familial hypercholesterolemia. *Am. J. Dis. Child. 129:*83.

Tyroler, H. A., Heyden, S., Bartel, A., Cassel, J., Cornoni, J. C., Hames, C. G., and Kleinbaum, D. 1971. Blood pressure and cholesterol as coronary heart disease risk factors. *Arch. Intern. Med. 128:*907.

Tyroler, H. A., Hames, C. G., Krishan, I., Heyden, S., Cooper, G., and Cassel, J. C. 1975. Black-white differences in serum lipids and lipoproteins in Evans County. *Prev. Med. 4:*541.

United States Department of Agriculture. 1969. Food intake and nutritive value of diets of men, women and children in the United States, Spring 1965. ARS-62-18, March. Beltsville, Md.: Agricultural Research Service.

United States Department of Agriculture. 1974. Dietary levels of households in the United States, seasons and year 1965–1966. HFCS Report No 18. Washington: U.S. Government Printing Office.

United States Department of Agriculture Food and Nutrition Service. 1974. A menu planning guide for type A school lunches. PA-719, No. 0100-03254. Washington: U.S. Government Printing Office.

United States Department of Health, Education and Welfare. 1972. Ten State Nutrition Survey. DHEW Pub. No. (HSM) 72-8133. V. 101. Washington:U.S. Government Printing Office.

United States Department of Health, Education and Welfare. 1976a. Automated blood pressure measuring devices for mass screening—Report of the Task Force. DHEW Pub. No. (NIH) 76-929. Washington:U.S. Government Printing Office.

United States Department of Health, Education, and Welfare. 1976b. Task force on genetic factors in atherosclerotic diseases. Public Health Service, National Heart and Lung Institute. DHEW Pub. No. (NIH) 76-922. Washington:U.S. Government Printing Office.

United States Senate—Select Committee on Nutrition and Human Needs. 1977. *Dietary Goals for the United States,* 2nd ed. Pub. No. 052-070-04376-8. Washington:U.S. Government Printing Office.

Ur. A., and Gordon, M. 1970. Origin of Korotkoff sounds *Am. J. Physiol. 218:*524.

Van Bergen, F. H., Weatherhead, D. S., Treloar, A. E., Dobkin, A. B., and Buckley, J. J. 1954. Comparison of indirect and direct methods of measuring arterial blood pressure. *Circulation 10:*481.

VanDerHaar, F., and Kromhout, D. 1978. *Food Intake, Nutritional Anthropometry and Blood Chemical Parameters in Three Selected Dutch School Children Populations.* Wageningeu, Netherlands: H. Veenman and B. V. Zonen

Veterans Administration Cooperative Study Group on Antihypertensive Agents. 1967. Effects of treatment on morbidity in hypertension. I. Results in patients with diastolic blood pressure averaging 115 through 129 mm Hg. *J.A.M.A. 202:*1028.

Veterans Administration Cooperative Study Group on Antihypertensive Agents. 1970. Effects of treatment on morbidity in hypertension: Results in patients with diastolic blood pressure averaging 90 through 114 mm Hg. *J.A.M.A. 213:*1143.

Von Behren, P. A., and Lauer, R. M. 1977. Blood pressure measurements in children. *Pediatr. Ann. 6:*33.

Voors, A. W. 1975. Cuff bladder size in a blood pressure survey of children. *Am. J. Epidemiol. 101:*489.

Voors, A. W., Foster, T. A., Frerichs, R. R., Webber, L. S., and Berenson, G. S. 1976. Studies of blood pressures in children, ages 5–14 years, in a total biracial community—The Bogalusa Heart Study. *Circulation 54:*319.

Voors, A. W., Webber, L. S., and Berenson, G. S. 1977a. A consideration of essential hypertension in the pediatric age. *Practical Cardiology 3:*29.

Voors, A. W., Webber, L. S., Frerichs, R. R., and Berenson, G. S. 1977b. Body height and body mass as determinants of basal blood pressure in children—the Bogalusa Heart Study. *Am. J. Epidemiol. 106:*101.

Voors, A. W., Webber, L. S., and Berenson, G. S. 1979a. Time-course studies of blood pressure in children—the Bogalusa Heart Study. *Am. J. Epidemiol., 109:*320.

Voors, A. W., Berenson, G. S., Dalferes, E. R., Jr., Webber, L. S., and Shuler, S. E. 1979b. Racial differences in blood pressure control. *Science, 204:*1091.

Voors, A. W., Webber, L. S., and Berenson, G. S. 1979c. A choice of diastolic Korotkoff phases in mercury sphygmomanometry of children. *Prev. Med., 8:*492.

Walker, A. R. P., and Walker, B. F. 1978. High high-density-lipoprotein cholesterol in African children and adults in a population free of coronary heart disease. *Br. Med. J. 2:*1336.

Webber, L. S., Voors, A. W., Foster, T. A., and Berenson, G. S. 1977. A study of instruments in preparation for a blood pressure survey of children. *Circulation 56:*651.

Webber, L. S., Srinivasan, S. R., Frerichs, R. R., and Berenson, G. S. 1978. Serum lipids and lipoproteins in the first year of life—the Bogalusa Heart Study. *18th Annual Conference on Cardiovascular Disease Epidemiology Newsletter*, p. 32.

Webber, L. S., Voors, A. W., Srinivasan, S. R., Frerichs, R. R., and Berenson, G. S. 1979a. Occurrence in children of multiple risk factors for coronary artery disease. *Prev. Med., 8:*407.

Webber, L. S., Voors, A. W., and Berenson, G. S. 1979b. A remarkable tracking of blood pressure in children—the Bogalusa Heart Study. *Nineteenth Conference on Cardiovascular Disease Epidemiology Newsletter 26:*51.

Webber, L. S., Srinivasan, S. R., Voors, A. W., and Berenson, G. S., 1979c. Persistence of levels for risk factor variables during the first year of life—The Bogalusa Heart Study. *J. Chronic Dis.,* In press,

Weinberg, R., Avet, L. M., and Gardner, M. J. 1976. Estimates of heritability of serum lipoprotein and lipid concentrations. *Clin. Genet.* 9:588.

Weiss, N. S., Hamill, P. V. V., and Drizd, T. 1973. Blood pressure levels of children 6–11 years. Relationship to age, sex, race, and socioeconomic status. *Vital Health Stat.*, series 11, No. 135. DHEW Pub. No. (HRA) 74-1617. Publish Health Service. Washington: U.S. Government Printing Office.

Werner, G. T., and Sareen, D. K. 1978. Serum cholesterol levels in the population of Punjab in northwest India. *Am. J. Clin. Nutr.* 31:1479.

Whitcher, C. 1969. Blood pressure measurement. In *Techniques in Clinical Physiology: A Survey of Measurements in Anesthesiology*, J. W. Bellville and C. S. Weaver, eds., p. 85. New York: McMillan.

Wiese, H. F., Bennet, M. J. Braun, H. G., Yamanaka, W., and Coon, E. 1966. Blood serum lipid patterns during infancy and childhood. *Am. J. Clin. Nutr.* 18:155.

Wilhelmj, C. M., Waldmann, E. B., McGuire, T. F., Yamanaka, W., and Coon, E. 1951. Basal blood pressure of normal dogs determined by an auscultatory method and a study of the effect of fasting. *Am. J. Physiol.* 166:296.

Wilmore, J. H., and McNamara, J. J. 1974. Prevalence of coronary heart disease risk factors in boys, 8 to 12 years of age. *Pediatrics 84*:527.

Winer, B. J. 1971. *Statistical Principles in Experimental Design*. New York: McGraw-Hill.

Winkelstein, W., Jr., Kantor, S., and Ibrahim, M. A. 1969. Remarks on the analysis of familial aggregation of blood pressure in the Alameda County blood pressure study. *Am. J. Epidemiol.* 89:615.

Wissler, R. W. 1978. Progression and regression of atherosclerotic lesions. In *The Thrombotic Process in Atherogenesis*, A. B. Chandler, K. Eurenius, G. C. McMillan, C. B. Nelson, C. J. Schwartz, and S. Wessler. eds., p. 77. New York: Plenum Press.

Wissler, R. W., and Vesselinovitch, D. 1977. Regression of atherosclerosis in experimental animals and man. *Mod. Concepts Cardiovasc. Dis. 46*:27.

Wolff, O. H. 1955. Obesity in childhood: a study of the birth weight, the height, and the onset of puberty. *Q. J. Med. 24*:109, new series.

Wood, J. E., and Cash, J. R. 1939. Obesity and hypertension: clinical and experimental observations. *Ann. Intern. Med. 13*:81.

Wright, B. M., and Dore, C. F. 1970. A random-zero sphygmomanometer. *Lancet 1*:337.

Yankauer, A., and Lawrence, R. A. 1955. A study of periodic school medical examinations. 1. Methodology and initial findings. *Am. J. Public Health 45*:71.

Youden, W. J. 1951. *Statistical Methods for Chemists*. New York: Wiley-Interscience.

Young, C. M., Hagan, G. C., Tucker, R. E., and Foster, W. D. 1952. A comparison of dietary study methods. 2. Dietary history vs. seven-day record vs. 24-hr. recall. *J. Am. Diet. Assoc. 28*:218.

Yudkin, J. 1972. Sucrose and cardiovascular disease. *Proc. Nutr. Soc. 31:*331.

Zacharias, L., Wurtman, R. J., and Schatzoff, M. 1970. Sexual maturation in contemporary American girls. *Am. J. Obstet. Gynecol. 108:*833.

Zeek, P. 1930. Juvenile arteriosclerosis. *Arch. Pathol. 10:*417.

Zinner, S. H., Levy, P. S., and Kass, E. H. 1971. Familial aggregation of blood pressure in childhood. *N. Engl. J. Med. 284:*401.

Zinner, S. H., Martin, L. F., Sacks, F., Rosner, B., and Kass, E. H. 1974. A longitudinal study of blood pressure in childhood. *Am. J. Epidemiol. 100:*437.

Index

Activity, physical, 394. *See also* Exercise
Adipose tissue, 138–39, 342–45. *See also* Body composition
Advisory group, 25
Age. *See also* Blood pressure, levels by age
  and atherosclerotic involvement, 6, 17
  and coronary artery disease, 10–12
  as general risk factor, 319
  and height, 131, 132, 136
  and lipids, serum, 155–58, 160–61, 181, 190, 193–94
  and lipoproteins, serum, 155–58, 160, 181, 201, 205
  and weight, 131, 132, 133, 137
Albumin, 362
Alpha lipoproteins. *See* Lipoproteins, HDL
Anthropometry, 31, 127–47. *See also* Arm measurements; Body composition; Height; Sexual maturation; Skinfold thickness; Weight
Aorta, atherosclerotic lesions, 17
  fatty streaks, 10
  fibrous plaques, raised lesions, 5, 10
Apoproteins, 152–53, 155
Arm measurements, 31, 129, 134

Arm measurements—*continued*
  circumference, 32, 129, 134, 141
  length, 32, 129, 134, 140
  See also Blood pressure, cuff selection
Arteriosclerosis, 4, 17. *See also* Hypertension
Atherosclerosis, 3–7, 17
  anatomic changes linked with clinical observations, 6–7
  childhood, 10
  clinical variables, 7
  early natural history, 11
  family history, 389–90
  geographic, 8–10
  mechanisms, multifactorial, 5
  and nutrition, 8–9, 289, 382, 391–93
  pathogenetic considerations, 4
  prevention, 391–94
  racial differences, 385
  regression, 379
  relation to hypertension, 4–7, 16
  relation to serum lipids, 7–8, 16
  sex differences, 6
Automatic data processing, 26, 44
Awards and prizes, 34

Behavior, 394
  and coronary artery disease, 16

Credits

We would like to thank the authors, journals, and publishers for their permission to reprint the following figures and tables in this text:

Figure 1–1. R. W. Wissler, in *The Thrombotic Process in Atherogenesis*, ed. by A. B. Chandler, K. Eurenius, G. C. McMillan, C. B. Nelson, C. J. Schwartz, and S. Wessler. Plenum Press (New York) 1978

Figure 1–3. J. P. Strong, *J. Atheroscler. Res. 10*:303 (1969). The Wistar Institute

Figure 1–4. W. E. Connor, and S. L. Connor, *Prev. Med. 1*:49 (1972). © Academic Press, Inc.

Figure 1–5. H. C. McGill, Jr., in *Atherosclerosis and Its Origin*, ed. by M. Sandler and G. H. Bourne. Academic Press (New York) 1963

Figures 1–6, 1–7, 24–2. G. S. Berenson, in *Atherosclerosis IV*, ed. by G. Schettler, Y. Goto, Y. Hata, and G. Klose. Springer-Verlag (Berlin) 1977

Figure 1–8. G. S. Berenson, E. R. Dalferes, Jr., R. Robin, and J. P. Strong, in *Evolution of the Atherosclerotic Plaque*. Univ. Chicago Press (Chicago) 1964. © 1964 by the University of Chicago

Table 1–1. G. S. Berenson, B. Radhakrishnamurthy, S. R. Srinivasan, and E. R. Dalferes, Jr., in *Nutrition and Metabolism in Medical Practice*, ed. by S. L. Halpern, A. L. Luhby, and G. S. Berenson. Futura Publ. Co., Inc. (Mt. Kisco, New York) 1973. Reprinted by permission of Symposia Specialists, Inc., P. O. Box 610397, Miami, FL 33161